Progress in Drug Research

Vol. 54

Edited by Ernst Jucker, Basel

Springer Basel AG

Editor

Dr. E. Jucker
Steinweg 28
CH-4107 Ettingen
Switzerland
e-mail: jucker.pdr@bluewin.ch

Visit our PDR homepage: http://www.birkhauser.ch/books/biosc/pdr

© 2000 Springer Basel AG

Originally published by Birkhäuser Verlag, Basel, Switzerland in 2000

Printed on acid-free paper produced from chlorine-free pulp. TCF ∞
Cover design and layout: Gröflin Graphic Design, Basel

ISBN 978-3-0348-9546-0   ISBN 978-3-0348-8391-7 (eBook)
DOI 10.1007/978-3-0348-8391-7

9 8 7 6 5 4 3 2 1

Contents

Contents

Foreword by the Editor

Volume 54 of *Progress in Drug Research* contains seven review articles and various indices which facilitate the use of these monographs and also help to establish PDR as an encyclopaedic source of information. The individual articles contain innumerable references and help the active researcher in finding the information he or she is interested in.

The first article of this volume deals with the Caco-2 cell permeability and human gastrointestinal absorption. Other contributions are devoted to pharmacology of appetite suppression – a problem of great actuality – or present an overview on progress made in the research of serotonin, dopamine and norepinephrine transporters in the central nervous system. Also, neuropeptides, which are summarily treated in view of the search for novel pharmaceutically active substances, is dealt with as well as regulation of NMDA receptors by ethanol. Troglitazone and emerging glitazones show new avenues for potential therapeutic benefits beyond glycemic control. The corresponding review is of great interest in the field of diabetic disorders. A final chapter on application of developmental biology to medicine and animal agriculture demonstrates the practical importance of modern genetic research

In summary, all chapters in this volume prove to be a valuable impulse for further research leading to new drugs.

In the 41 years of PDR's existence, drug research has undergone drastic changes; the original purpose of these monographs, however, remained unchanged: dissemination of information about actual trends and crucial points in drug research. In line with modern drug research, PDR now covers almost all scientific disciplines.

The editor is anxious to maintain the high standards of PDR and is grateful to the authors for their comprehensively written review articles. I would also like to thank the members of the Board of Advisors for their advice and for suggesting current topics. The reviewers have greatly helped to improve these monographs, and I am grateful to them as well.

I would also like to thank Birkhäuser Publishing Inc., and in particular Daniela Brunner, Ruedi Jappert, Bernd Luchner, Eduard Mazenauer and Gregor Messmer, with whom I have a harmonious and rewarding relationship. My very special thanks go to Mr. Hans-Peter Thür, Birkhäuser

Publishing's CEO. Over a few decades I have and still do enjoy Mr. Thür's constant support and encouragement to continue the editorship of PDR.

Basel, May 2000   Dr. E. Jucker

Progress in Drug Research, Vol. 54 (E. Jucker, Ed.)
© 2000 Birkhäuser Verlag, Basel (Switzerland)

Caco-2 cell permeability vs human gastro-intestinal absorption: QSPR analysis[1]

By Shijun Ren and Eric J. Lien

Department of Pharmaceutical
Sciences, School of Pharmacy,
University of Southern California,
1985 Zonal Ave., Los Angeles,
CA 90033, USA

[1]Part of this work has been presented
at a poster session of the AAPS Western Regional Meeting, San Diego,
California, USA, April 29–30, 1999

Shijun Ren

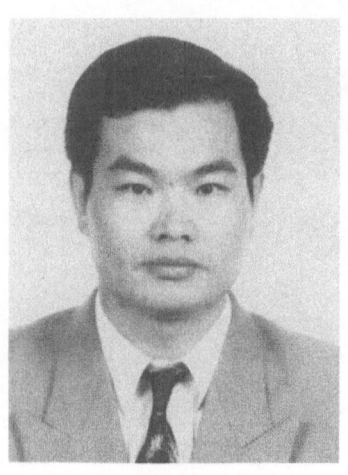

received his B.S. in pharmacy from Shandong Medical University in 1987. He joined the Institute of Pharmaceutical Research, Shandong Academy of Medical Sciences as a research assistant in 1987. From 1995 to 1997, he was a visiting research scholar in the School of Pharmacy, University of Southern California under the guidance of Dr. Eric J. Lien. In 1997, he was admitted to the School of Pharmacy, University of Southern California as a Ph.D. student. His research interests include structure-activity/permeability relationship and molecular modeling, cancer chemopreventive natural products, as well as anticancer and antiviral drug design and synthesis. He has published several book chapters and articles in various pharmaceutical journals.

Eric J. Lien

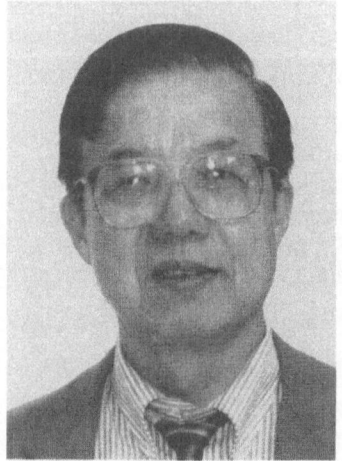

received his Ph.D. from the University of California San Francisco Medical Center in 1966. After his postdoctoral training at Pomona College, he joined the University of Southern California in 1968 as a faculty member. Professor Lien's research interests include structure-activity relationship and drug design, physical organic chemistry and natural products. He has served as a consultant to various government agencies, universities and private cooperations. His most recent work deals with the evolution of biomacromolecules, from thermoneutrons to living organisms.

Summary

The aim of this study is to elucidate quantitative structure-permeability relationship (QSPR) of various organic molecules through Caco-2 cells, and to ascertain the relationship between gastrointestinal (GI) absorption in humans and Caco-2 cell permeability. Caco-2 cell permeability and human GI absorption data were obtained from the literature. The maximum hydrogen bond-forming capacity corrected for intra-molecular H-bonding ($H_b{}^c$) and Lien's QSAR model were used in this study. The latest CQSAR software was utilized in calculating the logarithm of partition coefficient in octanol/water (Clog P) and in deriving all regression equations. For 51 compounds, a significant correlation was obtained between Caco-2 cell permeability (log P_{caco-2}) and $H_b{}^c$, octanol/PBS (phosphate buffered saline, pH 7.4) distribution coefficient (log D_{oct}), log MW and an indicator variable (I) for the charge, with a correlation coefficient of 0.797. When these compounds were divided into three subgroups, namely neutral, cationic and anionic compounds, much better correlations ($r = 0.968$, 0.915 and 0.931, respectively) were obtained using different combinations of various physicochemical parameters. A plot of human GI absorption vs. Caco-2 cell permeability obtained from different laboratories reveals that Caco-2 cell permeability cannot be used to precisely predict human GI absorption for compounds with P_{caco-2} below 5×10^{-6} cm/s, due to interlaboratory and experimental variabilities, and the lack of a simple correlation between human GI absorption and Caco-2 cell permeability. Caco-2 cell permeability may be estimated from the structures of drug molecules using the above-mentioned physicochemical parameters. In general, for compounds with P_{caco-2} above 5×10^{-6} cm/s, human GI absorption ranges from 50 to 100%. This is generally acceptable for development into oral dosage form. For the compounds with P_{caco-2} below 5×10^{-6} cm/s, careful interpretation of caco-2 cell permeability and use of internal standard for comparison are recommended. Otherwise, good drug candidates may be excluded due to incorrectly predicted poor absorption.

Contents

Shijun Ren and Eric J. Lien

Keywords

Caco-2 cells; calculated partition coefficient (Clog P); distribution coefficient (log D_{oct}); hydrogen bonding; oral absorption; permeability; QSAR

Glossary of abbreviations

Clog P, calculated log P; GI, gastrointestinal; H_b^c, the maximum hydrogen bond-forming capacity corrected for intra-molecular hydrogen bonding; log D_{oct}, logarithm of octanol/PBS (phophate buffered saline, pH 7.4) distribution coefficient; log P, logarithm of octanol/water partition coefficient; MW, molecular weight; P_{caco-2}, Caco-2 cell apparent permeability coefficient; QSAR, quantitative structure-activity relationship; QSPR, quantitative structure-permeability relationship

1   Introduction

Oral administration is the most important and preferred route for low molecular weight (< 500 Da) conventional drugs. The overall bioavailability of an orally administered drug depends on many factors, including physicochemical properties of the drug as well as various physiological and biochemical barriers (such as metabolic enzymes, drug transporters, and the presence of multidrug resistance (MDR) P-glycoprotein). In recent years, in order to elucidate the role of various physiological and biochemical barriers to drug absorption, and to rapidly predict human gastrointestinal (GI) absorption in high throughput screening (HTS), Caco-2 cell line (a cell line derived from a human colorectal carcinoma) has been used as an *in vitro* model to study human GI absorption of drugs which cross the intestinal epithelium by transcellular or paracellular passive diffusion [1–6]. The demonstration of a good correlation between the extent of oral drug absorption in humans and rates of transport across the Caco-2 cell monolayers by Artursson and Karlsson [2] has further contributed to the widespread use of these cells as an *in vitro* model for GI drug absorption. This suggests that human GI absorption may be "predicted" by using *in vitro* Caco-2 permeability. Furthermore, methods for predicting Caco-2 cell permeability or drug GI absorption using different physicochemical properties of the drugs have been examined [7–13]. Lien's group has also reported a general model to correlate membrane permeability with physicochemical properties, namely hydrophobicity as measured by octanol/water partition coefficient (log P), molecular weight (MW) as a measurement of molecular size, and hydrogen bonding capacity (H_b) [14–20].

$$\text{Log (permeability)} = -k_1 \cdot (\log P)^2 + k_2 \cdot \log P + n \cdot \log MW + q \cdot H_b + k_3 \quad (1)$$

In Eq. 1, when log P values lie in a relatively narrow range, the $-k_1 \cdot (\log P)^2$ term approaches zero, then log (permeability) becomes linearly dependent on log P, log MW and H_b. Van de Waterbeemd and Camenisch [11] have used a similar function to represent permeability-physicochemical property relationship.

$$\text{Permeability} = f \text{ (lipophilicity, molecular size, H-bonding capacity, charge)} \quad (2)$$

When distribution coefficients (log D) or apparent partition coefficients (log P′) instead of log P are used, the effect of difference in charge is included in the lipophilicity term (log D or log P′). When charge is a constant for all compounds analyzed, the charge term becomes part of the constant term.

Figure 1 shows the inter-relationships among physicochemical properties, Caco-2 cell permeability and human GI absorption in drug design and development.

Studies by Chiou et al. [21–23] demonstrated that rat may serve as a useful animal model to predict the extent of GI absorption in humans following oral administration of drugs in a solution or rapidly released dosage form. Recently, Caco-2 cell monolayers have been generally accepted as a primary absorption screening tool in the early stage of drug development. There are several examples of successful application of Caco-2 cell for prediction of or correlation with human GI absorption [2, 7]. However, different laboratories have reported very different threshold values of apparent permeability coefficients (P_{caco-2}) for poorly and well-absorbed compounds, and quite different P_{caco-2} values for the same compound. These prompted this systematic investigation.

The purpose of this study is to elucidate QSPR of diverse organic compounds through Caco-2 cell monolayers, and to ascertain the relationship between Caco-2 cell permeability and human GI absorption. A more coherent cutoff threshold value of P_{caco-2} for poorly and well-absorbed compounds will be suggested.

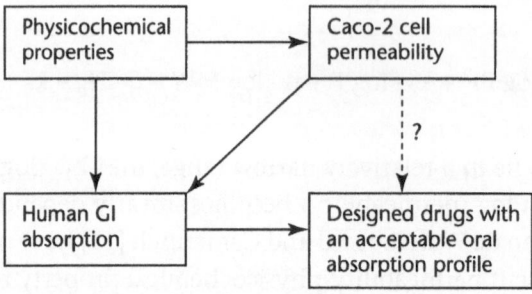

Fig. 1.
The interrelationships among physicochemical properties, Caco-2 cell permeability and human GI absorption in drug design and development.

2   Methods

Caco-2 cell permeability and human GI absorption data were obtained from the literature [2, 7, 24–29]. The latest CQSAR program [30] was utilized in calculating the Clog P (calculated log P) values, and in deriving all regression equations.

The maximum hydrogen bonding capacity corrected for intramolecular hydrogen-bonding (H_b^c) was calculated based on the following rules [14–20]: (a) the number of hydrogen donors is equal to the number of hydrogen atoms which can form hydrogen bonds as donors; (b) the number of hydrogen acceptors is equal to the lone electron pairs of a given group. For example, for –ỌH group the number of hydrogen donor is one, and there are two lone electron pairs on oxygen. Therefore, the total hydrogen bonding for –ỌH group is equal to 3; (c) if there are any intramolecular hydrogen bonds within a molecule, the number of intra-molecular hydrogen bonding will be subtracted from the total number of hydrogen bonding. For example, salicylic acid has one intramolecular hydrogen bond involving one hydrogen donor and one hydrogen acceptor, by subtracting 2 from the total number of 8, H_b^c of 6 is obtained. The atomic distances were obtained by using the Hyper-Chem program [31] after performing geometry optimization and energy minimization for the molecule. If the hydrogen donor and acceptor form a five- or six-member pseudo-ring and the atomic distance between two hetero-atoms (N, O) is around 2.63 to 3.10 Å [32], the intramolecular hydrogen bonding is assigned for the molecule.

3   Results and discussion

3.1 Correlation of Caco-2 cell permeability with physicochemical properties

Physicochemical properties (MW, H_b^c, log D_{oct}, Clog P, log P and pK_a), Caco-2 cell apparent permeability coefficients, and percent human GI absorption are presented in Table 1. For 51 diverse compounds, the following stepwise equations were obtained from the regression analysis.

Log P_{caco-2} = –0.126 (0.042) H_b^c + 1.900 (0.400)   (3)
   $n = 51$, $r = 0.648$, $r^2 = 0.420$, $s = 0.567$, $F_{1,49} = 35.53$, $p < 0.0005$

Log P_{caco-2} = –0.142 (0.038) H_b^c – 0.374 (0.195) I + 2.169 (0.381)   (4)
   $n = 51$, $r = 0.746$, $r^2 = 0.556$, $s = 0.502$, $F_{2,48} = 30.07$, $p < 0.0005$;
   $F_{1,48} = 14.68$, $p < 0.0005$

Log P_{caco-2} = –0.111 (0.042) H_b^c – 0.326 (0.185) I + 0.151 (0.104)
   log D_{oct} + 1.819 (0.428)   (5)
   $n = 51$, $r = 0.790$, $r^2 = 0.624$, $s = 0.467$, $F_{3,47} = 25.99$, $p < 0.0005$;
   $F_{1,47} = 8.47$, $p < 0.01$

Log P_{caco-2} = –0.094 (0.050) H_b^c – 0.334 (0.185) I + 0.202 (0.136) log D_{oct}
   – 0.679 (1.168) log MW + 3.304 (2.589)   (6)
   $n = 51$, $r = 0.797$, $r^2 = 0.635$, $s = 0.465$, $F_{4,46} = 19.98$, $p < 0.0005$;
   $F_{1,46} = 1.35$, $p < 0.25$

Log P_{caco-2} = –0.109 (0.039) H_b^c – 0.358 (0.150) I + 0.310 (0.111) log D_{oct}
   – 1.349 (0.924) log MW + 4.949 (2.062)   (7)
   $n = 46$, $r = 0.893$, $r^2 = 0.798$, $s = 0.357$, $F_{4,41} = 40.37$, $p < 0.0005$;
   $F_{1,41} = 8.52$, $p < 0.01$

Log P_{caco-2} = –0.146 (0.073) H_b^c – 0.342 (0.235) I – 0.002 (0.140) Clog P
   + 0.509 (1.462) log MW + 0.970 (2.987)   (8)
   $n = 50$, $r = 0.749$, $r^2 = 0.561$, $s = 0.506$, $F_{4,45} = 14.40$, $p < 0.0005$

Table 1.
The physicochemical properties, Caco-2 cell permeability (log P_{caco-2}) and percent GI absorption for 51 compounds.

	Compounds	Log P_{caco-2} obsd.[a]	Log P_{caco-2} calcd.	% absorbed[a]	MW	H_b^c	Clog P^e	Log D_{oct}^a	I	log P^f	pKa[g]
1	Griseofulvin	1.563	1.346[b]	Irregular	352.8	12	1.52	2.47	0	2.18	
2	Aminopyrine	1.562	1.722[b]	100	231.3	5	1.00	0.63	0	1.00	5.0
3	Piroxicam	1.551	1.189[c]	100	331.4	11	1.89	-0.07	-1	1.98	2.33, 5.07
4	Diazepam	1.524	1.687[b]	100	284.8	4	3.16	2.58	0	2.99	3.4
5	Caffeine	1.489	0.996[b]	100	194.2	8	-0.06	0.02	0	-0.07	0.6, 14.0
6	Nevirapine	1.479	1.373[b]	> 90	266.3	7	2.53	1.81	0		
7	Phenytoin	1.427	1.558[d]	90	252.3	8	2.09	2.26	1	2.47	8.3
8	Alprenolol	1.403	1.357[d]	93	249.3	5	2.65	1.38	1	2.89	9.7
9	Testosterone	1.396	1.457[b]	100	288.4	5	3.22	2.91	0	3.32	
10	Phencyclidine	1.393	1.593[d]		248.4	1	5.10	1.31	1	3.63	8.5[i]
11	Desipramine	1.387	1.528[d]	> 95	266.4	3	4.47	1.57	1	4.90	10.2
12	Metoprolol	1.375	0.763[d]	95	267.4	7	1.35	0.51	1	1.88	9.7
13	Progesterone	1.375	1.393[b]		314.5	4	3.78	3.48	0	3.87	
14	Salicylic acid	1.342	1.035[c]	100	138.1	6	2.19	-1.44	-1	2.26	3.0
15	Clonidine	1.338	1.138[d]	100	230.1	5	1.41	0.78	1	1.43	8.1
16	Propranolol	1.338	1.406[d]	90	259.3	5	2.19	1.55	1	2.98	9.5
17	Corticosterone	1.326	1.318[b]	100	346.5	8	2.32	1.78	0	1.94	
18	Warfarin	1.324	1.418[c]	98	308.3	9	2.62	0.64	-1	2.70	5.1
19	Indomethacin	1.310	1.352[c]	100	357.7	10	3.88	1.00	-1	4.27	4.5
20	Chlorpromazine	1.299	1.591[d]	Erratic	318.9	2	5.78	1.86	1	5.19	9.3
21	Meloxicam	1.290	1.189[c]	90	351.4	11	2.28	0.03	-1	3.01	3.4
22	Nicotine	1.288	1.435[d]	100	162.2	2	0.90	0.41	1	1.17	3.1, 8.2
23	Estradiol	1.229	1.044[b]	Rapidly metabolized	272.4	6	3.73	2.24	0	4.01	
24	Pindolol	1.223	0.671[d]	95	248.3	7	1.11	0.19	1	1.75	9.5
25	Telmisartan	1.179	1.418[c]	90	514.6	9	7.26	2.41	-1		
26	Hydrocortisone	1.146	1.301[b]	89	362.5	11	1.70	1.48	0	1.61	

Tasble 1 continued

27	Timolol	1.107	0.181dh	72	328.4	10	1.53	0.03	1	1.83	9.2
28	Dexamethasone	1.086	1.300b	100	392.5	11	1.75	2.16	0	2.01	
29	Scopolamine	1.072	0.326d	100	303.4	10	0.30	0.21	1		7.6
30	Dopamine	0.970	0.581d		153.2	7	0.17	-0.80	1		8.87, 10.63
31	Labetalol	0.969	0.841d	90	316.4	9	2.50	1.24	1		9.5
32	Acetylsalicylic acid	0.959	1.259c	100	180.2	7	1.02	-2.25	-1	1.19	3.50
33	Bremazocine	0.904	0.888b		351.9	7	3.77	1.66	0		
34	Zidovudine	0.841	0.952b	100	267.2	10	0.04	-0.58	0	0.05	
35	Urea	0.659	0.844d		60.1	8	-2.11	-1.64	1	-2.11	
36	Uracil	0.627	0.611d		112.1	8	-1.06	-1.11	1	-1.07	9.45
37	Nadolol	0.589	0.597d		309.4	9	0.33	0.68	1	0.71	9.67
38	Sucrose	0.233	0.106b		342.3	20	-3.09	-3.34	0	-3.01	
39	Cimetidine	0.137	0.269d	95	252.3	9	0.35	-0.36	1	0.40	6.9
40	Methylscopolamine	-0.161	-0.341d	90	318.5	10	-5.48j	-1.14	1	-0.07	7.9, 9.2
41	Hydrochlorothiazide	-0.292	-0.147d	90	297.7	15	-0.40	-0.12	1	0.16	9.6
42	Atenolol	-0.276	-0.273d	50	266.3	10	-0.11	-1.29	1	1.71	9.4
43	Acebutalol	-0.292	0.040d	90	336.4	11	1.70	-0.09	1	0.08	8.8, 10.1, 11.2
44	Terbutaline	-0.328	0.025d	73	225.3	9	0.48	-1.07	1	0.27	8.2
45	Ranitidine	-0.310	0.145d	50	314.4	10	0.63	-0.12	1		
46	Pirenzepine	-0.357	-0.245d	Poor	424.3	10	-0.89	-0.46	1		
47	Mannitol	-0.420	-0.436b	16	182.2	12	-2.05	-2.65	0	-3.10	
48	Ganciclovir	-0.420	-0.409b	3	255.2	16	-2.56	-0.10	0	-2.07	
49	Sulfasalazine	-0.523	-0.429c	13	394.4	15	3.83	-0.42	-1		2.4, 9.7, 11.8
50	Acyclovir	-0.602	-0.325b	20	225.2	15	-2.30	-0.35	0	-1.56	2.3, 9.3i
51	Chlorothiazide	-0.721	-0.555d	Dose-dependent	295.7	14	-0.31	-1.15	1	-0.24	6.7, 9.5

aFrom [24]; bcalculated from Eq. (11); ccalculated from Eq. (20); dcalculated from Eq. (16); ecalculated using the CQSAR database [30]; fmeasured log P values from the CQSAR database [30]; gfrom the CQSAR database [30]; ha statistical outlier, excluded from Eq. (16); ifrom [33]; jestimated value using the fragment constant (π) values of –N(CH$_3$)$_2$ and –N$^+$(CH$_3$)$_3$ in [34] and Clog P value of scopolamine.

The statistical parameters describing the regression are n, the number of data points; r, the correlation coefficient; and s, the standard deviation. The numbers in parentheses are 95% confidence intervals of coefficients in the equations. I is an indicator variable for the charge (I = 1 for the positively charged compounds; I = 0 for the neutral compounds; I = -1 for the negatively charged compounds). From Eqs. (3–6), one can see that the use of H_b^c, I, log D_{oct} and log MW does not give a very high correlation coefficient ($r = 0.797$). H_b^c is the most important contributor to Caco-2 cell permeability, followed by I, log D_{oct} and log MW. Log P_{caco-2} negatively depends on H_b^c, I and log MW and positively depends on log D_{oct}. Upon deletion of five statistical outliers (residual > 2s), namely sucrose (No. 38), timolol (No. 27), scopolamine (No. 29), piroxicam (No. 3) and progesterone (No. 13), Eq. (7) was obtained with an improved r and a decreased s. The use of Clog P instead of log D_{oct} resulted in Eq. (8) ($n = 50$ due to one missing fragment constant for Clog P) with a decreased r as compared to Eq. (6), indicating that log D_{oct} is a better descriptor than Clog P in correlating with Caco-2 permeability of diverse molecules. The squared correlation matrix of the parameters used in the regression analysis is shown in Table 2.

When 51 compounds were divided into three subgroups, namely neutral, cationic and anionic compounds, the following equations were obtained.

Neutral compounds

$$\text{Log } P_{caco-2} = 0.253 \ (0.105) \ \text{Clog P} + 0.650 \ (0.267) \tag{9}$$
$$n = 17, r = 0.797, r^2 = 0.636, s = 0.467, F_{1,15} = 26.17, p < 0.0005$$

$$\text{Log } P_{caco-2} = 0.313 \ (0.096) \ \text{Clog P} - 0.065 \ (0.047) \ (\text{Clog P})^2 + 1.004 \ (0.334) \tag{10}$$
$$n = 17, r = 0.882, r^2 = 0.778, s = 0.378, F_{2,14} = 24.51, p < 0.0005$$
$$\text{Clog } P_0 = 2.400 \ (1.438 - 7.460)$$

$$\text{Log } P_{caco-2} = 0.430 \ (0.119) \ \text{Clog P} - 0.130 \ (0.038) \ (\text{Clog P})^2 - 0.370 \ (0.154) \ H_b^c + 0.018 \ (0.007) \ (H_b^c)^2 + 2.817 \ (0.906) \tag{11}$$
$$n = 17, r = 0.968, r^2 = 0.937, s = 0.217, F_{4,12} = 44.54, p < 0.0005$$
$$\text{Clog } P_0 = 1.651 \ (1.265 - 2.180), \ H_b^c{}_0 = 10.190 \ (8.659 - 11.774)$$

$$\text{Log } P_{caco-2} = 0.142 \ (0.234) \ \log D_{oct} + 0.006 \ (0.098) \ (\log D_{oct})^2 - 0.113 \ (0.369) \ H_b^c + 0.002 \ (0.017) \ (H_b^c)^2 + 1.660 \ (2.091) \tag{12}$$
$$n = 17, r = 0.781, r^2 = 0.610, s = 0.540, F_{4,12} = 4.70, p < 0.025$$

Table 2.
The squared correlation matrix showing covariance (r^2) between the physicochemical parameters used in the regression analysis for 51 compounds.

	Clog P	log D_{oct}	log MW	H_b^c	I
Clog P	1.000	0.520	0.180	0.326	0.069
log D_{oct}		1.000	0.178	0.244	0.002
log MW			1.000	0.068	0.048
H_b^c				1.000	0.046
I					1.000

Cationic compounds

$$\text{Log } P_{caco\text{-}2} = -0.165 \ (0.058) \ H_b^c + 1.945 \ (0.498) \tag{13}$$
$$n = 26, \ r = 0.767, \ r^2 = 0.588, \ s = 0.487, \ F_{1,24} = 34.24, \ p < 0.0005$$

$$\text{Log } P_{caco\text{-}2} = 0.609 \ (0.159) \ \log D_{oct} - 2.248 \ (1.007) \ \log \text{MW} +$$
$$5.919 \ (2.406) \tag{14}$$
$$n = 26, \ r = 0.862, \ r^2 = 0.743, \ s = 0.393, \ F_{2,23} = 33.24, \ p < 0.0005$$

$$\text{Log } P_{caco\text{-}2} = -0.063 \ (0.066) \ H_b^c + 0.461 \ (0.217) \ \log D_{oct} - 1.627 \ (1.155)$$
$$\log \text{MW} + 4.952 \ (2.492) \tag{15}$$
$$n = 26, \ r = 0.884, \ r^2 = 0.781, \ s = 0.370, \ F_{3,22} = 26.22, \ p < 0.0005;$$
$$F_{1,22} = 3.88, \ p < 0.1$$

$$\underline{\text{Log } P_{caco\text{-}2} = -0.067 \ (0.058) \ H_b^c + 0.467 \ (0.191) \ \log D_{oct} - 1.775 \ (1.023)}$$
$$\underline{\log \text{MW} + 5.301 \ (2.209)} \tag{16}$$
$$\underline{n = 25, \ r = 0.915, \ r^2 = 0.837, \ s = 0.325, \ F_{3,21} = 35.87, \ p < 0.0005}$$

$$\text{Log } P_{caco\text{-}2} = -0.055 \ (0.064) \ H_b^c + 0.564 \ (0.238) \ \log D_{oct} - 0.126 \ (0.143)$$
$$(\log D_{oct})^2 - 2.085 \ (1.218) \ \log \text{MW} + 6.120 \ (2.722) \tag{17}$$
$$n = 26, \ r = 0.901, \ r^2 = 0.811, \ s = 0.352, \ F_{4,21} = 22.60, \ p < 0.0005$$

$$\text{Log } D_{oct_0} = 2.239 \pm \text{infinity}$$

$$\text{Log } P_{caco\text{-}2} = -0.102 \ (0.103) \ H_b^c + 0.367 \ (0.300) \ \text{Clog P} - 0.054 \ (0.047)$$
$$(\text{Clog P})^2 - 1.622 \ (1.772) \ \log \text{MW} + 5.152 \ (3.607) \tag{18}$$
$$n = 26, \ r = 0.831, \ r^2 = 0.691, \ s = 0.451, \ F_{4,21} = 11.73, \ p < 0.0005$$

$$\text{Clog } P_0 = 3.417 \ (1.364 - 12.717)$$

Anionic compounds

$$\text{Log } P_{caco\text{-}2} = -0.157 \ (0.179) \ H_b^c + 2.587 \ (1.803) \tag{19}$$
$$n = 8, \ r = 0.660, \ r^2 = 0.436, \ s = 0.534, \ F_{1,6} = 4.64, \ p < 0.1$$

Table 3.
The squared correlation matrix (r^2) of the physicochemical parameters used in the regression analysis for 17 neutral compounds.

	Clog P	log D_{oct}	log MW	$H_b{}^c$
Clog P	1.000	0.787	0.191	0.729
log D_{oct}		1.000	0.203	0.531
log MW			1.000	0.001
$H_b{}^c$				1.000

Table 4.
The squared correlation matrix (r^2) of the physicochemical parameters used in the regression analysis for 26 cationic compounds.

	$H_b{}^c$	log D_{oct}	log MW
Hb^c	1.000	0.331	0.054
log D_{oct}		1.000	0.124
log MW			1.000

$$\text{Log } P_{caco-2} = 0.854 \, (0.651) \, H_b{}^c - 0.048 \, (0.031) \, (H_b{}^c)^2$$
$$- 2.345 \, (3.298) \tag{20}$$
$$n = 8, \; r = 0.931, \; r^2 = 0.868, \; s = 0.284, \; F_{2,5} = 16.38, \; p < 0.01$$
$$H_b{}^c{}_0 = 8.819 \, (5.518 - 9.905)$$

From Eqs. (9–12), one can see that after correcting for the differences in $H_b{}^c$, log P_{caco-2} for the neutral compounds parabolically depends on hydrophobicity (Clog P). The optimal hydrophobicity (Clog P_0) is around 1.651 (from 1.265 to 2.180) (see Eq. (11) and Fig. 2). For this set of neutral compounds, Clog P is a better descriptor than log D_{oct}, as indicated by Eqs. (11) and (12). The squared correlation matrix (r^2) summarized in Table 3 indicates that Clog P shows covariance ($r = -0.854$, $r^2 = 0.729$) with $H_b{}^c$.

Caco-2 cell permeabilities (log P_{caco-2}) of 26 cationic compounds are positively dependent on log D_{oct} and negatively dependent on $H_b{}^c$ and log MW (see Eq. (15)). In contrast to the neutral compounds, log D_{oct} is a better descriptor than Clog P in predicting Caco-2 cell permeability for the cationic compounds. For eight anionic compounds, log P_{caco-2} highly significantly depends on the single parameter $H_b{}^c$. Due to the limited number of data points, this relationship may not be extrapolated to other data sets. Plots of

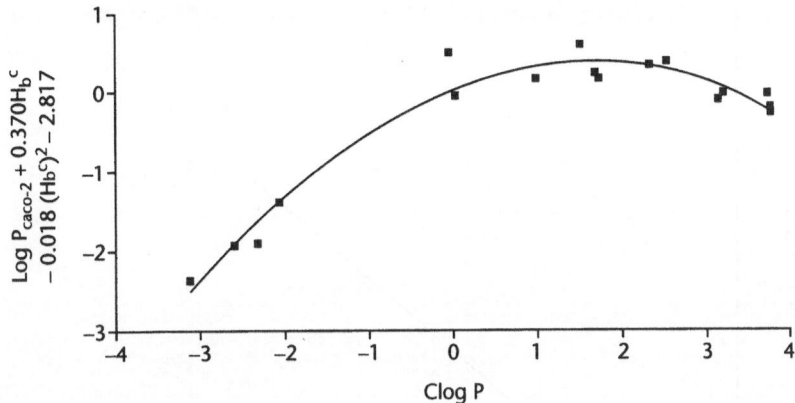

Fig. 2
A plot of log P_{caco-2} (after correcting for differences in H_b^c) vs. Clog P for 17 neutral compounds (Eq. (11), $n = 17$, $r = 0.968$)

calculated log P_{caco-2} values vs. observed log P_{caco-2} values for neutral and cationic compounds are shown in Figures 3 and 4.

The low correlation coefficient ($r = 0.797$) for 51 compounds indicates that other factors, such as metabolic enzymes, drug transporters, transcytosis/ endocytosis, as well as MDR P-glycoprotein may be involved in the transport of some of 51 compounds through Caco-2 cell monolayers. There are no simple mathematical correlations between Caco-2 cell permeability coefficients and any single physicochemical parameter. Therefore, any single parameter, for example log D_{oct} or log P can only be used to qualitatively determine Caco-2 cell permeability. Combination of different physicochemical parameters, like log MW (or any other parameters describing molecular size), and H_b^c, as well as other biochemical descriptors is needed to improve the correlation. Improvement of correlation by separating 51 diverse compounds into neutral, cationic and anionic subgroups shows that three types of compounds have different structural requirements in penetrating Caco-2 cell monolayers. In this study, we did not attempt to correlate the percent human GI absorption with the physicochemical properties of 51 compounds, because of variables involved in the drug absorption, e.g., the different time period required to reach the same percent GI absorption,

13

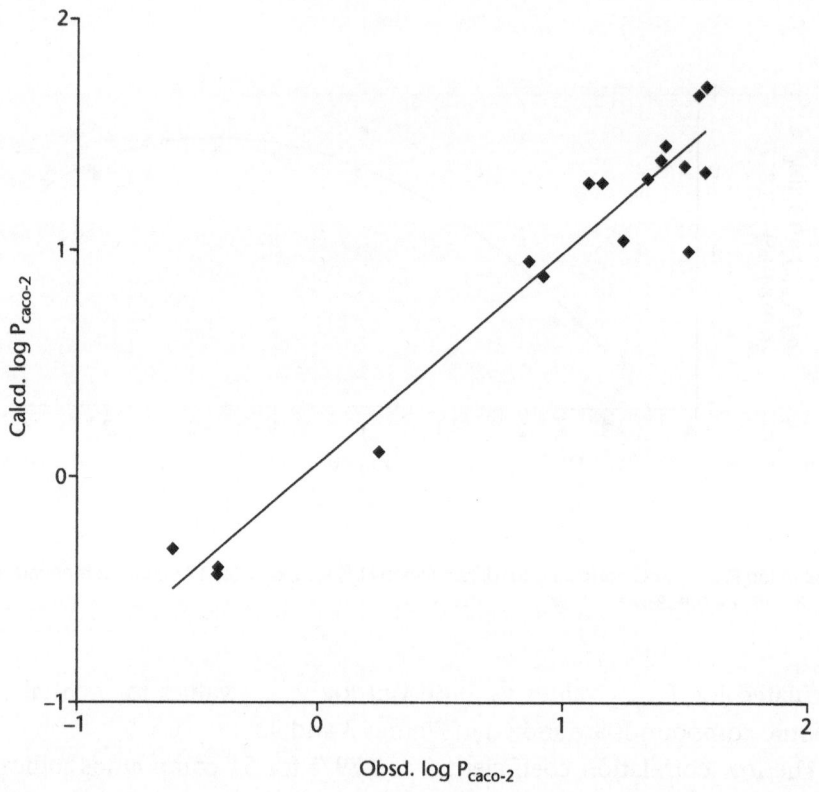

Fig. 3
A plot of calculated log P_{caco-2} vs. observed P_{caco-2} for 17 neutral compounds (Eq. (11), $n = 17$, $r = 0.968$).

formulation, intersubject variability, different experimental conditions and analytical methods used. Since different compounds with 100% human GI absorption appear to have very different physicochemical properties, no good correlation between human GI absorption and physicochemical properties can be obtained.

It has been reported that transport of quaternary ammonium compounds across rat small intestine is affected by the presence of alkylsulfate, due to the ion pair formation. This indicates that not only cation itself but also the presence of counter anion may affect the transport of cationic compounds through small intestine by forming ion pair [35].

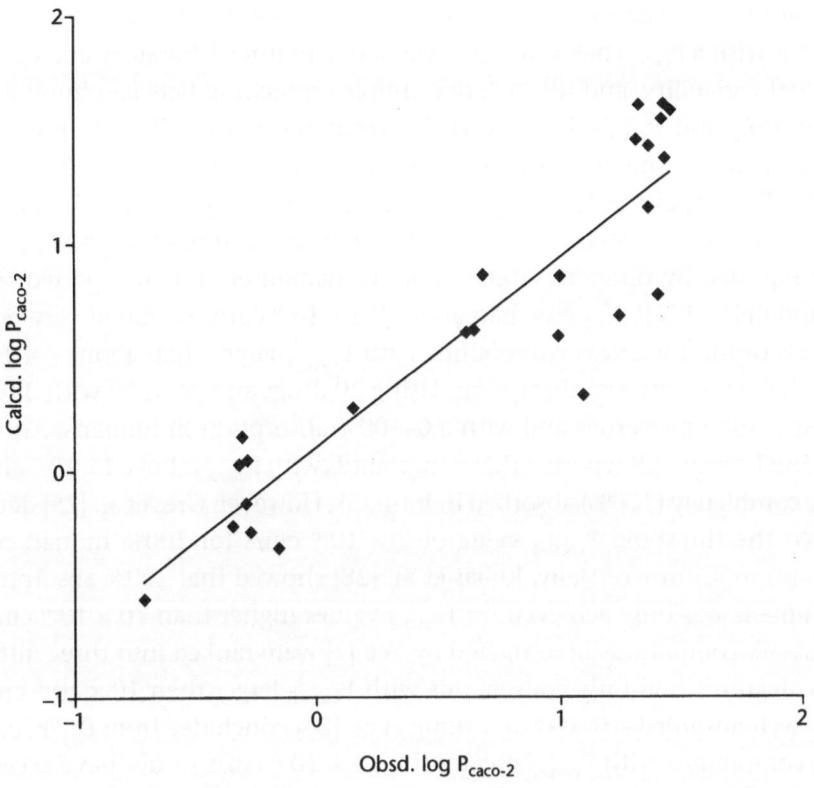

Fig. 4
A plot of calculated log P_{caco-2} vs. observed P_{caco-2} for 25 cationic compounds (Eq. (16), $n = 25$, $r = 0.915$).

3.2 Relationship of human GI absorption and Caco-2 cell permeability

The percent human GI absorption and Caco-2 cell permeability coefficients from currently available publications are summarized in Table 5 in order of decreasing permeability coefficients. A total of 138 pairs of percent GI absorption and P_{caco-2} data were systematically collected from the literature [2, 7, 24–29] for comparison in this study. For compounds with several different percent GI absorption data, an average value was used in the analysis. A plot of human GI absorption vs. P_{caco-2} (see Fig. 5) reveals that Caco-2 cell permeability cannot be used to predict precisely human GI absorption for compounds with a P_{caco-2} below 5×10^{-6} cm/s, due to inter-laboratory and experimental variability, and the lack of a simple correlation between human GI absorption and P_{caco-2}. In general, 76 compounds with P_{caco-2} above 5×10^{-6} cm/s have human GI absorption ranging from 50 to 100%, only six out of the 76 compounds have a percent human GI absorption less than 80%. The literature analysis demonstrates that there are controversies among the data reported by different laboratories. Yazdanian et al. [24] reported that compounds with P_{caco-2} less than about 0.4×10^{-6} cm/s exhibited very poor oral absorption whereas compounds with P_{caco-2} larger than about 7×10^{-6} cm/s had excellent oral absorption. Using 20 drugs and peptides with different structural properties and with a 0–100% absorption in humans, Artursson and Karlsson [2] reported that compounds with P_{caco-2} above 1×10^{-6} cm/s were completely (100%) absorbed in humans. However, Gres et al. [25] determined the threshold P_{caco-2} value of 2×10^{-6} cm/s for 100% human oral absorption. Controversially, Rubas et al. [28] showed that 100% absorption in humans was only achieved for P_{caco-2} values higher than 70×10^{-6} cm/s. Thirty-six compounds investigated by Yee [7] were ranked into three different categories, and only compounds with P_{caco-2} larger than 10×10^{-6} cm/s were well-absorbed (70–100%). Chong et al. [26] concluded from their study that compounds with P_{caco-2} greater than 1×10^{-6} cm/s would have acceptable absorption in humans (> 20%). Careful comparison reveals that P_{caco-2} values vary as much as one order of magnitude from one another for some compounds (see Table 6 for details).

The differences in the permeability coefficients reported from various laboratories may be due to variations in cell culture conditions such as passage number, type of medium, and days in culture, as well as the experimental conditions used for their measurement.

4   Conclusion

In conclusion, Caco-2 cell permeability may be estimated from the structures of drug molecules by combination of different physicochemical parameters (log D_{oct}, Clog P, $H_b{}^c$ and log MW), and by classification of diverse compounds into three categories (neutral, cationic and anionic). QSPR analysis demonstrates that there are different structural requirements to achieve the optimal

Table 5.
Percent GI absorption in humans and Caco-2 cell permeability coefficients from the different reports in decreasing order of permeability coefficients.

Compounds	$P_{caco-2} \times 10^{-6}$ (cm/s)	% Absorbed	Ref.
Phenytoin	89.83	100	[29]
Caffeine	84.29	100	[25]
Glycine	80.00	100	[7]
Progesterone	78.93	100	[28]
Naproxen	74.17	100	[28
Testosterone	72.27	100	[7]
Diazepam	70.97	100	[7]
Corticosterone	54.50	100	[2]
Ibuprofen	52.50	100	[7]
Testosterone	51.80	100	[2]
Tenidap	51.20	90	[7]
Caffeine	50.50	100	[7]
Antipyrine	49.01	97	25]
Valproic acid	48.00	100	[7]
Hydrocortisone	44.67	95	[29]
Testosterone	44.50	100	[25]
D-Phe-L-Pro	44.30	100	[7]
Salicylic acid	41.90	100	[26]
Propranolol	41.90	90	[2]
Alprenonol	40.50	93	[2]
Warfarin	38.30	98	[2]
Aminopyrine	36.50	100	[24]
Piroxicam	35.60	100	[24]
Hydrocortisone	35.40	80	[28]
Propranolol	34.43	90	[25]
CP-X	34.15	> 50	[7]
Diazepam	33.40	100	[24]
Caffeine	30.80	100	[24]
Acetylsalicylic acid	30.67	68	[7]
Trovoflaxicin	30.23	88	[7]
Nevirapine	30.10	> 90	[24]
Clonidine	30.10	95	[7]
Fluconazole	29.80	100	[7]
L-Phenylalanine	29.50	100	[29]
Noloxone	28.20	91	[7]
Propranolol	27.50	90	[7]
Metoprolol	27.00	95	[2]
Phenytoin	26.70	90	[24]
Alprenolol	25.30	93	[24]
Testosterone	24.90	100	[24]
Desipramine	24.40	> 95	[24]
Metoprolol	23.70	95	[24]
Dexamethasone	23.40	92	[7]
Felodipine	22.70	100	[2]
Salicylic acid	22.00	100	[24]
Clonidine	21.80	100	[24]

Table 5. (continued)

Compounds	$P_{caco-2} \times 10^{-6}$ (cm/s)	% Absorbed	Ref.
Propranolol	21.80	90	[24]
Desipramine	21.60	100	[7]
Hydrocortisone	21.50	89	[2]
Caffeine	21.40	100	[26]
Corticosterone	21.20	100	[24]
Warfarin	21.10	98	[24]
Guanabenz	20.90	79	[26]
Chloramphenicol	20.60	90	[7]
Indomethacin	20.40	100	[24]
Meloxicam	19.50	90	[24]
Nicotine	19.40	100	[24]
Metoprolol	18.00	95	[25]
Pindolol	16.70	95	[24]
Telmisartan	15.10	90	[24]
Propranolol	14.80	90	[26]
Imipramine	14.10	100	[7]
Hydrocortisone	14.00	89	[24]
Timolol	12.80	72	[24]
Dexamethasone	12.50	100	[2]
Ziprasidone	12.30	60	[7]
Dexamethasone	12.20	100	[24]
Hydrocortisone	12.19	80, 89, 95 (88[a])	[25]
PEG900	12.10	10	[28]
Salicylic acid	11.90	100	[2]
Scopolamine	11.80	100	[24]
Propranolol	11.20	95	[27]
Labetalol	9.31	90	[24]
Acetylsalicylic acid	9.09	100	[24]
Zidovudine	6.93	100	[24]
L-Phenylalanine	6.91	100	[25]
Nadolol	4.50	35	[26]
Gabapentin	4.33	74	[29]
Taurocholate	4.02	100	[25]
BVaraU	4.00	82	[26]
Atenolol	4.00	50	[26]
Mannitol	3.23	17	[28]
CP-W	3.12	50	[7]
Cimetidine	3.06	62	[7]
Sumatriptan	3.00	55	[7]
Cephalexin	2.69	100	[25]
Ganciclovir	2.67	8	[28]
Acetylsalicylic acid	2.40	100	[2]
Pravastatin	2.30	34	[26]
Acyclovir	2.00	30	[7]
Benzyl penicillins	1.96	30	[7]
Gabapentin	1.50	36	[29]

Table 5. (continued)

Compounds	$P_{caco-2} \times 10^{-6}$ (cm/s)	% Absorbed	Ref.
Cimetidine	1.37	95	[24]
Methotrexate	1.20	20	[7]
Mannitol	1.17	5, 16, 17 (12.7[a])	[25]
Atenolol	1.16	40–70, 50 (52.5[a])	[25]
Inuline	1.04	<1	[25]
Terbutaline	1.04	25–80, 73 (62.8[a])	[25]
PEG4000	0.97	0	[28]
Practolol	0.90	100	[2]
Cyclosporin A	0.86	30	[25]
L-Glutamine	0.85	60–90 (75[a])	[25]
PEG900	0.83	10	[7]
Mannitol	0.83	5	[29]
Amoxicillin	0.80	100	[26]
PEG4000	0.78	0	[7]
Sucrose	0.71	42	[25]
Mannitol	0.65	16	[7]
Enalaprilate	0.62	<10	[25]
Atenolol	0.53	50	[24]
Hydrochlorothiazide	0.51	90	[24]
Acebutalol	0.51	90	[24]
Mannitol	0.50	16	[26]
Cephalexin	0.50	100	[26]
Ranitidine	0.49	50	[24]
PEG400	0.48	8–52, 55.6 (42.8[a])	[25]
Terbutaline	0.47	73	[24]
Mannitol	0.38	16	[24]
Ganciclovir	0.38	3	[24]
Terbutaline	0.38	73	[2]
Amoxicillin	0.33	100	[25]
Sulfasalazine	0.30	13	[24]
Acyclovir	0.25	20	[24]
Atenolol	0.20	50	[2]
Cephalexin	0.18	95	[27]
Mannitol	0.18	16	[2]
Doxorubicin	0.16	5	[7]
PEG4000	0.15	<1	[25]
AVP	0.14	0	[2]
Sulphasalazine	0.13	13	[2]
dDAVP	0.13	1	[2]
Atenolol	0.13	40	[27]
Olsalazine	0.11	2	[2]
PEG4000	0.08	<1	[26]
PEG4000	0.05	0	[2]
Lisinopril	0.05	25	[26]
SQ-29852	0.02	60	[26]
CP-Z	0.00	0.003	[7]

[a]An averaged value.

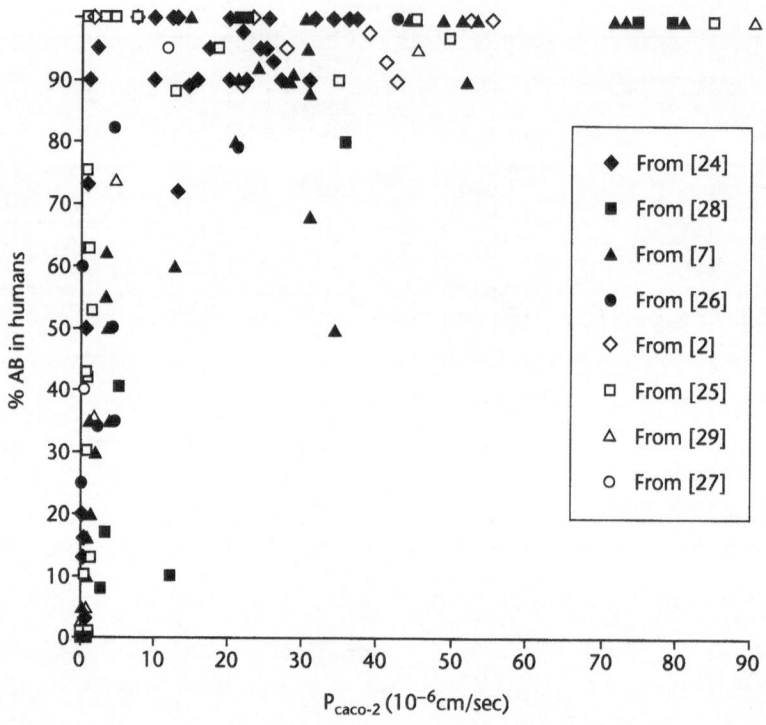

Fig. 5
A plot of percent GI absorption in humans vs. Caco-2 cell permeability coefficients.

human GI absorption for neutral, cationic, and anionic compounds. In general, for compounds with P_{caco-2} above 5×10^{-6} cm/s, human GI absorption ranges from 50 to 100%. This is generally acceptable for development into oral dosage form. A plot of human GI absorption vs. Caco-2 cell permeability reveals that Caco-2 cell permeability cannot be used as a surrogate marker of *in vivo* GI absorption for the compounds with P_{caco-2} below 5×10^{-6} cm/s, because of the interlaboratory and experimental variability, and the lack of a simple correlation between human GI absorption and Caco-2 cell permeability. Therefore, careful interpretation of Caco-2 cell permeability and use of internal standard for comparison are recommended. Otherwise, good drug candidates may be missed out due to incorrectly predicted poor absorption. Also, Caco-2 cell permeability (in a range of $0–5 \times 10^{-6}$ cm/s) estimated from

Table 6.
Comparison of human GI absorption and Caco-2 cell permeability data for the commonly tested compounds (see Table 5 for references).

Compounds	$P_{caco-2} \times 10^{-6}$ (cm/s)	% Absorbed
Acetylsalicylic acid	30.67	68
Acetylsalicylic acid	9.09	100
Acetylsalicylic acid	2.40	100
Atenolol	4.00	50
Atenolol	1.16	40–70, 50 (52.5[a])
Atenolol	0.53	50
Atenolol	0.20	50
Atenolol	0.13	40
Caffeine	84.29	100
Caffeine	50.50	100
Caffeine	30.80	100
Caffeine	21.40	100
Cephalexin	2.69	100
Cephalexin	0.18	95
Cephalexin	0.50	100
Dexamethasone	23.40	92
Dexamethasone	12.50	100
Dexamethasone	12.20	100
Hydrocortisone	44.67	95
Hydrocortisone	35.40	80
Hydrocortisone	21.50	89
Hydrocortisone	14.00	89
Hydrocortisone	12.19	80, 89, 95 (88[a])
Mannitol	3.23	17
Mannitol	1.17	5, 16, 17 (12.7[a])
Mannitol	0.83	5
Mannitol	0.65	16
Mannitol	0.50	16
Mannitol	0.38	16
Mannitol	0.18	16
Metoprolol	27.00	95
Metoprolol	23.70	95
Metoprolol	18.00	95
PEG4000	0.97	0
PEG4000	0.78	0
PEG4000	0.15	<1
PEG4000	0.08	<1
PEG4000	0.05	0
Propranolol	41.90	90
Propranolol	34.43	90
Propranolol	27.50	90
Propranolol	21.80	90
Propranolol	14.80	90

Table 6. (continued)

Compounds	$P_{caco-2} \times 10^{-6}$ (cm/s)	% Absorbed
Propranolol	11.20	95
Salicylic acid	41.90	100
Salicylic acid	22.00	100
Salicylic acid	11.90	100
Terbutaline	1.04	25-80, 73 (62.8[a])
Terbutaline	0.47	73
Terbutaline	0.38	73
Testosterone	72.27	100
Testosterone	51.80	100
Testosterone	44.50	100
Testosterone	24.90	100

[a]An averaged value.

physicochemical properties cannot be used as a surrogate for *in vivo* GI absorption. This finding may be useful in drug discovery setting where little is known about the new compound.

Acknowledgements

This work was supported in part by the H & L foundation. The authors would like to thank Dr. Corwin Hansch of Pomona College for providing us with an access to the CQSAR program.

References

1   Hidalgo J., Raub T.J. and Birchardt R.T.: Gastroenterology *96*, 736–749 (1989).
2   Artursson P. and Karlsson J.: Biochem. Biophys. Res. Commun. *175*, 880–885 (1991).
3   Artursson P.: J. Pharm. Sci. *79*, 476–482 (1990).
4   Wilson G., Hassan I., Dix C., Williamson I., Shah R., Mackay M. and Artursson P.: J. Control. Release *11*, 25–40 (1990).
5   Hilgers A., Conradi R. and Burton P.: Pharm. Res. *7*, 902–910 (1990).
6   Cogburn J., Donovan M. and Schasteen C.: Pharm. Res. *8*, 210–216 (1991).
7   Yee S.: Pharm. Res. *14*, 763–766 (1997).
8   Sugawara M., Takekuma Y., Yamada H., Kobayashi M., Iseki K. and Miyazaki K.: J. Pharm. Sci. *87*, 960–966 (1998).
9   Burton P.S., Conradi R.A., Ho N.F.H., Hilgers A.R. and Borchardt R.T.: J. Pharm. Sci. *85*, 1336–1340 (1996).

10   Norinder U., Osterberg T. and Artursson P.: Pharm. Res. *14*, 1786–1791 (1997).

11   van de Waterbeemd H. and Camenisch G.: Quant. Struct.-Act. Relat. *15*, 480–490 (1996).

12   Palm K., Luthman K., Ungell A., Strandlund G. and Artursson P.: J. Pharm. Sci. *85*, 32–39 (1996).

13   Krarup L.H., Christensen I.T., Hovgaard L. and Frokjaer S.: Pharm. Res. *15*, 972–978 (1998).

14   Lien E.J.: Drug Intell. Clin. Pharmacol. *4*, 7–9 (1970).

15   Lien E.J., in: J. Maas (ed.): Medicinal Chemistry IV. Proceedings of the 4th international symposium on medicinal chemistry. Amsterdam 1974, 319–342.

16   Lien E.J., in: E.J. Ariens (ed.): Drug Design. Academic Press, New York 1976, 81–132.

17   Lien E.J.: Prog. Drug Res. *29*, 67–95 (1985).

18   Lien E.J.: SAR Side Effects and Drug Design. Marcel Dekker, Inc., New York and Basel 1987, 92–154.

19   Lien E.J. and Gao H.: Pharm. Res. *12*, 583–587 (1995).

20   Ren S., Das A. and Lien E.J.: J. Drug Target. *4*, 103–107 (1996).

21   Chiou W.L. and Barve A.: Pharm. Res. *15*, 1792–1795 (1998).

22   Chiou W.L., Robbie G., Chung S.M., Wu T.C. and Ma C.: Pharm. Res. *15*, 1474–1479 (1998).

23   Chiou W.L.: Biopharm. Drug Disp. *16*, 71–75 (1995).

24   Yazdanian M., Glynn S.L., Wright J.L. and Hawi A.: Pharm. Res. *15*, 1490–1494 (1998).

25   Gres M., Julian B., Bourrie M., Meunier V., Roques C., Berger M., Boulenc X., Berger Y. and Fabre G.: Pharm. Res. *15*, 726–733 (1998).

26   Chong S., Dando S.A., Soucek K.M. and Morrison R.A.: Pharm. Res. *13*, 120–123 (1996).

27   Walter E., Janich S., Roessler B.J., Hilfinger J.M. and Amidon G.L.: J. Pharm. Sci. *85*, 1070–1076 (1996).

28   Rubas W., Jezyk N. and Grass G.M.: Pharm. Res. *10*, 113–118 (1993).

29   Stewart B.H., Chan O.H., Lu R.H., Reyner E.L., Schmid H.L., Hamilton H.W., Steinbaugn B.A. and Taylor M.D.: Pharm. Res. *12*, 693–699 (1995).

30   BioByte Corp.: CQSAR database, 201 W 4th Street, Suite 204, Claremont, CA 91711, USA (1999).

31   Hypercube, Inc.: HyperChem for Window, Version 5.0, 1115 NW 4th Street, Gainesville, FL 32601, USA (1996).

32   Stryer L.: Biochemistry, 3rd edition. W. H. Freeman and Company, New York 1988, 7–8.

33   Foye W.O., Lemke T.L. and Williams D.A.: Principles of Medicinal Chemistry. Williams & Wilkins, Media, PA 1995, 948–961.

34   Lien E.J., in: J. Swarbrick and J.C. Boylan (eds.): Encyclopedia of Pharmaceutical Technology. Marcel Dekker, New York 1995, Vol. 11, 293–307.

35   Masaki B.W., Lien E.J. and Biles J.A.: Acta Pharm. Suecica *10*, 43–52 (1973).

Progress in Drug Research, Vol. 54 (E. Jucker, Ed.)
©2000 Birkhäuser Verlag, Basel (Switzerland)

Pharmacology of appetite suppression

By Jason C.G. Halford[1] and John E. Blundell[2]

[1]Department of Psychology, Eleanor Rathbone Building, University of Liverpool, Liverpool, L69 3BX, UK, and [2]Biopsychology Group, School of Psychology, University of Leeds, Leeds, LS2 9JT, UK

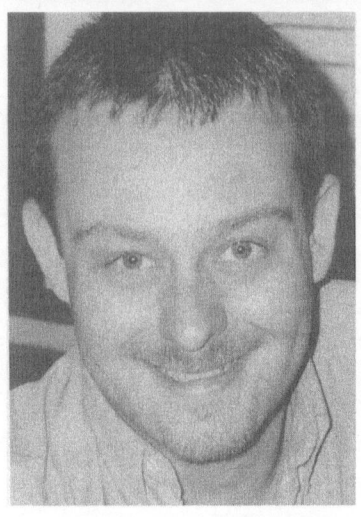

Jason C.G. Halford

gained his Ph.D. under the supervision of Professor Blundell at the University of Leeds in 1994. He was a member of Professors Blundell's biopsychology group between 1991–1996. He also worked in the Laboratory for the Study of Human Feeding Behaviour, Pennsylvania State University, between 1996–1997. Currently, Jason Halford is a lecturer in human ingestive behaviour, and Assistant Director of the Kissileff Laboratory for the study of ingestive behaviour, at the Department of Psychology, University of Liverpool.

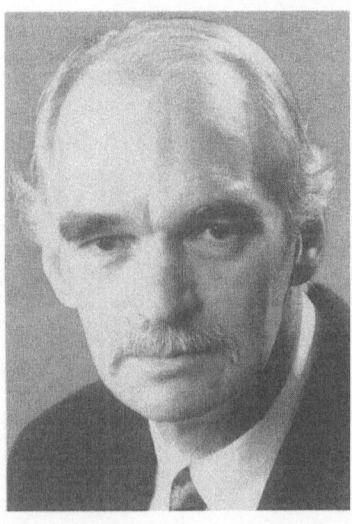

John E. Blundell

is Professor of Psychobiology and Head of the School of Psychology at the University of Leeds, England. Professor Blundell has published numerous articles and reviews in the area of appetite regulation and obesity. His specific interests include the psychopharmacology of appetite regulation, pharmacotherapy of human obesity and the impact of diet on energy regulation.

Summary

Despite a rising worldwide epidemic of obesity there is currently only a very small number of anti-obesity drugs available to manage the problem. Large numbers of differing pharmacological agents reliably produce a reduction in food intake when administered acutely to animals, and when administered chronically they result in a significant decrease in body mass. Behavioural analysis of drug-induced anorexia in animals demonstrates that various compounds profoundly effect feeding behaviour in differing ways. This indicates the variety of mechanisms by which pharmacological agents can induce changes in food intake, body weight and eventually body composition. Some of the same drugs produce decreases in food intake and weight loss in humans. Some of these drugs do so by modifying the functioning of the appetite system as measured by subjective changes in feelings of hunger and fullness (indices of satiety). Such drugs can be considered as "appetite suppressants" with clinical potential as anti-obesity agents. Other drugs induce changes in food intake and body weight through various physiological mechanisms inducing feelings of nausea or even by side effect related malaise. Of the drugs considered suitable candidates for appetite suppressants are agents which act via peripherally satiety peptide systems (such as CCK, Bombesin/GRP, Enterostatin and GLP-1), or alter the CNS levels of various hypothalamic neuropeptides (NPY, Galanin, Orexin and Melanocortins) or levels of the key CNS appetite monoamine neurotransmitters such as serotonin (5-HT) and noradrenaline (NA). Recently, the hormone leptin has been regarded as a hormonal signal linking adipose tissue status with a number of key central nervous system circuits. The peptide itself stimulates leptin receptors and it links with POMC and MC-4 receptors. These receptors may also provide drug targets for the control of appetite. Any changes induced by a potential appetite suppressant should be considered in terms of the (i) psychological experience and behavioural expression of appetite, (ii) metabolism and peripheral physiology, and (iii) functioning of CNS neural pathways. In humans, modulation of appetite may involve changes in total caloric consumption, subjective changes in feelings of hunger and fullness, preferences for specific food items, and general macronutrient preferences. These may be expressed behaviourally as changes in meal patterns, snacking behaviour and food choice. Within the next 20 years it is certain that clinicians will have a new range of anti-obesity compounds available to choose from. Such novel compounds may act on a single component of the appetite system or target a combination of these components detailed in this review. Such compounds used in combination with lifestyle changes and dietary intervention may be useful in dealing with the rising world epidemic of obesity.

Jason C.G. Halford and John E. Blundell

Contents

Keywords

Appetite, satiety, hunger, obesity, food intake, behaviour, CCK, bombesin, enterostatin, GLP-1, 5-HT, NA, NPY, galanin, CRF, orexin, melanocortin, leptin

Glossary of abbreviations

5-HT, serotonin-5-hydroytryptamine; 5-HTP, 5-hydroytryptophan; ARC, Arcuate nucleus; AP, Area postrema; CART, cocaine and amphetamine regulated transcript; CCK, cholecystokinin; CRF, corticotrophin-releasing factor; CNS, central nervous system; DA, dopamine; GLP-1, glucagon-like peptide-1; GRP, gastrin releasing peptide; HPA, hypothalamic pituitary adrenal axis; IL-6, interleukin-6; LH, lateral hypothalamus; LNAAs, large neutral amino acids; MC, melanocortin; MCH, melanin-concentrating hormone; αMSH, α melanocyte-stimulating hormone; NA, noradrenaline; NAc, nucleus accumbens; NPY, neuropeptide Y; NTS, nucleus tractus solitarius; POMC, pro-opiomelanocortin; PPA, phenylpropanolamine; PVN, para ventricular nucleus; SNRI, serotonin and noradrenaline re-uptake inhibitor; SSRI, selective serotonin re-uptake inhibitor; TNFα, tumour-necrosis factor α; VMH, ventromedical hypothalamus

1   Introduction

The expression of appetite can be considered to result from the dynamic interaction between the biological status of the organism and various aspects of its environment. The organism's biology determines the homeostatic systems that maintain the body's levels of energy. Energy needs initiate a drive to acquire energy (hunger). The environment determines the source and availability of energy, and therefore satisfaction of the drive (satiation). In the late twentieth century food unavailability is no longer the major determining environmental factor in most cultures. Many of us live in a calorie-rich environment with a vast array of pleasurable food items "freely" available. In such situations the determining environmental factors become (i) social and cultural norms, and (ii) the range, composition and quality of food items on offer. Under these circumstances any functioning anti-obesity drug should control the impact of such stimulating environmental factors on appetite. The functioning of the appetite system is not strictly homeostatic. Signals of energy surplus appear less potent than those of energy deficit. The appetite system defends well against energy deficit (brought about by under-consumption), but not against energy excess (overconsumption). Thus, homeostatic control of food intake and appetite is asymmetrical. This asymmetry may be critical in explaining the prevalence of adiposity and obesity in human populations. This in turn has generated particular interest in appetite suppression drugs.

A vast number of pharmacologically active agents can induce anorexia in rodents. The literature is full of experiments demonstrating that various chemicals, when given to fasted rats, prevent the restriction-induced food binge (large meal) observed in placebo treated animals. Such agents may produce substantial reductions in immediate energy intake, but these studies often use unrealistically large and biologically inappropriate doses of test compound. Additionally, these studies do not provide us with the most important data on the nature of the appetite suppression. Is the reduction in food (in terms of energy) due to the drug acting on the natural process of energy regulation? Or is the drug effect the result of a non specific blockage of, or impediment to, the expression of feeding behaviour? This failure to define the nature of drug induced anorexia precludes the disclosure of information relevant to the mechanism of action on the drug.

1.1 The expression of appetite

The biopsychological system underlying the expression of appetite can be conceptualised as having three domains:

1. The domain of psychological events (e.g. sensations of hunger, satiety, hedonics and cravings), accompanying behavioural operations (meal intake, snacking behaviour, food choice) and their consequences (energy intake and macronutrient composition).
2. The domain of peripheral physiology and metabolic events related to the effect of absorbed nutrients and their utilisation or subsequent conversion for storage (i.e. the changes in body due to either energy intake and/or energy deficit).
3. The domain of neurochemical (classic neurotransmitters, neuropeptides and hormones) and metabolic interactions within the CNS (i.e. how various signals of the body's energy status are detected in the brain).

The expression of appetite reflects the synchronous operation of events and processes in all three domains [1]. Neural events trigger and guide food seeking and consummatory behaviour. These neural events (initiating the drive to eat) are a direct response to the demands of peripheral physiology (the need for energy). Thus, events in physiology are translated into changes in the brain neurochemical activity and trigger feeding behaviour. Conversely, satisfaction of the body's demands leads to physiological and metabolic changes which trigger different neural events inhibiting the hunger drive and consummatory behaviour. Thus, CNS activity ultimately represents the presence or absence of the motivation to feed (see Fig. 1).

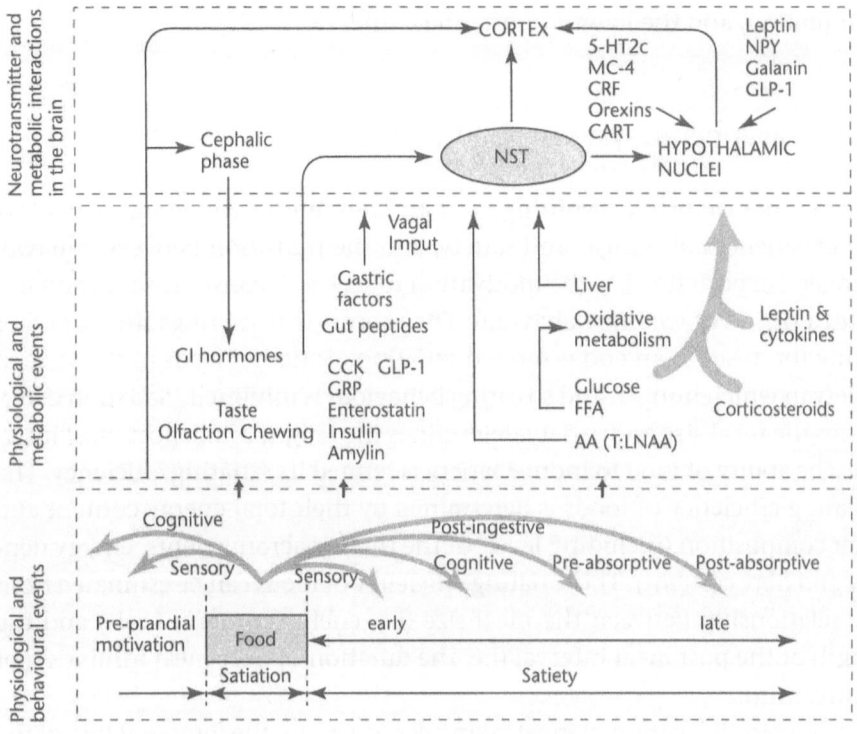

Fig. 1
Diagram showing the expression of appetite reflected in the relationship between the three levels of operation (i) domain of psychological events and behaviour, (ii) domain of peripheral physiology and metabolism and (iii) domain of neurochemistry and metabolic interactions within the CNS (AA, amino acid; FFA, free fatty acids; see glossary of abbreviations)

The appetite system can be considered purely in terms of the amount of energy consumed or in terms of macronutrient content (calories from protein, carbohydrate and fat). However, beyond the physical and biochemical parameters of food intake, eating is also a distinct and measurable behavioural event. Eating behaviour has a definable structure, and eating events fall into a distinct pattern. Omnivorous mammalian feeding (in rodents, some primates and most humans) is characterised by discontinuous or bout feeding. Periods of eating are separated generally by longer periods of non eating. These periods can be termed meals (and snacks) and intermeal intervals respectively. But what internal processes determine meal initiation and termination, and the length of intermeal intervals?

1.2 The appetite system – Hunger and satiety

The internal factors determining meal and non meal periods are psychological experiences of hunger and satiety, and the transition between the two. Hunger can be defined as the motivation to seek and consume food, and initiates a period of feeding behaviour. The process which brings this period of eating (or meal) to an end is termed satiation. Satiation leads to the state of satiety in which hunger, and so eating behaviour is inhibited. Satiation determines the meal size and satiety determines the length of the post meal interval. The ability of food to induce satiety is termed its satiating efficiency. The satiating efficiency of foods is determined by their total energy content and their composition (including levels of the three macronutrients, energy density and fibre content). The satiating efficiency of foods can be estimated from the relationship between the meal size (i.e. energy content: kcals) and the length of the post meal interval (i.e. the duration of post-meal inhibition of eating: min).

This episodic pattern of meal taking demonstrates the temporal flux of the physiological systems underpinning hunger and satiety. The net effect of these systems can be considered before (pre prandial), during (prandial) and after (post prandial) a meal. One of the key pre prandial features is the cephalic phase. The cephalic phase is characterised by pre consummatory physiological signals generated by the sight and smell of the food. Its function is to prepare the body for the ingestion of food. Afferent sensory information provided by sight and smell (carried to the brain stem via cranial nerves) stimulates hunger before eating, and also into the initial stages of consumption. This stimulatory force continues to act as a positive reinforcer of consumption during the prandial phase.

1.3 Prandial phase

During the prandial phase the CNS receives sensory afferent input reflecting the amount of food eaten and initial estimations of its nutrient content. This involves the interaction of psychological and physiological processes. We are able to cognitively judge how much food we have eaten and estimate whether it may satisfy us. Mechano-receptors in the gut detect the distension of gut lining caused by the presence of food. This aids the estimation of the volume of food consumed. In addition, chemo-receptors detect the chemical presence of various nutrient in the gastro intestinal tract. These provide information on the composition (and possible energy content) of the food consumed. Both, mechano- and chemo-receptors generate afferent signals which reach the CNS via the vagal nerve. These signals can be collectively termed post-ingestive satiety signals.

1.4 Post-prandial phase

A distinction should be drawn between pre- and post-absorptive satiety signals. Post-absorptive satiety signals which are generated by the detection of nutrients which have been absorbed from the gastro intestinal tract and entered circulation in the periphery. Circulating nutrients are either metabolised by the various tissues and organs of the periphery, activate CNS receptors, or they enter the brain directly. Either of these outcomes appear to generate post-absorptive metabolic satiety signals. Circulating nutrients affect liver function which generates afferent vagal satiety signals detected in the CNS. Fluctuations in the levels of circulating nutrients, and their metabolites, may be directly detected by CNS receptors in the various areas of the brain stem (e.g. nucleus of the solitary tract (NTS), and the adjacent area postrema (AP)). Additionally, nutrients or their metabolites may affect CNS neurotransmitter and neuropeptides synthesis and so have a direct impact on CNS neurochemical activity.

1.5 Factors derived from energy metabolism and storage

Long-term control of the expression of appetite is derived from the processes of energy storage and the status of the body's energy stores. Blood carries various substances other than nutrients which reflect the body's energy status. Such factors would probably be generated in organs implicated in nutrient metabolism and energy storage such as the liver, the pancreas and in adipose tissue layers. For example, both insulin and leptin (indicators of glucose metabolism, and fat storage respectively) have been shown to have potent effects on food intake. These may provide the most potent determinant of food intake and the expression of appetite in the long term (either promoting satiety and potently inhibiting food intake, or stimulating hunger and initiating food intake). The number of potential active metabolites and bi-products produced by energy metabolism of differing nutrients is vast, providing a wide range of potential indicator substances (e.g. satietin, adipsin or cytokine signals such as interleukins and tumour-necrosis factors). Such long-term factors could act in a similar manner to the circulating hormone leptin which is released by the fat cells of adipose tissue. Released leptin in the blood stream is detected by leptin receptors in the CNS. Stimulation of leptin receptors has been shown to have potent effects on brain neurochemistry (see later).

1.6   Neural control of appetite

The CNS receives information generated by the sensory experience of eating, and from the periphery indicating the ingestion, absorption, metabolism and storage of energy. This information reaches the CNS via three main routes.

1. Peripheral receptors in gut (distension and chemo-receptors) and metabolic changes in the liver (energy conversion and energy status) send afferent signals via vagus to AP/NTS complex in the brain stem.
2. Receptors in the CNS, particularly in the brain stem detect circulating levels of nutrients, their metabolites and other factors.
3. Factors such as neurotransmitter precursors crossing the blood brain barrier and directly alter CNS neurochemical activity particularly in key hypothalamic nuclei and associated limbic areas.

To regulate appetite a variety of structures within the CNS integrate multiple signals, to assess the biological need for energy, to generate or inhibit conscious experiences of hunger, and subsequently to initiate the appropriate behavioural action. Original theories of the neural control of appetite were based around a dual centre hypothesis in which the opposing action of two hypothalamic nuclei controlling hunger and satiety ultimately determined the expression of appetite and the occurrence of feeding behaviour. This "dual-centre" theory was based on early studies demonstrating that lesions and stimulation of the lateral hypothalamus (LH) and ventral medical hypothalamus (VMH) caused marked and opposing effects on rodent food intake. Much research has subsequently concentrated on another key hypothalamic site, the paraventricular nucleus (PVN). Infusions of various agents in or near the PVN produce either marked increases or decreases in food intake, and of specific macronutrients (see later). Other key limbic sites identified as playing critical roles in appetite regulation include the arcuate nucleus (ARC), nucleus accumbens (NAc), the amygdala, posterior hypothalamus and the dorsal medial hypothalamus [1].

More recently the roles of non hypothalamic/limbic sites in the expression of appetite have increasingly been recognised. Much attention has been paid to the tracts which run from the brain stem in to the limbic system. For example the NTS/AP (nucleus of the solitary tract/area postrema) adjacent areas in the hind brain relay vagal afferent satiety signals from the periphery (particularly receptors in the gastrointestinal tract and liver) to the hypothalamus. This area of the brain stem appears to possess receptors sensitive to levels of circulating nutrients (see later). Additionally, it should also be noted that afferent sensory information from the mouth including taste (carried by cranial nerves) is relayed to the cortex via the NTS. The NTS sends neural projections into key areas like the hypothalamic and other limbic sites associated with appetite control. These inter-linked sites contain the key neurotransmitters and neuropeptides associated with the expression of appetite.

To summarise, for pharmacologists wishing to alter appetite for therapeutic reasons there are numerous biological systems underpinning the natural control of food intake which could be pharmacologically targeted. Reductions in food intake could be achieved by enhancing satiety and/or inhibiting hunger or by altering food selection away from high fat (high energy dense) foods and toward lower fat (lower energy dense) items. These target systems can been divided into three broad categories; short-term peripheral satiety factors, central hunger and satiety factors, and long-term circulatory factors.

2 Short-term peripheral satiety factors

Peripheral satiety factors are released in response to the physical and chemical presence of food in the gastrointestinal tract. The release of the gastrointestinal factors such as cholecystokinin (CCK), bombesin, gastrin releasing peptide (GRP), glucagon, glucagon like pepetide-1 (GLP-1) and enterostatin inform the brain that both the stomach is full and that the gut contains nutrients. These agents enhance satiety. Of these factors the gut peptide CCK has been the most extensively researched.

2.1 Cholecystokinin

The gut hormone CCK was initially shown to dose dependently reduce food intake in rodents and monkeys, and was consequently identified as a potential satiety agent by Gibbs et al. [2, 3]. Exogenous doses of CCK adjusted rodent eating behaviour in a manner consistent with a satiety enhancing action [4]. Additionally, pharmacologically blocking the action of endogenous CCK reversed both the hypophagic and satiety enhancing CCK effects (see [5, 6] for reviews). CCK-8 (octapeptide CCK variant) also produces similar effects on food intake and satiety in humans, although it can also induce feelings of nausea and/or anxiety in some subjects [7, 8].

Endogenous CCK is a gastrointestinal peptide which varies in chain length (from 4 peptides to 33). Most exogenous studies have used CCK-8 (octopeptide) to produce changes in feeding behaviour. The actual effects of endogenous CCK may be due to both CCK-8 and/or CCK-33 variations of the peptide. Peripheral CCK appears to induce satiety via two distinct mechanisms, via direct stimulation of vagal CCK receptors and via prolonging gastric distension (which also results in increased vagal activation). CCK is released from the intestinal tract into the blood stream in response to ingested fat and protein [9] and stimulates CCK_A receptors on vagal afferents in the periphery. These vagal afferent fibres in the gut terminate in the NTS. Stimulation of other CCK_A receptors on the pyloric sphincter results in an inhibition of stomach emptying. This has the net result of enhancing gastric distension, and so increasing afferent signals from mechano-receptors in the stomach wall. Distension signals also appear to be relayed by the vagus to the

CNS. Efferent as well as afferent vagal fibres may be critical in peripheral CCK satiety effects [10].

The relative contribution of both the direct and the indirect peripheral CCK mechanisms to the net effect of endogenous CCK has not yet been fully determined. However, much research has also focused on the effects of CCK in the CNS. Corp et al. [11] using antagonists administered directly into the CNS suggest that CCK released CNS is not necessary for the satiating effect of peripherally administered CCK-8 in rats. This is confirmed, as intracerebroventricular CCK_A receptor antagonists do not reduce satiation by induced by endogenous CCK [12]. However, other evidence does exist suggesting central CCK_B receptors may be critical in mediating satiety. Antagonism of CNS CCK_B receptors does increases food intake [13].

Endogenous CCK release in the gut may, or may not, directly stimulate CNS mechanisms but peripheral CCK does have a marked effect on CNS neurochemistry. Peripheral administration of CCK-8 has been shown to stimulate the release of 5-HT within the hypothalamic areas such as the PVN [14, 15]. However, blocking CNS 5-HT transmission does not completely block CCK-8 induced reduction in food intake suggesting the hypophagic effects of endogenous CCK may not be totally dependent on its action on CNS 5-HT. There is the possibility that circulating CCK may be directly detected by brain stem receptors, possibly in the AP next to NTS. Additionally, the role of CCK_B receptors, located within the CNS, in the regulation of food intake and the expression of appetite (hunger and satiety) has yet to be fully investigated.

2.2 Bombesin/GRP

Similar to CCK, the intestinal hormone bombesin has been shown to reduce food intake without disrupting the structure of feeding behaviour [16]. The full role of the bombesin polypeptide and its analogue (gastrin releasing peptide (GRP)) in human appetite has still to be determined. It is important to note that although both bombesin and GRP block normal food intake, GRP fails to block sham feeding, suggesting its precise mechanism action may not be identical to bombesin [17]. Both central and peripheral administration of bombesin blocks feeding responses in animals [16, 18]. Bombesin may mediate its hypophagic affects via neuromedin B-10 and/or GRP preferring receptors [19, 20]. Direct stimulation of both these receptors produces an additive reduction on food intake, suggesting a role for both in the endogenous action of bombesin. A key site in bombesin action appears to be the AP/NTS complex in the brain stem. High concentrations of bombesin are not only found in the gastrointestinal tract, but can be found in key hypothalamic areas associated with feeding control (see [21] for review). Moreover, definitive meal related flux in endogenous levels of CRF- and BN-like peptides in a variety of hypothalamic nuclei are observed before, during and after a spontaneous meal in rodents [22]. This suggests CNS levels of bombesin-like peptides are intimately linked to meal taking behaviour. This evidence also suggests a critical link between bombesin and CRF functioning. CRF receptor antagonists block the effects of centrally administered bombesin on food intake and satiety [23]. Therefore, bombesin induced hypophagia may partly be mediated through interactions with CRF.

Bombesin appears to reduce human food intake in a similar manner (i.e. satiety enhancing). However, whether bombesin related compounds would be useful in treating obesity remains questionable. Infusion of bombesin, when combined with a gastric preload, inhibits food intake and increases satiety in lean women. However, when the same procedure is employed with obese women they do not respond in the same way to the infused bombesin. Thus, the obese may be insensitive to bombesin induced satiety [24].

2.3   Enterostatin

The pentapeptide enterostatin has been shown to specifically reduce the intake of fat, rather than protein or carbohydrate in animals offered a choice, or in other selection paradigms [25–28]. Enterostatin (peptide structure Val-Pro-Asp-Pro-Arg) is produced by the cleavage of pancreatic procolipase to colipase in the gut [29]. Enterostatin's effect of food intake is accompanied by non disruptive changes in feeding behaviour which are consistent with the operation of satiety, and the inhibition of hunger [30, 31]. These satiety enhancing effects are not related to enterostatin's effects on gastric emptying [32], but do require the consumption of a high fat diet for expression [27, 28]. The response to enterostatin is believed to be biphasic with lower doses having the most potent effect on food intake [25]. Enterostatin induced reductions in food intake are observed when the peptide is either administered chronically or acutely into the CNS [26, 32, 33] or peripherally [25–27, 30]. Particular CNS sites implicated in the action of enterostatin are the PVN and the amygdala [31, 34].

2.4 Glucagon-like peptide-1

Glucagon-like peptide (GLP)-1 (also produced in response to nutrient stimulation from the gut) produces a potent reduction in food intake when administered into the CNS of the rat. Both brain stem AP/NTS sites and hypothalamic ARC and PVN sites have been implicated in this GLP-1 hypophagic response [35–39]. C-fos procedures indicate that GLP-1 administered into the CNS activates neurones in the PVN and the amygdala [35]. No disruptions in feeding behaviour or illness appear to be associated with this effect [38]. If given chronically via the same intracerebroventricular route, GLP-1 produces a significant decrease in rodent body weight [40]. In men duodenal infusions of glucose produce corresponding decreases in appetite and increases in blood GLP-1, leading the authors to speculate on the role of GLP-1 in mediating the effects of glucose on appetite [41]. In obese men GLP-1 infusions increase feelings of fullness, and inhibit feelings of hunger [42]. In lean men GLP-1 infusions have been reported to reduce food intake and overall energy consumption with similar effects on hunger and fullness [43].

3 Central hunger and satiety factors – Monoamines

The role of monoamines in appetite control is well established by the numerous monoamine-active appetite suppressant drugs, both historically and those currently available (e.g. amphetamine, manzidol, phentamine, phenylpropanolamine (PPA), fenfluramine, d-fenfluramine and sibutramine). Such compounds reduce food intake (via satiety and/or non satiety mechanisms) and/or increase energy expenditure (via hyperactivity and/or thermogenesis) through a variety of differing mechanisms from sympathetic arousal to direct effects on hunger and satiety. Amphetamine with its dopaminergic (DA) and noradrenergic (NA) action, has been used as a weight reducing agent since the 1920s. Amphetamine is no longer widely used to treat obesity because of its side effects and addictive potential. However, such side-effects are not a necessary accompaniment of the hypophagic action of all monoaminergic drugs. In particular, the monoamine serotonin (5-HT) has been closely linked with the process of satiation and the state of satiety [44]. Serotoninergic drugs such as d-fenfluramine and the selective serotonin re-uptake inhibitors (SSRI) fluoxetine and sertraline have also be shown to potently reduce food intake and induce weight loss in animals and in humans (see [45] for review). The combination of fenfluramine and phentamine (DA and NA active) also proved to be an effective anti-obesity treatment (Phen-Fen combination). However, the combination also produced unacceptable effects on heart valvular function. Additionally sibutramine, a serotonin and noradrenaline reuptake inhibitor (SNRI), has also proved to be an effective hypophagic and anti-obesity compound. This would indicate monoamine systems in general, and 5-HT in particular, may be critical in the regulation of food intake.

3.1   Serotonin (5-HT)

The first studies to demonstrate a link between 5-HT and food intake were performed over 20 years ago (see [44–46] for reviews). To summarise, when 5-HT or its precursors, tryptophan and 5-HTP, are administered to rodents, food intake, eating rate and meals size are all significant reduced. Additionally, drugs which increased synaptic 5-HT (5-HT release or 5-HT re-uptake inhibition) produced similar changes to food intake without any apparent disruption to the structure of feeding behaviour. Conversely, blocking the synthesis of neuronal 5-HT (with p-chlorophenylalanine) or neurotoxically lesioning 5-HT neurons increased food intake. Consequently, it was proposed that the serotoninergic system was directly implicated in the control of food intake [44].

At the present time 14 different sub-types of 5-HT receptor have been identified: those most directly implicated in appetite regulation appear to be presynaptic 5-HT_{1A} and post synaptic 5-HT_{1B} ($5\text{-HT}_{1D\beta}$ in humans) and the 5-HT_{2C} receptor [45]. A large body of data has arisen from examining the effect of 5-HT functioning on food intake: most data have come from studies using serotoninergic drugs such as d-fenfluramine and its less specific predecessor fenfluramine, and SSRIs such as fluoxetine and sertraline. These drugs in combination with selective antagonists of the various 5-HT receptors subtypes indicate that 5-HT_{1B} and/or 5-HT_{2C} receptors are responsible for the satiety enhancing effects of CNS 5-HT.

Direct agonists of 5-HT receptors also reliably produce reductions in food intake. However, only agonists of 5-HT_{1B} and/or 5-HT_{2C} receptors subtypes produce the changes in feeding behaviour consistent with the operation of satiety [45–47]. Such agonists include mCPP ($5\text{-HT}_{1B/2C}$ agonist), TFMPP ($5\text{-HT}_{1B/2C}$ agonist) and CP-94 253 (5-HT_{1B} agonist). The direct action of the presynaptic 5-HT_{1A} receptor produces an increase in food intake consistent with its role as a presynaptic autoreceptor. Activation of the 5-HT_{2A} also produces a marked reduction in food intake but the alteration in feeding behaviour produced by 5-HT_{2A} activation is not consistent with satiety. Further evidence for the role of 5-HT_{2C} receptors in the control of food intake comes from 5-HT knockout transgenic mice. Tecott et al. [48] successfully produced a breed of mice that possessed no functional 5-HT_{2C} receptors. These 5-HT_{2C} knockout mice demonstrated marked hyperphagia and obesity.

The data from a limited number of human studies employing selective 5-HT agonists appears to confirm that agonism of 5-HT_{2C} and 5-HT_{1B} receptors produces reliable reductions in food intake, hunger and/or body weight consistent with a satiety enhancing action. mCPP has been shown to reduce food intake and hunger in lean women and reduce body weight in the obese [49, 50], and the novel $5\text{-HT}_{1B/1D}$ agonist sumatriptan has also been shown to reduce food intake (specifically of high fat food) in lean women [51].

Contradictory data exists on whether 5-HT_{1B} receptor-induced hypophagia is mediated in the PVN [52] or in adjacent hypothalamic nuclei [53, 54]. This debate is based on the accuracy of drug administration and/or PVN lesions procedures in the early studies. However, 5-HT drugs appear to potently affect levels of neuropeptide Y in the PVN. Blocking 5-HT synthesis or antagonising 5-HT receptor results in increases in NPY functioning in the PVN [55–57]. Additionally, 5-HT and CCK functioning have been experimentally linked. The actions of 5-HT drugs can be blocked by CCK-A antagonists. Conversely, anorexia induced by CCK-8 can be blocked by selective 5-HT agonists indicating the critical role of 5-HT_{2C} receptors in this mechanism. However, such interactions need careful interpretation as not all apparent blockades will necessarily involve a common receptor [45].

Much research on the role of 5-HT in appetite regulation has concentrated on whether CNS 5-HT functioning causes changes in the intake of specific macronutrients. It has been demonstrated that changes in dietary carbohydrate can have potent effects on 5-HT synthesis in the brain. CNS levels of dietary tryptophan, the penultimate precursor of 5-HT are effected by the competition from other large neutral amino acids (LNAAs) to cross the blood brain barrier. Dietary carbohydrate indirectly influences this competition to favour tryptophan by increasing the tryptophan:LNAA ratio [58]. Some authors have argued that raised CNS 5-HT levels subsequently determine carbohydrate intake (through selective suppression) whilst having little effect on the intake of other macronutrients (a sparing effect), thus forming a theoretical 5-HT carbohydrate intake feedback loop. Animal and human experiments testing this feedback loop have produced somewhat contradictory data. Many studies have demonstrated some degree of selective carbohydrate suppression supporting this theoretical system. However, enhanced 5-HT functioning has also been shown to have no macronutrient selective effects, or to even selectively reduce the intake of macronutrients other than carbohydrate. Assessment of the theoretical 5-HT carbohydrate intake feedback loop theory is further complicated by the methodological problems associated with diet selection studies in both animals and humans (such methodological problems are not restricted to 5-HT studies!).

However, there is accumulating evidence that 5-HT may influence the consumption of dietary fat [45, 59]. In addition, some recent animals studies have demonstrated that 5-HT, and 5-HT active drugs, selectively suppresses fat intake in fat preferring rats [60, 61]. This is consistent with human evidence demonstrating that the most potent effects of the 5-HT anti-obesity compound d-fenfluramine is on the intake of high fat snack foods [45, 62], and the effects of the 5-HT$_{1B/1D}$ agonist sumatriptan on fat intake [51]. This evidence is reviewed in more detail else where [62]. To summarise, it is likely that the 5-HT system exerts both general inhibitory effect over the pattern of food intake (by modulating hunger and satiety), and also has a selective effect on the consumption of macronutrients (fat, carbohydrate and protein).

3.2 Noradrenaline (NA)

Compared to 5-HT the role of the catecholamines, noradrenaline and dopamine in appetite regulation is comparatively less well defined. It has been demonstrated that activation of α_2 adrenoceptors in the PVN stimulates feeding behaviour, and this is associated with an endogenous releases of noradrenaline [63, 64]. Consequently, it could be supposed that hypothalamic NA and 5-HT acted in an antagonist manner to control food intake. However, agents which activate adrenergic β_2 receptors in the LH have been shown to produce a marked decrease in food intake [65]. Additionally, the effects of the over-the-counter weight loss medication phenylpropanolamine (PPA) appear to be mediated by α_1 adrenoceptors in the PVN [66]. Wellman et al. [67, 68] have subsequently proposed that the NA component of feeding control is mediated by the antagonistic action of α_1 and α_2 adrenoceptors within the PVN. Sibutramine, now licensed in the USA and in some parts of Europe, as a novel anti-obesity compound, has a potent noradrenergic action. Jackson et al. [69, 70] have suggested that NA mechanisms, rather than 5-HT mechanisms are responsible for the drug's initial action on food intake. These antagonist studies implicated α_1 and β_1 adrenoceptors, and possibly 5-HT$_{2C}$ receptors in the action of sibutramine. If this is the case, then this NA-mediated action of sibutramine appears to alter feeding behaviour in a manner consistent with satiety and in a similar manner to that produced by 5-HT drugs [71].

3.3 Dopamine (DA)

Like 5-HT, dopamine activation has been associated with decreases in food intake. However, the direct effect of DA on levels of activity could account for some of the observed hypophagic effects. Despite this, a large number of studies using drugs which selectively stimulate D_1 and/or D_2 receptors have shown that DA may play a role in the regulation of food intake. This may be related to the role of the CNS dopamine system in pleasure and/or directly in satiety. Moreover, the stimulation D1 receptors with low doses of selective agonists produce reductions in food intake with little evidence of behavioural disruption [65, 72, 73]. The particular role of the dopamine D_1 receptors in the natural control of food intake and satiety deserves further study. Because of dopamine's intimate role in limbic hedonic systems, dopaminergic weight control drugs may have addictive potential. It is worth noting that alpha-ergo bromocriptine, a dopamine agonist known as "Ergoset" has been proposed as a potential drug treatment for obesity.

Short-term clinical trials (18 weeks) have demonstrated Ergoset's effect on body weight and body fat [74].

4   Central hunger and satiety factors – Neuropeptides and other factors

A number of peptides which act as short-term peripheral satiety factors also have potent effects on feeding behaviour and food intake when directly administered into various regions of the CNS associated with appetite regulation. In addition, it should not always be assumed that the effects of these substances administered into the CNS will be identical to that produced by peripheral administration. The same hypothalamic areas identified as critical in appetite regulation by monoamines have been subsequently shown to contain a number of neuropeptides, most of which are appetite stimulants of varying potency.

4.1   Neuropeptide Y (NPY)

The role of hypothalamic neuropeptide Y (NPY) which produces the most marked stimulation of appetite, has come under particular focus. NPY is a 36 amino acid peptide found throughout the CNS. The hypothalamic NPY neurons implicated in appetite regulation project from the Arcuate Nucleus (ARC) into the PVN [75]. Increased levels of NPY in the PVN produce a potent stimulation of appetite resulting in an immediate and marked increase in food intake (see later). Deprivation augments endogenous NPY secretion which is normalised by subsequent feeding. Additionally, like food deprivation, NPY appears to increase food intake by promoting meal initiation and delaying meal termination, which is consistent with an increase in hunger [76]. Thus, CNS levels of NPY, like 5-HT, appear to be sensitive to the body's nutritional status.

NPY action in the PVN appears to oppose the effect of endogenous 5-HT in the same location. The fact that 5-HT functioning in the PVN inhibits NPY (by acting in the ARC) and vice versa would appear to confirm this close antagonist relationship [55–57]. The 5-HT$_{1B}$ receptor subtype in particular may be critical in this relationship [77]. Agonism of 5-HT$_2$ receptors also blocks the hyperphagic response elicited by NPY infusion into the PVN, but does not block the effects of NPY infusions at other sites [78]. It is the 5-HT_{2A} receptor subtype, rather than the 5-HT_{2C} classically associated with satiety, which appears to mediate this effect [79]. The antagonistic relationship between NPY and 5-HT in the PVN may be critical in the ultimate expression of appetite regulation and energy balance.

If hypothalamic NPY is critical in appetite regulation then its secretion should be determined by changes in peripheral physiology and metabolism related to short- and long-term energy balance. As noted earlier, food deprivation stimulates mRNA-NPY expression, but also energy excess should inhibit NPY functioning. Indeed, hypothalamic NPY does appear to be sensitive to levels of circulating insulin [80–82] and the *ob* protein leptin (signals of carbohydrate and fat storage respectively). The obese *ob/ob* mice which have no functioning leptin system, or the obese *db/db* mice which have no sensitivity to circulating *ob* protein leptin both possess increased levels of hypothalamic NPY mRNA. Moreover, CNS administration of leptin in leptin deficient ob/ob mice blocks the feeding response induced by exogenous NPY [75, 83–85]. Therefore NPY, along with galanin, may be one of a number of excitatory neuropeptides which leptin inhibits to reduce food intake and body weight [86–88].

Currently, at least five differing NPY receptors exist and are termed Y_1 to Y_5 [89]. A variety of studies employing receptor specific NPY ligands and selective NPY receptor subtype antagonists appear to indicate both Y_1 [90–92] and Y_5 [93, 94] receptors are critical in mediating the exogenous NPY hyperphagic response. Moreover, the Y_1 receptors have been implicated in the selective stimulation of carbohydrate intake [95]. However, the role of NPY Y_1 and Y_5 in the endogenous effects of NPY has yet to be determined [93]. NPY knock-out mice (no functioning NPY system), or mice bred with knockout Y_1 or Y_5 receptors do not display marked differences in body weight from the norm (i.e. the expected decrease) and can even develop obesity [96, 97]. In non-transgenic animals both high and low levels of NPY can result in hyperphagia and increased body weight. This is attributed to a rapid development of NPY Y_1 receptor hypersensitivity [98]. However, excessive and "anarchic" levels of NPY are associated with the dys-regulated feeding behaviour and hyperphagia observed in obese Zucker rats [99, 100]. Initial human genetic data suggests that endogenous NPY and the functioning of NPY Y_1 and Y_5 receptors are unlikely to be implicated in the development of human morbid obesity [101]. However, this does not mean that NPY blocking drugs may not be potentially useful anti-obesity compounds.

4.2 Galanin

Galanin, a 29 amino acid peptide found in both the gut and the brain, also produces a powerful feeding response when injected into the PVN of the rat. Some authors have further suggested that natural galanin functioning in the PVN may selectively stimulate the intake of dietary fat [102–104]. Hyperphagic effects are also observed if galanin is injected into the brain stem (at the site of the NTS) [105]. PVN lesions do not abolish CNS galanin induced feeding responses suggesting it is the NTS region that may be important in the galanin induced feeding response [106]. It is possible that galanin is one of the excitatory neuropeptides which the ob protein leptin may inhibit to reduce food intake and decrease body weight [87, 88]. Obviously blocking a system which selectively stimulates fat intake would have potential as an anti-obesity drug treatment.

4.3 Corticotrophin-releasing factor (CRF)

Corticotrophin-releasing factor (CRF), which is synthesised in the key areas of the forebrain such as the PVN, may mediate the effects of NPY, other neurochemical appetite factors, and peripheral satiety and adiposity signals [107]. Exogenous CNS CRF itself potently decreases food intake. Moreover, it is implicated in mediating the hypophagic effects of both bombesin [22, 23] and leptin [86, 108]. Because of the critical role of CRF in the hypothalamic pituitary adrenal axis (HPA) it has been difficult to separate its role in appetite regulation and the stress response. Consequently, the integral role of CRF in appetite regulation is still to be fully determined [37]. Urocortin, a neuropeptide related to CRF, binds with high affinity to CRF_2 receptors. Urocortin appears to be more potent than CRF itself at suppressing food intake and less implicated than CRF in the stress response [109]. Both CNS administration of CRF and urocortin appear to alter food intake via CRF_2 receptors. This receptor may be partially responsible for mediating the effects of stress on appetite [110].

4.4 Orexin

In 1998, Sakuria and colleagues identified two novel peptides in hypothalamic areas of adult rats associated with appetite regulation (the lateral (LH) and posterior hypothalamus). These two neuropeptides were named orexin A and orexin B. When either of the orexin peptides were administered into the CNS they stimulated food intake. This is consistent with activation of the LH. Moreover, when the rats were fasted orexin mRNA levels were up-regulated demonstrating the orexin system is sensitive to the nutritional status of the rodent [111]. Orexins (also termed hypocretins) appear to have potent effects on both pre and post synaptic receptors of neurons in these areas [112]. Two orexin receptors have been identified. Orexin OX_1 receptors are most abundant in the VMH whereas orexin OX_2 receptors are most abundant in the PVN [113]. The locus coeruleus (LC) and nucleus accumbens (NAc) may also be critical parts of the orexin appetitive system [113, 114]. Centrally administered orexin A produces a consistent increased food intake but this effect is less pronounced than NPY induced orexegenisis. Activation of neurones in the PVN and ARC are associated with this effect [115]. Orexin would appear to be another excitatory neuropeptide implicated in hunger (like NPY and galanin). However, the selectivity of the effects of orexins on food intake and/or energy balance and its integration into the other systems of appetite regulation remains to be determined, as does the effects of orexins on feeding behaviour.

4.5 Melanocortin (MC)

Much recent experimental research has focused on the identification of the mechanism responsible for the agouti gene mutation model of obesity in mice. Recent studies have shown that the agouti protein potently antagonises CNS melanocortin receptors and this may be critical in the aetiology of this mouse obesity phenotype. This is analogous to the effect of melanin-concentrating hormone (MCH) [116]. The net result of antagonising the hypothalamic melanocortin system appears to be increased food intake and/or body weight. Conversely, melanocortin peptides such as alpha melanocyte-stimulating hormone (αMSH) reduce food intake and reverse positive energy balance. αMSH and other melanocortin peptides are derived from pro-opiomelanocortin (POMC). Overfeeding appears to stimulate and starvation appears to inhibit endogenous mRNA expression of POMC [117, 118] suggesting the melanocortin system may be critical in the processes of satiety and long-term weight control (see [119] for review).

Studies have concentrated on the role of specific melanocortin receptors, particularly CNS MC_3-R MC_4-R receptors [120]. Inactivation of melanocortin-4 receptors (MC_4-R) by gene targeting results in mice that develop a maturity onset obesity syndrome associated with hyperphagia and diabetes which replicates the mouse agouti obesity syndrome mentioned previously [121]. CNS administration of melanocortin analogues which are potent agonists of neural melanocortin receptors inhibit the hyperphagia produced by fasting or NPY administration in mice [122]. This suggests that activation of CNS melanocortinergic neurones can potently inhibit feeding behaviour. Furthermore, POMC gene mutations preventing the production of endogenous melanocortin peptides have been implicated in the development of a specific childhood obesity syndrome [123]. It has also been found that MC_4-R agonists and antagonists have extremely potent effects on feeding when injected in the paraventricular nucleus (PVN), a site where MC_4-R gene expression is very high [124]. MC_4-R antagonist studies have also confirmed the contribution of the brain stem MC system in the control of feeding [125] and long-term weight regulation [126]. The hyperphagic effects of a selective MC_4-R antagonist can be blocked by NPY Y_1 receptor antagonist, suggesting that increased feeding induced by lack of MC_4-R activation may be mediated through activation of the NPY-ergic system [127]. The action of CNS Leptin on food intake and body weight is inhibited by selective MC_4-R antagonists suggesting that endogenous leptin inhibits food intake and lowers body weight via the melanocortin system [128]. Moreover, hypothalamic POMC mRNA is stimulated by leptin [118].

4.6   Other potent anorectic agents

A number of other substances act to produce potent decreases in food intake and/or body weight, which could be developed therapeutically. The cannabiniod receptor antagonist, SR141716 administered peripherally to normal weight rats dose dependently reduces food intake and body weight over a period of two weeks [129]. The role of endogenous cannabiniod receptors in the natural operation of the appetite has yet to be determined. Cocaine and amphetamine regulated transcript (CART) is a recently identified novel endogenous neuropeptide which acts as a satiety factor in the rat brain [130, 131]. CART functioning appears to be closely associated with the action of both leptin and NPY [130, 132]. In these studies CART induced c-fos expression has been observed in the PVN, ARC, amygdala and the NTS, further implicating it in appetite regulation [132].

5 Long-term circulatory factors

As noted earlier one of the classical theories of appetite control has involved the notion of a so-called long-term regulation involving a signal which informs the brain about the state of adipose tissue stores [133]. This idea has given rise to the notion of a lipostatic or ponderostatic mechanism. Indeed this is a specific example of a more general class of peripheral appetite (satiety) signals believed to circulate in the blood and reflecting the state of depletion or repletion of energy reserves which directly modulate brain mechanisms. Such substances may include satietin, adipsin or cytokine signals interleukin-6 (IL-6) tumour-necrosis factors (such as TNFα) [134].

5.1 Leptin (ob-protein)

In 1994, a landmark scientific event occurred with the discovery and identification of a mouse gene responsible for obesity [135]. A mutation of this gene in the *ob/ob* mouse produces a phenotype characterised by the behavioural trait of hyperphagia and the morphological trait of obesity. The *ob* gene controls the expression of a protein (the *ob*-protein) by adipose tissue and this protein can be measured in the peripheral circulation. The identification and synthesis of the protein made it possible to evaluate the effects of experimental administration of the protein either peripherally or centrally. Because the *ob*-protein caused a reduction in food intake as well as an increase in metabolic energy expenditure, it has been termed "leptin" from the Greek for thinness, leptos [136–138]. Whereas the *ob/ob* mouse lacked the *ob* protein leptin and so became obese, in another mouse obesity model the *db/db* mouse, the ability of adipose tissue to produce leptin did not appear critical. Further study of the leptin system in the *db/db* mouse demonstrated they were not leptin-deficient. However, a genetic defect in the *db/db* mouse rendered them insensitive to the newly identified adiposity signal [138–140]. The *db/db* mouse lacks the leptin receptor. With the identification of a human leptin analogue it was possible that either an inability to synthesise leptin in human adipose tissue and/or the insensitivity to released leptin may be a critical factor in the aetiology of human obesity. Since 1994, a proliferation of available data on the role of leptin has accrued. For a more detailed review of the neurobiology of leptin and the role of leptin in human appetite regulation see Campfield and Smith [141] and Coppack et al. [142].

There is evidence that leptin interacts with NPY, one of the brain's most potent neurochemicals involved in appetite [75, 83–85, 87, 88]. Together NPY and other neuromodulators (galanin, MC and CRF) may be involved in a peripheral-central circuit which links an adipose tissue signal with central appetite mechanisms and metabolic activity [86–88, 108, 127, 128] (see Fig. 2). Leptin probably acts in an analogous manner to insulin which has both central and peripheral actions; for some years it has been proposed that brain insulin represents a body weight signal with the capacity to control appetite. Like leptin, insulin also appears to inhibit NPY mRNA expression in the ARc [80–82].

The precise relationship between the *ob*-protein leptin and weight regulation remain to be fully determined. Circulating levels of leptin appear to reflect the current status of body fat deposition and increase with the degree of obesity [143, 144]. In animals and humans which are obese the measured amount of ob-protein (leptin) in the plasma is greater than in lean counterparts. Although the *ob*-protein is perfectly positioned to serve as a signal from adipose tissue to the brain, high levels of the protein obviously do not prevent obesity or weight gain. This may suggest instead some form of leptin insensitivity. However, in the obese the *ob*-protein certainly reflects the amount of adipose tissue in the body. Since the specific receptors for the protein (namely *ob*-receptors) have been identified in the brain (together with the gene responsible for its expression) a defect in body weight regulation could reside at the level of the receptor itself, or the integration of the subsequent signal into CNS appetite regulatory centres, rather than with the *ob*-protein. It is expected that drugs for the treatment of obesity based on the *ob*-protein concept will be developed within a few years.

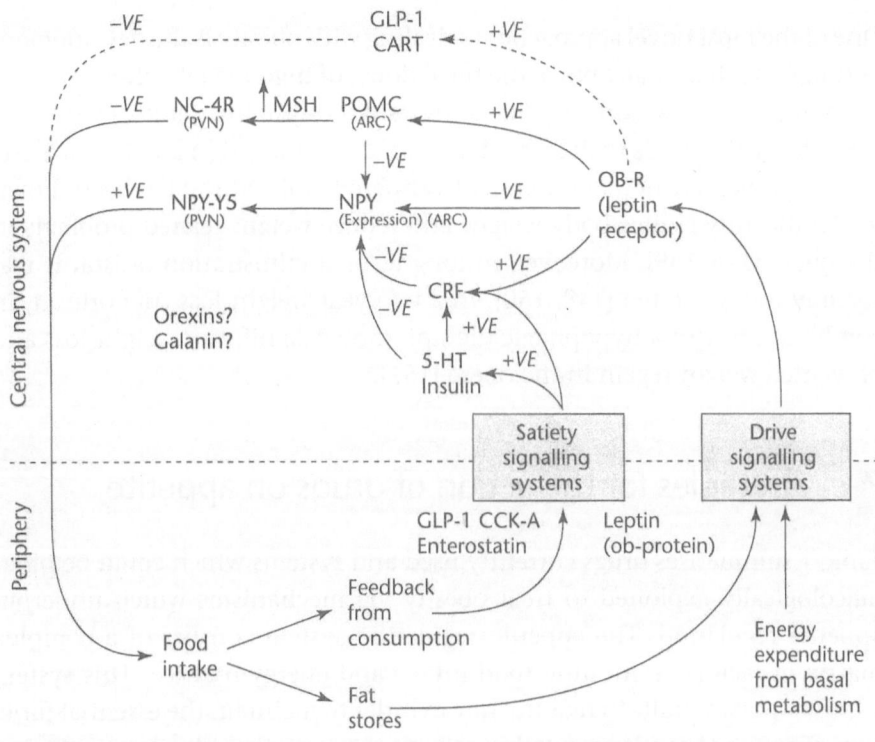

Fig. 2
Proposed interrelationship among agents known to exert effects on the expression of appetite. Scheme distinguishes between rapidly acting episodic satiety signalling systems and more slowly acting tonic signals reflecting need-induced drive for food (see glossary of abbreviations).

In a small number of individuals very severe obesity has been linked to leptin deficiency [145]. In turn the absence of leptin is caused by a mutation in the *ob* gene in these individuals. The extreme obesity can be treated by daily injections of leptin, and over the course of one year body weight was reduced by approximately 14 lbs. This is believed to be due to a suppression of energy intake. Very recently the first results of clinical trials with leptin have been published. Daily administration for 6 months produced a magnitude of weight loss comparable to that produced by other anti-obesity drugs such as d-fenfluramine (now withdrawn), sibutramine and xenical.

6   Other approaches

One of the most novel approaches to dealing with obesity is the development of drugs which partially block the breakdown of ingested fats, thus reducing the amount of fat absorbed. Orlistat (tetrahydrolipstatin, xenical) is a lipase inhibitor which leads to decreased intestinal fat absorption and has recently been approved as a new anti-obesity treatment [146]. Orlistat has been shown to significantly reduce body weight and reduce weight-related problems in the obese [146–149]. Moreover, in long-term administration orlistat is reasonably well tolerated [148, 150]. In a two-year weight loss trial orlistat, in combination with a hypophagic diet, promoted significant weight loss and prevented weight regain in the obese [151].

7   Strategies for the action of drugs on appetite

Table 1 summarises drugs currently used and systems which could be pharmacologically exploited to treat obesity via mechanisms which underpin appetite regulation. The appetite regulation system consists of a complex matrix of factors controlling food intake and energy balance. This system seems to possess built-in redundancy in order to maintain the essential function of eating. Appetite regulation reflects the operation of an asymmetrical system with a strong defence against energy deficit (weight loss) but only a weak protection against energy surplus (weight gain). At the present time the most potent drugs available can produce a maximal average weight loss of about 10 kg in clinical trials. Such a weight loss is suffcent to significantly improve metabolic risk factors and obesity-related disease such as diabetes, but clearly does not constitute a cure for obesity. It remains to be demonstrated whether the next generation of anti-obesity drugs can exert more potent and enduring effects on body weight.

Acknowledgements

We are grateful to Gill Thompson, Department of Psychology, University of Central Lancashire, Preston, PR1 2HE, UK, for her help in reviewing the literature.

Table 1.
Anti-obesity drugs (working mainly through appetite control) available or currently under testing, and potential future anti-obesity drugs

Current	Potential (some currently under development)
Sibutramine	$5\text{-}HT_{2C}$ agonists
[Xenical*]	$5\text{-}HT_{1B/1D}$ agonists
Leptin	Leptin sensitizers
Ergoset?	MC-4 agonists
Phentermine	CRF_2 agonists
	Enterostatin
	GLP-1
	GRP
	NPY Y_5 antagonists
	Galanin antagonists
	CBR-1 antagonists
	Orexin antagonists
	Opioid antagonists

*Xenical does not have a direct effect on appetite mechanisms but certainly exerts control over appetite via nutrient absorption.

References

1   Blundell J.E.: Trends Pharmacol. Sci. *12*, 147–157 (1991).

2   Gibbs J., Young R. and Smith G.P.: J. Comp. Physiol. *84*, 488–493 (1973).

3   Gibbs J., Falasco J.D. and McHugh P.R.: Am. J. Physiol. *230*, 12–18 (1976).

4   Antin J., Gibbs J., Holt J., Young R.C. and Smith G.P.: J. Comp. Physiol. Psychol. *89*, 784–790 (1975).

5   Dourish C.T., Rycroft W. and Iversen S.D.: Science *245*, 1509–1511 (1989).

6   Moran T.H. and Schwatz G.J.: Crit. Rev. Neurobiology. *9*, 1–28 (1994).

7   Kissileff H.R., Pi-Sunyer X., Thornton J. and Smith G.P.: Am. J. Clin. Nutr. *34*, 154–160 (1981).

8   Greenough A., Cole G., Lewis J., Lockton A. and Blundell J.: Physiol. Behav. *64* (1999, in press).

9   Hopman W.P.M., Jansen J.B. and Lamers C.B.: Scand. J. Gastroenterol. *20*, 843–847 (1985).

10   Moran T.H., Baldessarini A.R., Salorio C.F., Lowery T. and Schwartz G.J.: Amer. J. Physiol. *41*, R1245–R1251 (1997).

11   Corp E.S., Curcio M., Gibbs J. and Smith G.P.: Physiol. & Behav. *61*, 823–827 (1997).

12   Brenner L.A. and Ritter R.C.: Physiol. & Behav. *63*, 711–716 (1998).

13   Dorre D. and Smith G.P.: Physiol. Behav. *65*, 1–14 (1998).

14   Esfanhani N., Bedner I., Quershi G.A. and Sodersten P.: Biochem and Behav. *51*, 9–12 (1995).
15   Voigt J.P., Sohr R. and Fink H.: Pharm. Biochem. Behav. *59*, 179–182 (1998).
16   Gibbs J., Fauser E.A., Rowe B.J., Rolls E.T and, Maddison S.P.: Nature *282*, 208–210 (1979).
17   Smith J., Perez S., Rushing P.A., Smith G.P. and Gibbs J.: Peptides *18*, 1465–1467 (1997).
18   Stuckley J.A. and Gibbs J.: Brain Res. Bull. *8*, 617–621 (1982).
19   Stratford T.R., Gibbs J. and Smith G.P.: Peptides *17*, 107–110 (1996).
20   Flynn F.W.: Physiol & Behav *62*, 791–798 (1997).
21   McCoy J.G. and Avery D.D.: Peptides *11*, 595–697 (1990).
22   Plamondon H. and Merali Z.: Amer. J. Physiol. *41*, R268–R274 (1997a).
23   Plamondon H. and Merali Z.: Eur. J. Pharmacol. *340*, 99–109 (1997b).
24   Lieverse R.J., Mascle A.A.M., Jansen J.B.M.J., Lam W.F. and Lamers C.B.H.W.: Eur. J. Clin. Nutr. *52*, 207–212 (1998).
25   Erlanson-Ablertsson C., Mei J., Okada S., York D.A. and Bray G.A.: Physiol. Behav. *49*, 1191–1194 (1991).
26   Okada S., York D.A., Bray G.A., Erlanson-Albertsson C.: Physiol. Behav. *49*, 1185–1189 (1991).
27   Mei J. and Erlanson-Albertsson C.: Obes. Res. *4*, 161–165 (1996).
28   Lin L. and York D.A.: Amer. J. Physiol. *44*, R619–R623 (1998a).
29   Erlanson-Ablertsson C. and Larsson A.: Regul. Pept. *22*, 325–331 (1988).
30   Lin L., McClanahan S., York D.A. and Bray G.A.: Physiol. Behav. 53, 789–794 (1993).
31   Lin L. and York D.A.: Peptides *19*, 557–562 (1998b).
32   Lin L. and York D.A.: Brain Res. *745*, 205–209 (1997a).
33   Shargill N.S., Tsujii S., Bray G.A., Erlanson-Albertsson C.: Brain Res. *544*, 137–140 (1991).
34   Lin L. and York D.A.: Peptides *18*, 1341–1347 (1997b).
35   Turton M.D., O'Shea D., Gunn I., Beak S.A., Edwards C.M.B., Meeran K., Choi S.J., Taylor G.M., Heath M.M., Lambert P.D.et al.: Nature *379*, 6560, 69–72 (1998).
36   Tang-Christensen M., Larsen P.J. and Goke R.: Am. J. Physiol. *271*, R848–R856 (1996).
37   Rowland N.E. and Kalra S.P.: CNS Drugs *7*, 419–426 (1997).
38   McMahon L.R. and Wellman P.J.: Amer. J. Physiol. *43*, R23–R29 (1998).
39   Hwa J.J., Ghibaudi L., Williams P., Witten M.B., Tedesco R. and Strader C.D.: Peptides *19*, 869–875 (1998).
40   Meeran K., O'Shea D., Edwards C.M.B., Turton M.D., Heath M.M., Gunn I., Abusnana S., Rossi M., Small C.J., Goldstone A.P. and Taylor G.M.: Endocrinology *140*, 244–250 (1999).
41   Lavin J.H., Wittert G.A., Andrews J., Yeap B., Wishart J.M., Morris H.A., Morley J.E., Horowitz M. and Read N.W.: Amer. J. Clin. Nutr. *68*, 3 (1998).
42   Naslund E., Gutniak M., Skogar S., Rossner S. and Hellstrom P.M.: Amer. J. Clin. Nutr. *68*, 3 (1998).
43   Gutzwiller J.P., Goke B., Drewe J., Hildebrand P., Ketterer S., Handschin D., Winterhalder R., Conen D. and Beglinger C.: Gut *44*, 81–86 (1999).
44   Blundell J.E.: Int. J. Obes. *1*, 15–42 (1977).
45   Blundell J.E. and Halford J.C.G.: CNS Drugs *9*, 473–495 (1998).
46   Blundell J.E.: Am. J. Clin. Nutr. *55*, 1555–1595 (1992).
47   Halford J.C.G., Wanninayake S.C.D. and Blundell J.E.: Pharmacol. Biochem. Behav. *61*, 159–168 (1998).
48   Tecott L.H.,Sum L.M. and Akana S.F.: Nature *374*, 542–546 (1995).

49   Walsh A.E., Smith K.A. and Oldman A.D.: Psychopharmacology *116*, 120–122 (1994).

50   Sargent P.A., Sharpley A.L. and Williams C.: Psychopharmacology *133*, 309–312 (1997).

51   Boeles S., Williams C. and Campling GM.: Psychopharmacology *129*, 179–182 (1997).

52   Hutson P.H., Donohoe T.P. and Curzon G.: Psychopharmacology *97*, 550–552 (1988).

53   Fletcher P.J. and Coscina D.V.: Pharmacol. Biochem. Behav. *46*, 487–491 (1993).

54   Coscina D.V., Feifel D., Norbrega J.N.: Am. J. Physiol. *266*, R1562–R1567 (1994).

55   Dryden S., Wang Q. and Frankish H.M.: Brain Res. *699*, 12–18 (1995).

56   Dryden S., Frankish H.M. and Wang Q.: Brain Res. *724*, 232–237 (1996).

57   Dryden S., Frankish H.M. and Wang Q.: Neuroscience *72*, 557–566 (1996).

58   Fernstorm J.D.: Appetite *8*, 163 (1987).

59   Blundell J.E., Lawton C.L. and Halford J.C.G.: Obesity Res. *3*, 471–476 (1995).

60   Smith B.K., York D.A. and Bray G.A.: Pharmacol. Biochem. Behav. 60, 105 (1998a).

61   Smith B.K., York .DA. and Bray G.A.: Am. J. Physiol. (1999, in press)

62   Halford J.C.G., Smith B.K. and Blundell J.E.: In: Neural Control of Macronutrient Selection (1999).

63   Leibowitz S.F.: Pharmacol. Biochem. Behav. *8*, 163–175 (1978).

64   Leibowitz S.F.: Neurosci. Biobehav. Rev. *12*, 101–109 (1988).

65   Angel I.: Clin. Neuropharmacol. *13*, 361–391 (1990).

66   Wellman P.J.: Am. J. Clin. Nutr. *55*, 193s–198s (1992).

67   Wellman P.J., Davies B.T., Morien A. and McMahon L.: Life Sciences *53*, 669–679 (1993).

68   Wellman P.J., McMahon L.R., Green T. and Tole A.: Pharmacol. Biochem. Behav. *57*, 281–284 (1997).

69   Heal D.J., Aspley S., Prow M.R., Jackson H.C. and Cheetham S.C.: Int. J. Obesity 22 (1), s18–s28 (1998).

70   Jackson H.C., Nearham M.C., Hutchins L., Mazurkiewicz S.E., Needham A.M., Heal D.J.: Brit. J. Pharmacology *121*, 1613–1618 (1997).

71   Halford J.C.G., Heal D.J. and Blundell J.E.: Br. J. Pharamcology *114*, 378p (1995).

72   Terry P., Gilbert D.B. and Cooper S.J.: Obes. Res. *3*, s515–s524 (1995).

73   Phillips G.D., Howes S.R., Whitelaw R.B., Robbins T.W. and Everitt B.J.: Psychopharmacology *117*, 82–90 (1995).

74   Cincotta A.H. and Meier A.H.: Diabetes Care *19*, 667–679 (1996).

75   Dryden S. and Williams G.: Curr. Opin. Endo. Diab. *3*, 51–58 (1996).

76   Bivens C.L.M., Thomas W.J. and Stanley B.G.: Brain Res. *782*, 271–280 (1998).

77   Grignaschi G., Sironi F. and Samanin R.: Eur. J. Pharmacol. *274*, 221–224 (1995).

78   Currie P.J. and Coscina D.V.: Neuroreport *8*, 3759–3762 (1997).

79   Currie P.J. and Coscina D.V.: Brain Res. *803*, 212–217 (1998).

80   Schwartz M.W., Marks J., Sipols A.J., Baskin D.B., Wood S.C., Kahn S.E. and Porte J.D.: Endocrinology *128*, 2645–2647 (1991).

81   Schwartz M.W., Figlewicz D.P., Baskin D.G., Woods S.C., Kahn S.E. and Porte J.D.: Endocrine Rev. *2*, 109–113 (1994).

82   Woods S.C., Seeley R.J., Porte D. and Schwartz M.W.: Science *280*, 1378–1383 (1998).

83   Erickson J.C., Clegg K.E. and Palmiter R.D.: Nature *381*, 415–418 (1996).

84   Erickson J.C., Hollopetter G. and Palmiter R.D.: Science *274*, 1704–1707 (1996).

85   Smith F.J., Campfield L.A., Moschera J.A., Bailon P.S. and Burn P.: Reg. Peptides. *75*, 433–439 (1998).

86   Schwartz M.W., Seeley R.J., Campfield L.A., Burn P. and Baskin D.G.: J. Clin. Inv. *98*, 1101–1106 (1996).

87   Sahu A.: Endocrin. *139*, 795–798 (1998).

88   Sahu A.: Endocrin. *139*, 4739–4742 (1998).

89   Balashubramaniam A.: Peptides *18*, 445–457 (1997).

90   Lopez-Valpuesta F.J., Nyce J.W. and Myers R.D.: Neuroreport *7*, 2781–2784 (1996).

91   Kask A., Rago L and, Harro J.: Brit. J. Pharmacol. *124*, 1507–1515 (1998).

92   Wieland H.A., Engel W., Eberlein W., Rudolf K., Doods H.N.: Brit. J. Pharmacol. *125*, 549–560 (1998).

93   Marsh D.J., Hollopeter G., Kafer K.E. and Palmiter R.D.: Nature Medicine *4*, 718–721 (1998)

94   Tang-Christensen M., Kristensen P., Stidsen C.E., Brand C.L. and Larsen P.J.: Endocrin. *159*, 307–312 (1998).

95   Leibowitz S.F. and Alexander J.T.: Peptides *12*, 1251–1260 (1991).

96   Hollopeter G., Erickson J.C. and Palmiter R.D.: Int. J. Obes. *22*, 506–512 (1998).

97   Woldbye D.P.D. and Larsen P.J.: Nature Medicine *4* (6), 671–672 (1998).

98   Kalra P.S., Dube M.G., Xu B. and Kalra S.P.: Reg. Peptides *72*, 121–130 (1997).

99   Stricker-Krongrad A., Kozak R., Burlet C., Nicolas J.P. and Beck B.: Amer. J. Physiol. *43*, R2112–R2116 (1997).

100   Ishihara A., Tanaka T., Kanatani A., Fukami T., Ihara M. and Fukuroda T.: Amer. J. Physiol. *43*, R1500–R1504 (1998).

101   Roche C., Boutin P., Dina C., Gyapay G., Basdevent A., Hager J., Guy-Grand B., Clement K. and Froguel: Diabetologic *40*, 671–675 (1997).

102   Leibowitz S.F.: Obes. Res. *3* (suppl 4), 573–589s (1995).

103   Leibowitz S.F., Akabayashi A., Alexander J.T. and Wang J.: Endocrinol. *139*, 1771–1780 (1998).

104   Lin L., York D.A. and Bray G.A.: Obes. Res. *4*, 117–123 (1996).

105   Koegler F.H. and Ritter S.: Obes. Res. *4*, 329–336 (1996).

106   Koegler F.H. and Ritter S.: Physiol. Behav. *63*, 521–527 (1998).

107   Menzaghi F., Heinrichs S.C. and Pich E.M.: Brain Res. *618*, 76–82 (1993).

108   Gardner J.D., Rothwell N.J. and Luheshi G.N.: Nature Neurosci. *1*, 103 (1998).

109   Spina M., Merlo-Pich E., Chan R.K.W., Basso A.M., Rivier J., Vale W. and Koob G.F.: Science *273* (5281), 1561–1564 (1996).

110   Smagin G.N., Howell L.A., Ryan D.H., DeSouza E.B. and Harris R.B.S.: Neurorep.*7*, 1601–1606 (1998).

111   Sakurai T., Amemiya A., Ishii M., Matsuzaki I., Chemelli R.M., Tanaka H., Williams S.C., Richardson J.A., Kozlowski G.P., Wilson S. et al.: Cell *92*, 573–585 (1998).

112   van den Pol A.N., Gao X.B., Obrietan K., Kilduff T.S. and Belousov A.B.: J. Neurosci. *18*, 7962–7971 (1998).

113   Trivedi P., Yu H., MacNeil D.J., Vander Ploeg L.H.T. and Guan X.M.: FEBS Letters *438*, 71–75 (1998).

114   Peyron C., Tighe D.K., van den Pol A.N., de Lecea L., Heller H.C., Sutcliffe J.G. and Kilduff T.S.: J. Neurosci. *18*, 9996–10015 (1998).

115   Edwards C.M.B., Abusnana S., Sunter D., Murphy K.G., Ghatel M.A. and Bloom S.R.: J. Endocrinology *160*, R7–R12 (1999).

116   Ludwig D.S., Mountjoy K.G., Tatro J.B., Gillette J.A., Frederich R.C., Flier J.S. and Maratos-Flier E.: Amer. J. Physiol. *37*, E627–E633 (1998).

117   Hagan M.M., Rushing P.A., Schwartz M.W., Yagaloff K.A., Burn P., Woods S.C. and Seeley R.J.: J. Neurosceince *19*, 2362–2367 (1999).

118   Mizuno T.M., Kleopoulos S.P., Bergen H.T., Roberts J.L., Priest C.A. and Mobbs C.V.: Diabetes *47*, 294–297 (1998).

119   Fisher S.L., Yagaloff K.A. and Burn P.: Int. J. Obesity *23*, s54–s58 (1999).

120   Kiefer L.L., Ittoop O.R.R., Bunce K., Truesdale A.T., Willard D.H., Nichols J.S., Blanchard S.G., Mountjoy K., Chen W.J. and Wilkison W.O.: Biochemistry *36*, 2084–2090 (1997)

121   Huszar D., Lynch C.A., Fairchild-Huntress V., Dunmore J.H., Fang Q., Berkemeier L.R., Gu W., Kesterson R.A., Boston B.A., Cone R.D. et al.: Cell *88*, 131–141 (1997).

122   Fan W., Boston B.A., Kesterson R.A., Hruby V.J. and Cone R.D.: Nature *385*, 6612, 165–168 (1997).

123   Krude H., Biebermann H., Luck W., Horn R., Brabant G. and Gruters A.: Nature Genetics *19*, 155–157 (1998).

124   Giraudo S.Q., Billington C.J. and Levine AS.: Brain Res. *809*, 302–306 (1998).

125   Grill H.J., Ginsberg A.B., Seeley R.J. and Kaplan J.M.: J. Neuroscience *18*, 10128–10135 (1998).

126   Skuladottir G.V., Jonsson L., Skarphedinsson J.O., Mutulis F., Muceniece R., Raine A., Mutule I., Helgason J., Prusis P., Wikberg J.E.S. and Schioth H.B.: Brit J. Pharmacol. *126*, 27–34 (1999).

127   Kask A., Rago L., Korrovits P., Wikberg J.E.S. and Schioth H.B.: Biochem. Biophys. Res. Com. *248*, 245–249 (1998).

128   Kask A., Rago L., Wikberg J.E.S. and Schioth H.B.: Eur. J. Pharmacol. *360*, 15–19 (1998).

129   Colombo G., Agabio R., Diaz G., Lobina C., Reali R. and Gessa G.L.: Life Sci. *63*, 113–117 (1998).

130   Kristenbesen P., Judge ME., Thim L., Ribel U., Christjansen K.N., Wulff B.S., Clausen J.T., Jensen P.B., Madsen O.D., Vrang N., Larsen P.J. and Hastrup S.: Nature *393*, 72–76 (1998).

131   Lambert P.D., Couceyro P.R., McGirr K.M., Vechia S.E.D., Smith Y. and Kuhar M.J.: Synapse *29*, 293–298 (1998).

132   Vrang N., Tang Christensen M., Larsen P.J. and Kristensen P.: Brain Res. *818*, 499–509 (1999).

133   Kennady J.C.: Proc. R. Soc. London (Biol.) *140*, 578 (1953).

134   Mohamed-Ali V., Pinkney J.H. and Coppack S.W.: Int. J. Obes. *22*, 1145–1158 (1998).

135   Zhang Y., Proenca R., Maffei M., Barone M. and Friedman J.M.: Nature *372*, 425–432 (1994)

136   Pelleymounter M.A., Cillen M.J., Baker M.B., Hecht R., Winters D., Boone T. and Collins F.: Science *269*, 540–543 (1995).

137   Halaas J.L., Gajiwala K.S., Maffei M., Cohen S.L., Chati B.T., Rabiowitx D., Lallone R.L., Burley S.K. and Friedman J.M.: Science *269*, 543–546 (1995).

138   Campfield L.A., Smith F.J., Guisez Y., Devos R. and Burn P.: Science *269*, 546–549 (1995).

139   Chen H., Charlet O., Tartaglia L.A., Woolf E.A., Weng X., Ellis S.J., Lakey N.D., Culpapper J., Moore K.J., Breibart R.F. et al.: Cell *84*, 491–495 (1996).

140   Lee G., Proenca R., Montez J.M., Carrol K.M., Darvishzadeh J.G., Leed J.I. and Freidman J.M.: Nature *379*, 632–635 (1996).

141   Campfield L.A. and Smith F.J.: Proc. Nutr. Soc. *57*, 429–440 (1998).

142   Coppack S.W., Pinkney J.H. and Mohamed-Ali V.: Proc. Nutr. Soc. *57*, 461–470 (1998).

143   Maffei M., Halaas J., Ravussin E., Partley R.E., Lee G.H., Zhang Y., Fei H., Kim S., Lallone R., Ranganathan S., Kern P.A. and Friedman J.M.: Nature Medicine *1*, 1155–1161 (1995).

144   Considine R.V., Sinda M.K., Heiman M.L., Kriauciunas A., Stephens T.W., Nyce M.R.,

Ohannesian J.P., Marco C.C., McKee L.J., Baur T.L. and Caro J.F.: N. Engl. J. Med. *334*, 292–295 (1996).

145 Montague C.T., Farooqi I.S., Whitehead J.P., Soos M.A., Rau H., Wareham N.J., Sewter C.P., Digby J.E., Mohammed S.N., Hurst J.A. et al.: Nature *387*, 903–908 (1997).

146 Drent M.L. and van der Veen E.A.: Obes. Res. *3*, S623–S625 (1995).

147 James W.P.T., Avenell A., Broom J. and Whitehead J.: Int. J. Obes. *21*, S24–S30 (1997).

148 Van Gaal L.F., Broom J.I., Enzi G. and Toplak H.: Eur. J. Clin. Pharmacol. *54*, 125–132 (1998).

149 Davidson M.H., Hauptman J., Di Girolamo M., Foreyt J.P., Halsted C.H., Heber D., Heimburger D.C., Lucas C.P., Robbins D.C., Chung J. and Heymsfield S.B.: JAMA *281*, 235–242 (1999).

150 McNeely W. and Benfield P.: Drugs *56*, 241–249 (1998).

151 Sjostrom L., Rissen A., Anderson T., Boldrin M., Golay A., Koppeschaar H.P.F. and Kempf M.: Lancet *352*, 167–172 (1998).

Progress in Drug Research, Vol. 54 (E. Jucker, Ed.)
©2000 Birkhäuser Verlag, Basel (Switzerland)

Serotonin, dopamine and norepinephrine transporters in the central nervous system and their inhibitors

By Berend Olivier[1],
Willem Soudijn[2] and
Ineke van Wijngaarden[2]

[1]Dept. of Psychopharmacology,
Faculty of Pharmacy, Utrecht Uni-
versity, Sorbonnelaan 16, NL-3584
CA Utrecht; PsychoGenics Inc.,
4 Skyline Drive, Hawthorne, NY
10532, USA, and Dept. of Psychia-
try, Yale University School of
Medicine, 34 Park St., New Haven,
CT 06508, USA, and [2]Leiden/
Amsterdam Center for
Drug Research, P.O. Box 9502,
NL-2300 RA Leiden, The Nether-
lands

Berend Olivier

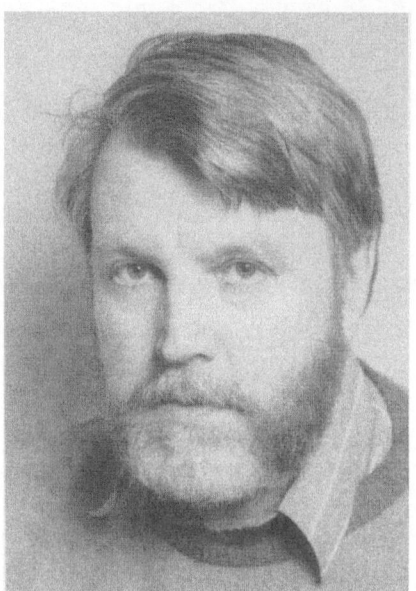

studied neurobiology (1967–1973) at the University of Groningen, leading to a PhD thesis (1977) on the role of the hypothalamus in rat social behaviour. In 1977, he started a new behavioural pharmacology group at Philips-Duphar in Weesp (now Solvay Pharmaceuticals), leading to the development of a new class of psychotropic drugs, serenics, against pathological aggression in psychiatric patients. In 1985, he became head of CNS-pharmacology and involved in research to find new chemical entities, including antidepressants, antipsychotics and anxiolytics. Since 1992, he has been professor of Psychopharmacology, Utrecht University, and a senior principal scientist at CNS-Research Solvay. Since April 1999 he is Vice-President of Research for PsychoGenics Inc., New York, and full adjunct professor at Yale University. His present interests are in the neurobiology and psychopharmacology of anxiety, depression, aggression and sexual behaviour. He leads an active research program in Utrecht, centering around serotonin and CRH, using animal models of psychiatric diseases.

Summary

An overview is presented on progress made in the research on neuronal transporters of serotonin, dopamine and norepinephrine in the central nervous system.

Tools developed by molecular biology, such as expression of cloned transporters, their mutants and chimera in non-neuronal cells offered the opportunity to study the putative domains for binding of substrates and uptake inhibitors and discover factors in the regulation of the transporter function. The study of the distribution of monoamine transporters in human brain became possible by the development of selective radiolabelled transport inhibitors.

The relationships between the chemical structure of the uptake inhibitors and the affinity for the monoamine transporters is reported, and the (potential) therapeutic applications of the compounds are discussed.

Contents

Keywords

Serotonin transporter, dopamine transporter, norepinephrine transporter, localization in CNS, structure, ligand binding domains, regulation, selective inhibitors, pharmacology, (potential) therapeutics.

Glossary of abbreviations

DAT, dopamine transporter; DA, dopamine; 5-HT, 5-hydroxytryptamine (serotonin); NET, norepinephrine transporter; NE, norepinephrine; PET, position emission tomography; SERT, serotonin transporter; SI, selectivity index; SPECT, single photon emission computed tomography; TM, transmembrane domain.

1   Introduction

Neuronal transmission in the central nervous system is effected by the release of neurotransmitters from the presynaptic neuron into the synaptic cleft where they stimulate receptors in the membrane of pre- and postsynaptic neurons.

Stimulation of these receptors is ended by re-uptake of the neurotransmitter into the presynaptic neuron where it is partly enzymatically inactivated and partly stored in presynaptic vesicles.

For a minor part the neurotransmitter may be taken up in glial cells where it is enzymatically destroyed.

The re-uptake mechanism is effected by neurotransmitter transporters located in the presynaptic membranes whereas the vesicular uptake of the neurotransmitter in the presynaptic neuron is caused by transporters in the vesicle membranes.

The serotonin transporters (SERT), the dopamine transporters (DAT) and the noradrenaline (= norepinephrine) transporters (NET) form a subfamily of the fairly large family of transporters that are dependent on extracellular Na^+-ions whereas the vesicular transporters are H^+-dependent.

The structural features (Fig. 1) common to the neurotransmitter transporters SERT, DAT and NET but also to many other Na^+-dependent transporters are:

- twelve putative membrane spanning domains (TMs) consisting of about 25 hydrophobic amino acids each;
- a large extra-cellular loop between TM3 and TM4 with potential sites for N-glycosylation;
- both rather large N- and C-terminal domains containing potential phosphorylation sites are situated at the intracellular side of the transporter.

The overall structure of the vesicular neurotransmitter transporter in the vesicle membrane is similar to that of the monoamine transporters SERT, DAT and NET but it has distinctive molecular features. The corresponding large

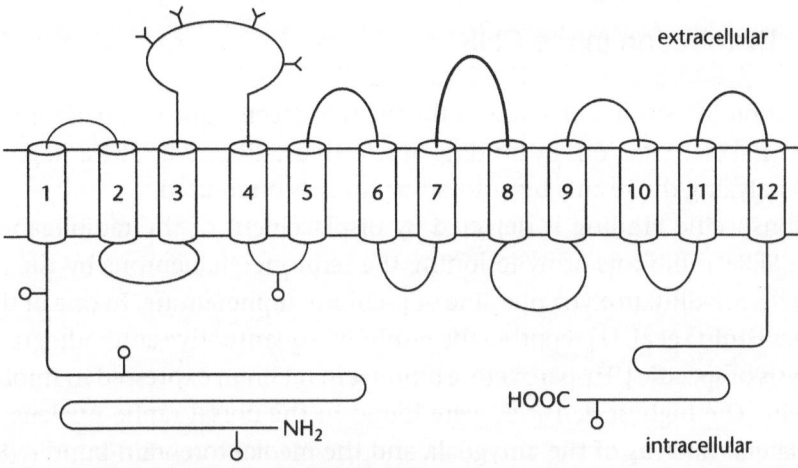

Fig. 1
Overall modell of the Na⁺Cl⁻ dependent monoamine transporters in the central nervous system. Y, N-glycosylation site; ꭤ, phosphorylation site.

N-glycosylation sites containing loop connects TM3 with TM4 and projects into the vesicular lumen, whereas the N-and C-terminals are oriented toward the cytoplasmatic side.

Re-uptake of neurotransmitters from the synaptic cleft is one important factor in the complex regulation mechanism of neuronal neurotransmission.

Inhibition of the re-uptake by selective inhibitors of the neurotransmitter transporter, thereby enhancing the concentration of neurotransmitter in the synaptic cleft, is a means of ameliorating the neurotransmission in a dysfunctioning neuronal population.

Thus SERT and/or NET inhibitors are useful drugs in the treatment of depression, obsessive compulsive disorder and panic disorder whereas DAT inhibitors may be useful in attention deficit/hyperactivity disorder.

DAT inhibitors can also be used as diagnostic tools when used as markers for deficits in the density of receptor populations, e.g. in Parkinson's disease or suspicion of Parkinson's disease using positron emission tomography (PET) or single photon emission computed tomography (SPECT).

The development of new SERT, DAT and NET inhibitors is still in progress.

2   The serotonin transporter (SERT)

2.1   Distribution in the CNS

In distribution studies of SERTs in the brain the technique of labelling SERTs in coronal brain sections by binding of selective radioactive SERT antagonists and analyzing the results by autoradiography is often used.

Nonspecific binding is detected by displacement of the radioligand by other SERT inhibitors or by lesioning the serotonergic neurons by the neurotoxins 5,7-dihydroxytryptamine or p-chloroamphetamine. In one of these studies Hrdina et al. [1] reported the results of a quantitative autoradiographic analysis of specific [³H]-paroxetine binding in rat brain expressed in fmol/mg protein. The highest densities were found in the dorsal raphe nucleus, the basolateral nucleus of the amygdala and the medial forebrain bundle (872, 632 and 506 fmol/mg protein, resp.).

High densities were found in several nuclei of the thalamus (about 400 fmol/mg protein), in the dorsal area and the dorsomedial nucleus of the hypothalamus (409 and 324 fmol/mg protein), and in several regions of the midbrain, including the median raphe nucleus and substantia nigra reticularis (470 and 437 fmol/mg protein resp.). In the pons, the locus coeruleus shows a high density of 423 fmol/mg protein. Lower densities ranging from 250-200 fmol/mg protein were found in the basal ganglia, the hippocampus and the temporal, perirhinal, and entorhinal cortex. The lowest density was found in the frontal cortex (60 fmol/mg protein).

A very similar distribution of [³H]paroxetine binding sites was found in *post mortem* human brain as reported by Cortés et al. [2]. The labelling of SERTs by the selective antagonist [³H]citalopram was used to analyze the neuroanatomical distribution of SERTs in the rat and human forebrain [3]. In general the densities of labelling of binding sites by [³H]citalopram in substructures of the hippocampus, hypothalamus and amygdala in human and rat brain tissue are identical. However, there are some striking differences. The ventromedial and arcuate nuclei of the hypothalamus and the cortical nucleus of the amygdala are densely labelled in the human brain tissue but sparsely labelled in the rat counterparts. The reverse holds true for the basolateral nucleus of the amygdala of the rat which is densely labelled whereas its human counterpart is sparsely labelled.

The expression of SERT messenger RNA in tissue sections of the human brainstem was reported by Austin et al. [4]. The *in situ* hybridization technique using an antisense oligonucleotide probe labelled with 35S-deoxy ATP revealed a dense hybridization signal in the median and dorsal raphe nuclei and a slightly lower signal in the caudal linear raphe nucleus. Hybridization was also detected in scattered cell groups in the B9 area in the supralemniscal cell group. No hybridization was found in the substantia nigra or the locus coeruleus. Similar results were found by Bengel et al. [5] using the same technique in mouse brain, by Fujita et al. in rat brain [6] and McLaughlin et al. in human brain stem raphe nuclei [7].

The distribution of SERTs in mouse brain was studied by incubation of brain sections with [^{125}I]RTI-55 to specifically label SERTs, together with LR1111 to prevent radioactive labelling of dopamine uptake sites [5].

Quantitative autoradiographic analysis of the specific [^{125}I]RTI-55 binding to SERTs showed that dorsal and median raphe nuclei were strongly labelled. This was probably caused by the binding of [^{125}I]RTI-55 to SERTs situated on serotonergic cell bodies and dendrites. High binding (12 ± 1.1 nCi/mg tissue) was also found in the substantia nigra, a region rich in serotonergic synapses. In the globus pallidus, superior colliculus and lateral geniculate nucleus a binding of 10 nCi/mg tissue was observed. Intermediate binding was detected in thalamus (dorsolateral), nucleus accumbens, caudate putamen and inferior colliculus. Low binding was found in all regions of the hippocampus (3.5–4.0 nCi/mg tissue). The technique of localization of SERTs by interaction with site-specific antibodies against the C-terminal [8] or N-terminal [9] of the SERT protein was recently described. In the study reported by Zhou et al. [10] a SERT-N terminal antibody against a 71 amino acid segment of the N-terminal protein of SERT was used for the recognition of SERT protein in serotonin (5-HT) neurons. It was found that SERTs were not only localized at synaptic junctions, varicosities, cell bodies and somatodendrites in the rat brain, but a high density of SERTs was also found at axonal fibres of 5-HT neurons such as the cingulum bundle and the medial forebrain bundle, the largest axonal bundle in the brain. High densities of SERTs were situated in the varicosity plasma membrane surrounding the presynaptic varicosity (perisynaptic area) which is filled with 5-HT containing vesicles. The perisynaptic SERTs are located near the synaptic cleft but not at the presynaptic membrane of the cleft. This suggests that 5-HT released in the synaptic cleft diffuses out of the cleft to be transported back into the 5-HT neuron by the perisynaptic SERTs or even by axonal SERTs situated at a longer distance from the synapse [10, 11]. The binding of [^{3}H]-citalopram matched the immunocytochemical staining of SERTs in coronal brain slices of the rat [10].

A voltammetric assay was used to study the high affinity uptake *in vivo* in rats of 5-HT by SERTs located on the axons of the medial forebrain bundle which bear few varicosities. 5-HT was locally applied by microinjection and the decay over time of the extracellular 5-HT was recorded. Local injections in cerebellum and capsula interna were used as controls. It was shown that the decay time of extracellular 5-HT in the median forebrain bundle but not in cerebellum or capsula interna was prolonged by the selective SERT inhibitors paroxetine and citalopram [10].

Further investigation is needed on the regulatory role of axonal SERTs distant from synapses and varicosities scavenging 5-HT released from distant sources and reaching the axonal SERTs by diffusion.

2.2 The structure of the serotonin transporter

The putative general structure of the SERT is shown in Figure 1. cDNA cloning strategies and expression of the cDNA encoding the amino acid sequence of rat [12–14], human [15, 16] and mouse [17] SERTs revealed the molecular structure and function of the cloned SERTs. After correction of some discrepancies in the early reports it was shown that rat, human and mouse SERTs consist of 630 amino acids and having a relative molecular mass of about 70 kD. The amino acid sequence homology of rat and human SERT is 92% with the differences largely occurring in the N-terminus, a region not expected to be essential in the recognition of substrate or antagonist [15]. The sequence homologies of mouse and human or rat SERTs are 94% and 97%, respectively [17]. Twenty out of 52 differences in amino acid composition are found in the N-terminal of human and rat SERTs which presumably is not involved in the binding of endogenous substrate or antagonists [15]. A single gene encoding the human SERT appears to be localized at chromosome 17 q 11.1–q 12 [15].

2.3 5-HT transport mechanism

The role of ions in the molecular mechanism of reuptake of neurotransmitters by monoamine transporters was comprehensively reviewed by Rudnick and Clark [18]. For the binding of 5-HT actions to the transporter, cobinding of extracellular sodium ions and chlorine ions is required for the formation of a quaternary complex with the transporter. After formation of the quaternary complex a conformational change of the transporter takes place, whereby 5-HT$^+$, Na$^+$, and Cl$^-$ are translocated from the exterior to the interior of the 5-HT neuron. The stoiochiometry of transport of 5-HT$^+$, Na$^+$ and Cl$^-$ = 1:1:1.

Mechanistic analysis of the ion dependence of the human SERT transfected in mouse fibroblast cells showed that the results are consistent with the predictions that the Cl$^-$-ion facilitates the binding of 5-HT and the Na$^+$-ion enables translocation of the bound 5-HT [19]. The return to the initial state of the transporter is K$^+$ dependent. After dissociation of 5-HT$^+$, Na$^+$ and Cl$^-$ from the transporter, intracellular K$^+$ is bound and translocated from the interior of the neuron to the exterior where it dissociates from the carrier complex. As the return to the initial state of the transporter is facilitated by intracellular K$^+$ the 5-HT reuptake will be accelerated.

Inhibition of 5-HT uptake is effected by competitive binding of a 5-HT uptake inhibitor to the SERT, thereby preventing the binding of 5-HT to its recognition site on the transporter. The binding of potent 5-HT selective inhibitors is monophasic, that is they bind with high affinity at a single site on the transporter.

The question is whether 5-HT uptake inhibitors of different chemical structures all will bind to the same site wholly or partially, overlapping the 5-HT recognition site or to totally different sites that all prevent competitively the binding of 5-HT.

2.4 Ligand binding domains of the 5-HT transporter

In order to obtain more detailed information on the features of the interaction sites that bind substrates and antagonistst several chimeras were constructed.

Three functional cross-species chimera between rat and human SERT transiently expressed in Hela cells were described by Barker et al. [20]. This is of interest because some ligands differ considerably in affinity for the SERT of both species and cross-chimeras species are used to try and explain these differences. For example the affinities of imipramine and other tricyclic SERT inhibitors are higher for the human than for the rat SERT, whereas the reverse is true for the substrate d-amphetamine. Serotonin and non-tricyclic antagonists tested exhibit no species preference. In the 5-HT uptake inhibition test in transiently transfected Hela cells the chimera R1-272 H273-630 (i.e. R$_{(rat)}$

amino acid sequence $H_{(human)}$ amino acid sequence) displays the same characteristics as the cloned human SERT with regard to the inhibition constants K_i of the tricyclic 5-HT uptake inhibitors and d-amphetamine. On the other hand the pharmacological properties of the chimera H1-362R363-630 and its ligands are identical to those of the cloned rat SERT in this test. The K_is of imipramine and d-amphetamine obtained with chimera H1-362R363-531H532-630 in the 5-HT uptake test indicate that this chimera and the human SERT are similar in this respect. The sequence H532-630 comprises transmembrane domains 11 and 12 and the intracellular carboxyl terminus. The latter region seems not involved in the discriminatory properties of the ligands as shown by testing the chimera H1-593 R594-630 [20]. So it is plausible that the cause of the species difference in affinities of the tricyclic uptake inhibitors is to be sought in species differences in the amino acid sequence 532-593. Barker and Blakely [21] showed that a single amino acid phenylalanine (F586) in human SERT is responsible for the higher affinity of the tricyclics. When in the human SERT F586 in transmembrane 12 was converted by site directed mutagenesis into the corresponding rat SERT valine 586 (V586) the affinities of the tricyclics were reduced. When on the other hand the rat SERT V586 was converted into the human SERT F586 the affinities of the tricyclics were increased. These results suggest that the amino acid F586 in the human SERT is implicated in the binding of tricyclics such as imipramine.

Chen et al. [22] investigated the role of the 20 amino acid residues in the TM3 domain on the 5-HT transporter activity by replacing the residues one at a time with cysteine and expressing the mutants in Intestine 407 cells. The majority of the mutants did not impair 5-HT transport. Only the mutants I179C and Y175C significantly decreased the 5-HT transport, whereas Y176C entirely blocked the transport (I = isoleucine, Y = tyrosine). Almost all mutants did not react with the impermeant cysteine reagent [2-(trimethyl-ammonium)ethyl]methanethiosulfonate (MTSET). The only two mutants that were readily inactivated by MTSET were I172C and I179C. The mutant I172C was protected from inactivation by MTSET by 5-HT or cocaine but I179C was not. The inactivation of both mutants by the small impermeant MTSET suggests that these residues are exposed to the external medium and are situated in a channel formed by the transmembrane domain of the SERT.

The binding of the high affinity analogue of cocaine, 2β-carbomethoxy-3β-(4-[^{125}I]iodophenyl)tropane (β-CIT) to the I172C mutant inactivated by MTSET is inhibited. This inhibition is much less pronounced in the I179C mutant. Taken together these observations strongly suggest that Ile-172 is close to the binding site of 5-HT and cocaine. Also Tyr176, a highly conserved residue, may contribute to the binding site of 5-HT and cocaine. When mutated to cysteine (Y176C), the transport of 5-HT is blocked and the affinity for 5-HT, cocaine and β-CIT is drastically diminished.

Sur et al. [23] substituted 16 cysteine residues of the rat SERT with either serine or alanine to study the effect on 5-HT transport and on inhibitor binding. The effect on 5-HT transport and on the binding of ^{3}H-citalopram of 12 mutants transfected in HEK 293 cells was comparable to that of the wild-type rSERT.

Mutants C147S located in the second internal loop, C200S located in the second external loop, C369A and C540A located in TM7 and TM11 of rSERT neither transported 5-HT nor bound the antidepressants. Immunocytochemical analyses showed that these mutants were not expressed at the cell surface. It was suggested that cysteines 369 and 540 could form an intramolecular S-S bridge required for cell surface expression [23]. Compared to the wild-type mutant, C209S suffers a 85% reduction in maximal transport rate and a loss of positive cooperativity (n_H = 1.05 vs 1.46). Also the binding affinities of ^{3}H-imipramine and ^{3}H-citalopram were reduced two- and three-fold, respectively.

The possibility that cysteine 209 is part of an S–S-bridge stabilizing homodimeric or homotetrameric oligomers is considered. Mutants of the three external cysteine residues of the SERT molecule were expressed in HeLa cells and their properties compared to those of the wildtype SERT [24]. Cysteine 109 located on the short (eight amino acids) first external loop between TM1 and 2 was substituted by alanine (C109A). 5-HT transport activity and membrane surface expression of mutant and wild-type were similar. Cysteine 200 and 209 in the large loop between TM3 and 4 were replaced by serine, one at a time, or both (C200S, C209S, C200S–C209S). The transport activity of mutants C200S and C200S-C209S was reduced to 19% whereas the activity of C209S was practically nil. The membrane surface expression of C209S and C200S was much less than that of the wild-type SERT or of the double mutant. The effect on transport activity of C200S and C209S is probably due to poor surface expression and that of the double mutant on a decreased intrinsic activity. The affinity of the cocaine analogue [^{125}I]β-CIT for the three mutants was significantly decreased relative to the wild-type especially for the C209S mutant. It is plausible that in the wild-type SERT C200 and C209 are linked by a disulfide bond.

A chimeric rat SERT was constructed by substituting about half of its external second loop by a corresponding 34 amino acid sequence of the human norepinephrine transporter NET [25].

Ten residues in the substituting NET region are the same as in the SERT and six residues are considered as functionally the same. The NET region is six residues longer than the corresponding SERT region. Both wild-type and chimera were transiently expressed in HeLa cells. It was found that the production and level at the surface membrane of wild-type SERT and chimera in HeLa cells are similar. However, the 5-HT transport by the chimera was drastically impaired. This was not caused by the longer loop length of the chimera as shortening the loop by deletion of the six extra amino acids only worsened the transport activity. Evidently there is a block in the translocation mechanism and further research on the role of the second extracellular loop in this mechanism is required.

It was shown by Sur et al. that serine 545 in TM11 is responsible for the Na^+ dependence of rat SERT for 5-HT transport [26]. Three serine residues located in TM11 were substituted by alanine and each mutant S545A, S555A and S559A was expressed in HEK 293 cells. The level of membrane surface expression of wild-type rSERT and of the three mutants did not differ. The kinetic parameters of 5-HT transport by S555A and S559A were similar to those of the wild-type SERT. In contrast, however, the apparent affinity of 5-HT for the S545A mutant is lower than for the wild-type transporter, but the maximal velocity of transport is about two-fold higher. The 5-HT transport by the S545A transporter is Na^+-independent in that 5-HT transport is not impaired if Na-cations are substituted by Li-cations. In the wild-type SERT the binding of a Na-atom has to precede the binding of 5-HT before translocation can take place. The authors of this study [26] propose that the conformation of the S545A mutant is such that binding of 5-HT is direct as in this case Na^+-ions are not essential for the initial phase of the transport cycle and the translocation step can be driven by Li-cations. If the binding of Na^+ and 5-HT causes a conformational change of the native SERT, leading to the opening of a permeation pathway, it is possible that mutant S545A is already in the activated conformation for the translocation of 5-HT [26]. The affinities of citalopram for the S545A mutant and the wild-type rat SERT are the same. The affinity of imipramine for the mutant is five times lower than for the wild-type rSERT. However, there are twice as many binding sites for imipramine on the S545A mutant than there are for citalopram. It was demonstrated that imipramine in contrast to citalopram has a high affinity and a low affinity binding site on rSERT [26–28]. The serine residue 545 in TM11 of rSERT is essential in the Na^+-dependence of 5-HT transport and imipramine binding. The translocation step is not selective for Na^+ as Li^+ can replace Na^+ in this phase of the mechanism of transport.

The human SERT (hSERT) and the SERT of the fruitfly *Drosophila melanogaster* (dSERT) differ in their affinity for monoamine transporter antagonists. Most hSERT antagonists such as paroxetine, fluoxetine, RTI-55, imipramine and citalopram have a significantly lower affinity for dSERTs than for hSERTs. However, the affinity of mazindol (a NET/DAT selective antagonist) for the dSERT is much higher than for the hSERT. Mazindol was a more potent inhibitor of 5-HT transport by dSERT (K_i = 6.6 nM) than by hSERT (K_i = 84 nM) [29]. By using the chimera D1-136 H137-625 and H1-118 D119-627, it was found that the determinants for the potencies of citalopram and mazindol antagonizing 5-HT transport are located in the TM1-TM2 region. In order to determine whether a single amino acid in this region determines the species difference in the potencies of mazindol or citalopram eight amino acids in the TM1-TM2 region of hSERT were substituted by nonconserved amino acids in corresponding positions in dSERT, using the mutants Y95F, L119V, T122C, I123L, M124F, A125L and I130L. Of all mutants Y95F was the only one which shifts the potencies of mazindol and citalopram from the potencies at the hSERT to the potencies at the dSERT. K_is of mazindol for the hSERT, the dSERT and the mutant are resp., 103 ± 4.7, 5.0 ± 0.5, 12 ± 0.6 nM; those for citalopram 2.5 ± 0.9, 32 ± 8.4, 21 ± 2.5 nM, resp. Thus a single amino acid Tyr95 in TM1 is crucial for the species-selective recognition of mazindol and citalopram.

2.5 Transporter regulation

One of the possible pathways of regulation of monoamine uptake transport is phosphorylation by phosphokinases of serine or threonine residues in the N- and C-terminals and/or internal loop between TM4 and 5 of the transporter.

Qian et al. [30] showed that cell surface expressed hSERT in HEK-293 cells was internalized and 5-HT uptake capacity was reduced after activation by phorbol esters of protein kinase C. This downregulation was blocked by the inhibitor of protein kinase C, staurosporine. In a later study by Ramamoorthy et al. [31] using HEK-293-hSERT cells, it was demonstrated that endogenous protein kinases C, A and G and probably other, yet unidentified protein kinases phosphorylate hSERT at distinct sites with different effects on 5-HT transport. Whereas phosphorylation of hSERT by activated protein kinase C leads to down regulation of 5-HT transport capacity, phosphorylation by activated protein kinase A or G has no effect. Phosphorylation and dephosphorylation are probably important mechanisms in the regulation of surface expression and internalization of monoamine transporters.

Upregulation of 5-HT transport probably by activation of cGMP dependent protein kinases was recently described. Millar and Hoffman showed that stimulation of the A_3 adenosine receptor in rat basophilic leukemia cells (RBL2H3) by 5'-N-carboxamidoadenosine (NECA) resulted in an increase in [^{3}H]5-HT uptake [32]. Stimulation of the A_3 receptor leads to an increase of the level of inositol triphosphate and Ca^{2+} which could activate various protein kinases. However the increase of 5-HT uptake is not induced by stimulation of phosphokinase C as phorbolesters reduce the uptake capacity of 5-HT transporters. It was found that the elevated Ca^{2+} level after activation of the A_3 receptor in RBL cells stimulates the nitricoxide (NO) production by nitricoxide synthetase (NOS) and that NO stimulates the production of cyclic guanylyl 3',5' monophosphate (cGMP) by soluble guanylylcyclase. cGMP could then activate a cGMP dependent kinase which could phosphorylate the 5-HT transporter. The response to A_3 receptor activation was blocked by NOS inhibitors and inhibitors of cGMP synthese.

In a study on the effect of N-glycosylation on the activity of rSERT expressed in insect Sf9 cells it appeared that the affinity K_d of the transport inhibitor [^{125}I]RT1 55 for the unglycosylated transporter is identical to that for the rSERT but that its binding capacity is 20-fold lower. The K_m for 5-HT transport by the unglycosylated transporter is identical to that of rSERT but the maximal transport rate is 34 times lower because of the low expression of the active form [33]. The active form is expressed at a 20-fold lower level than the native rSERT. The results show that N-linked glycosylation is not required for the 5-HT transport by rSERTs. It is possible that glycosylation of the transporter protein is also a factor in the regulatory process of 5-HT transport, for instance, by facilitating the transport of the transporter to the surface membrane of the neuron.

It is also possible that glycosylation prevents the transporter protein of misfolding to inactive products [33].

2.6   Selective inhibitors of the serotonin transporter

Fluoxetine (Tab. 1) was one of the first selective SERT inhibitors in clinical use as an antidepressant (for review see [34]). Fluoxetine displays a high affinity for the rat SERT (pK_i = 8.5), a moderate affinity for the rat NET (pK_i = 6.9) and hardly any affinity for the rat DAT (pKi=5.5) [35, 36]. The compound has little affinity for α- and β-adrenoceptors, dopamine, muscarine, histamine-H1, opiate, GABA, benzodiazepine and serotonin (5-HT$_{1A-D}$, 5-HT$_2$, 5-HT$_3$) receptors [37, 38].

Fluoxetine, belonging to the class of substituted 3-phenoxy-3-phenyl-propanamines, is a racemate. The racemate and both enantiomers display similar affinities for the rat SERT. However, the (S)-enantiomer is 6.5 times more selective for SERT than the (R)-enantiomer (selectivity index SERT/NET: (S) = 155; (R) = 24). Fluoxetine displays a high affinity for the human SERT (pK_i = 9.0) and a low affinity for the human NET (pK_i = 6.1) [39]. Norfluoxetine (N-demethyl fluoxetine), the major metabolite of fluoxetine in animals and humans is as potent but more selective than the parent compound (rat SERT: pK_i = 8.5; rat NET: pK_i = 5.8; human SERT: pK_i = 8.6; human NET: pK_i = 5.4) [35, 39]. In rats the (S)-enantiomer of norfluoxetine is about as potent as (S)-fluoxetine but three times more selective. The (R)-enantiomer of norfluoxetine is nine times less potent but as selective as (R)-fluoxetine [35].

The selectivity for SERT inhibition of the phenoxy-propanamines depends on the position of the substituent on the phenoxy moiety. Mono-substitution in the para position as in fluoxetine results in selective SERT inhibition, but monosubstitution in the ortho position results in selective NET inhibition as in nisoxetine (o-MeO) or tomoxetine (o-Me) (cf 4.6). Disubstitution in the ortho-para or meta-para positions has little effect on the SERT selectivity. The (R)-2-Me-4-iodo and (R) and (S)-3Me-4-iodo-phenoxy congeners are potent and selective SERT inhibitors (pK_i values: 9.2; 9.2 and 9.5 respectively) [40].

Selective SERT inhibition is maintained in MDL 28618A (Tab. 1), a semi-rigid analogue of fluoxetine. The absolute configuration of MDL 28618A is 1S,2S [41]. Although data are not reported, MDL 28618A seems ten times more potent than the cis(–)enantiomer [42].

Femoxetine and its close structural analogue, paroxetine (Tab. 1) are differently constrained analogues of fluoxetine. Both compounds are members of a series of 3-substituted 4-phenylpiperidines, existing as two diastereomers and four optical enantiomers. Femoxetine is the 3R,4S trans(+)-enantiomer.

Table 1.
Selective SERT inhibitors of the aryloxypropanamine type.

Fluoxetine pK$_i$ = 8.5   MDL 28618A   Femoxetine pK$_i$ = 7.7

Paroxetine pK$_i$ = 8.7   YM992 pK$_i$ = 7.7   Dapoxetine pIC$_{50}$ = 8.0

Femoxetine displays a good affinity for the rat SERT (pK$_i$ = 7.7) and is moderately selective with respect to the rat NET (pK$_i$ = 6.7) and highly selective with respect to the rat DAT (pK$_i$ = 5.8) [36]. N-demethyl femoxetine is about ten times more potent than femoxetine. The trans(–)enantiomer of femoxetine is a rather weak inhibitor of SERT (pK$_i$ = 6.5). N-demethylation increases the affinity significantly (pK$_i$ = 8.6) [43].

Paroxetine is one of the most potent and selective SERT inhibitors known (for review see [44]). The compound displays a very high affinity for the rat and human SERT (pK$_i$ values: 10.3 and 10.2, respectively).

Table 2.
SAR of paroxetine analogues for the rat SERT.

trans	R$_1$	R$_2$	R$_3$	R$_4$	R$_5$	R$_6$	R$_7$	pK$_i$
–				F				9.1[a]
–	Me			F				8.4
±				F				8.7
±				H				8.5
±		Me						8.0
±			Me					8.3
±				Me				8.4
±				F	Me			7.1
±				F		Me		6.8
±				F			Me	8.3

[a] paroxetine

Paroxetine is about three decades more selective with respect to NET [39]. The effect on DAT is virtually nil [36]. The drug has no or hardly any affinity for α- and β-adrenoceptors, histamine-H$_1$, serotonin and dopamine receptors and a low affinity for muscarine receptors [35, 39]. In contrast to femoxetine, paroxetine is the 3S,4R trans(–)enantiomer. However, in both compounds the large substituents are in the same diequatorial position [43]. Similar to the femoxetine series, N-methylation of paroxetine decreases the affinity for the rat SERT (Tab. 2). The 4-fluoro substituent of paroxetine is not essential for high affinity. The unsubstituted phenyl group in the trans (±) series has a similar activity for the rat SERT as the 4-fluoro derivative (Tab. 2). Methyl substitution of the phenyl group is well tolerated in the meta- and para positions. Ortho substitution decreases the activity by five times. Methyl substitution of the methylenedioxybenzene moiety is only tolerated at C-3. Substitution at the 5 or 6 position has a negative effect on the activity (pK$_i$ values: 7.1 and 6.8 respectively) [45].

Restriction of the conformation of paroxetine by substitution of the piperidine ring with an ethylene bridge is unfavourable for high affinity and selectivity for SERT. Only the (1R)-2β,3α-enantiomer, possessing the same stereochemistry as paroxetine displays a good affinity for the rat SERT (pIC$_{50}$ = 8.3). Similar to paroxetine, the (1R)-2β,3α-enantiomer exists in a flattened boat conformation with pseudo-equatorial substituents. Surprisingly, the high selectivity of paroxetine is not present in the (1R)-2β,3α-enantiomer. This tropane analogue displays a high affinity for the SERT (pIC$_{50}$ = 8.3),

NET (pIC_{50} = 7.8) and DAT (pIC_{50} = 8.4). N-methylation results in a compound with selectivity for DAT [46].

YM992 (Tab. 1) is a ring closed phenoxypropanamine, structurally related to viloxazine, a selective NET inhibitor. In contrast to viloxazine, YM 992 displays affinity for the SERT (pK_i = 7.7). YM992 is not selective with respect to 5-HT$_{2A}$ receptors and α_1-adrenoceptors [47].

Dapoxetine, a (1-naphthoxy)-1-phenylpropanamine compound is a selective inhibitor of SERT (pIC_{50} = 8.0) structurally related to fluoxetine. In dapoxetine, the phenyl group is shifted from the 3-position of the phenoxypropanamine chain in fluoxetine, to the 1-position, resulting in a benzylamine derivative (Tab. 1). Dapoxetine is the (S)-enantiomer. Its antipode is slightly less active (pIC_{50} = 7.5). Dapoxetine shows a ten-fold greater selectivity for SERT than fluoxetine [48]. The development of dapoxetine was stopped in 1995.

An example of a constrained benzylamine derivative is the aminotetralin sertraline (Tab. 3). The compound displays a high affinity for the rat and human SERT (pK_i values: 8.5 and 9.8 respectively). Sertraline is selective with respect to the rat NET (pK_i = 6.7), human NET (pK_i = 6.1) and rat DAT (pK_i = 6.6) [36, 39]. Sertraline has neither significant affinity for α- and β-adrenoceptors nor for muscarinic, histamine-H$_1$, serotonin 5-HT$_{1A-D}$, 5-HT$_{2-4}$ or dopamine D$_2$ receptors and only a weak affinity for the human α_1-adrenoceptors [49, 39]. Sertraline has the 1S,4S configuration. The cis(–)enantiomer is less potent and not selective with respect to rat NET and DAT.

The comparable trans-enantiomers are either NET selective or not selective at all [50]. Contraction of the non-aromatic ring of the aminotetralin moiety of sertaline into the corresponding indanamine enhances the SERT affinity (Tab. 3). The structure-activity relationships of the indanamines is very similar to that of the aminotetralins [51].

Zimeldine (Tab. 3) can be considered as a ring opened analogue of the indanamine compound 1. Zimeldine is a moderately potent inhibitor of the rat SERT (pK_i = 7.3) and human SERT (pK_i = 6.8). The compound is fairly selective with respect to NET (rat: pK_i = 5.7, human: pK_i = 5.0) and DAT (rat: pK_i = 4.6, human: pK_i = 4.9 [52, 53]. Zimeldine has the cis (Z) configuration. The trans-(E) isomer is a weak inhibitor of the rat SERT (Tab. 4) [54].

Norzimeldine (N-demethylzimeldine), the major metabolite of zimeldine is a potent and selective inhibitor of SERT (Tab. 4) [54, 52]. The primary amino analogue is a weak SERT inhibitor (pK_i = 6.4). The regio isomers of zimeldine and norzimeldine display a lower affinity for the SERT than their

Table 3.
Selective SERT inhibitors derived from aminotetralin and isoquinoline.

Sertraline pK$_i$ = 8.5   Compound 1 pIC$_{50}$ = 9.4   Zimeldine pK$_i$ = 7.3

McN 5652 - Z   pK$_i$ = 9.4   Venlafaxine pK$_i$ = 7.7   Compound 2 pK$_i$ = 8.6

Table 4.
SAR of zimeldine analogues for the rat SERT.

X	R	conf.	pK$_i$	X	R	conf.	pK$_i$
4-Br	Me	Z	7.4	4-Br	H	Z	8.5
4-Br	Me	E	6.5	4-Br	H	E	7.2
3-Br	Me	Z	6.9	3-Br	H	Z	7.2
2-Br	Me	Z	n.d	2-Br	H	Z	7.7
2.4-diCl	Me	Z	7.2	2.4-diCl	H	Z	8.4

parent compounds (Tab. 4). Ortho-para disubstitution with chlorine does not affect the potency for SERT [54]. Zimeldine proved to be a clinically effective antidepressant but was withdrawn because of its supposed implication in the occurrence of the Guillain-Barré syndrome in some patients.

Another example of a constrained benzylamine derivative is the hexahydro-pyrroloisoquinoline McN 5652-Z (Tab. 3). McN 5652-Z has a high affinity for the rat SERT (pK_i = 9.4). The compound is moderately selective with respect to NET and DAT (selectivity indices: 4.6 and 60.3 respectively). McN 5652-Z is the trans(+)enantiomer. The trans(–) and the cis(±) compounds are significantly less active [55]. After further studies on McN 5652-Z as a potential clinically useful antidepressant the development was halted.

Venlafaxine can be considered as a ring-opened analogue of McN 5652-Z (Tab. 3). Venlafaxine, a racemate, is marketed as a dual (5-HT and NE) uptake inhibitor (for review see [56]). In rat brain synaptosomes, venlafaxine has only a three-fold preference for 5-HT. The racemate and both enantiomers display similar activities for the SERT (pIC_{50} values: (RS) = 6.7; (R) = 6.7; (S) = 7.0). The (R)-enantiomer does not differ significantly from the racemate in selectivity. The (S)-enantiomer is more selective for SERT (selectivity index 31) [57]. The major metabolite (4-OH instead of 4-OC), having a similar potency for SERT as venlafaxine, tends to be more selective (Si = 6) [58]. Exchanging the 4-MeO group of venlafaxine for a CF_3 group results in an increase in selectivity index (Si = 7) with a concomitant twofold decrease in affinity for the SERT. Ring contraction of the cyclohexyl moiety into a cyclopentyl group results for venlafaxine and its CF_3 analogue in a considerable increase in selectivity index (Si = 14.5 and 20 respectively). The activity for SERT is hardly affected [57]. Recent radioligand binding studies show that venlafaxine is rather selective for SERT [39, 53, 59]. Venlafaxine and its major metabolite O-desmethylvenlafaxine bind with comparable affinity to the rat SERT (pK_i = 7.7) and human SERT (pK_i = 8.1). The affinity of both compounds for the NET is about 50 (rat) and 330 (human) times less. The effect on DAT is virtually nil [53, 36]. The low affinity of venlafaxine for the NET in the binding studies is in sharp contrast to the relatively high activity in the functional tests (*in vitro* and *in vivo* uptake experiments). These results suggest that venlafaxine and the radioligand [³H]-nisoxetine may bind to a (partly) different site on NET. Venlafaxine was used as lead compound for the design of compound 2 (Tab. 3). Compound 2 displays a high affinity for the rat SERT (pK_i = 8.6) and human SERT (pK_i = 8.9). The compound is less selective than venlafaxine for the human SERT [60].

Table 5.
Selective SERT inhibitors derived from tricyclics (TCAs).

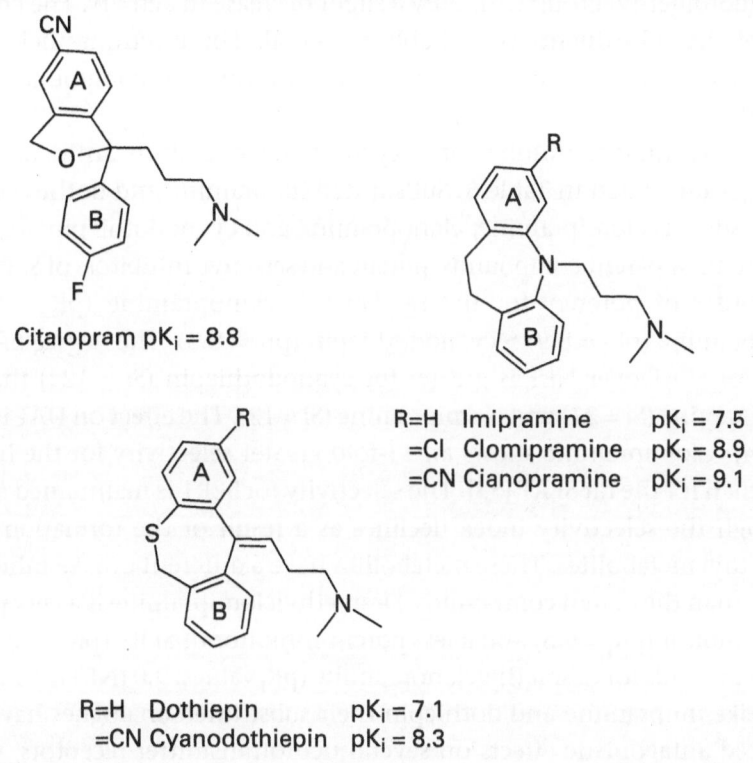

Citalopram pK$_i$ = 8.8

R=H Imipramine   pK$_i$ = 7.5
=Cl Clomipramine   pK$_i$ = 8.9
=CN Cianopramine   pK$_i$ = 9.1

R=H   Dothiepin   pK$_i$ = 7.1
=CN Cyanodothiepin   pK$_i$ = 8.3

Citalopram (Tab. 5) is a potent and highly selective inhibitor of SERT (for review see [61]). The compound displays a high affinity for the rat SERT (pK$_i$ = 8.8) and human SERT (pK$_i$ = 8.9) and hardly any affinity for NET (rat: pK$_i$ = 5.2; human: pK$_i$ = 5.4) and DAT (rat: pK$_i$ = 4.4; human: pK$_i$ = 4.6) [52, 53].

Citalopram is a ring-opened analogue of the tricyclic first generation antidepressants (TCAs). But in contrast to the tricyclics, citalopram has little or no affinity for neurotransmitter receptors such as α_1- and α_2-adrenoceptors, muscarinic, dopaminergic, serotonergic (5-HT$_{1A-B}$, 5-HT$_2$) and histaminergic-H$_1$ receptors [62]. Citalopram is the most selective SERT inhibitor described yet. Citalopram is a racemate but no data are available on putative enantiomers. Demethylcitalopram, the major metabolite of citalopram is slightly less potent, but retains selectivity for SERT [52, 53]. Substitution on both aromatic moieties as illustrated in citalopram is essential for high activity. The para-fluoro atom on the B ring can be exchanged for a chloro atom or a cyano group, and the cyano group on the A ring for a fluoro, chloro, bromo atom or trifluoromethyl group with only a slight decrease in activity. The effect of bulk of the substituents is probably marginal. The electronic field effect seems to be a highly important factor in determining the compound's activity [63].

A representative number of tricyclic first generation antidepressants (TCAs) is illustrated in Table 5. Substituted imipramine and dothiepin congeners such as clomipramine, cianopramine and cyanodothiepin are, compared to their parent compounds, potent and selective inhibitors of SERT. The rank order of potency for the rat SERT is cianopramine (pK_i = 9.1) > clomipramine (pK_i = 8.9) > cyanodothiepin (pK_i = 8.3). The degree of selectivity for SERT over NET is greater for cyanodothiepin (Si = 124) than for cianopramine (Si = 21) and clomipramine (Si = 12). The effect on DAT is nihil [52, 64]. Clomipramine shows an 11-fold greater selectivity for the human SERT than for the rat SERT [53]. The selectivity for SERT is maintained *in vivo*, although the selectivity index declines as a result of the formation of N-desmethyl metabolites. These metabolites have a different uptake inhibitory profile than the parent compounds. Desmethylclomipramine is a very potent NET inhibitor (pK_i = 9.5) and a less potent inhibitor of SERT (pK_i = 7.5) [52]. The same holds for desmethylcianopramine (pK_i values: 9.0 (NET); 7.9 (SERT) [65]. Like imipramine and dothiepin their substituted analogues have pronounced antagonistic effects on several neurotransmitter receptors, which may contribute to the overall pharmacological effects or side-effects of the compounds. Clomipramine and cianopramine have a substantial affinity for α_1-adrenoceptors, $5\text{-}HT_2$, histamine-H_1, muscarinic and dopamine D_2 receptors [65]. Cyanodothiepin displays a moderate affinity for muscarine receptors and a weak affinity for the other receptors tested (α_1, $5\text{-}HT_2$, $D_{1,2}$) [64].

Fluvoxamine is a nontricyclic SERT inhibitor structurally related to the tricyclic antidepressant noxiptiline (Tab. 6). Fluvoxamine displays a high affinity and selectivity for the rat SERT (pK_i = 8.3; Si values 100 (NET)) and 1000 (DAT) [66] as well as for the human SERT (pK_i = 8.7; Si values 590 (NET)) and 4180 (DAT) [53]. Fluvoxamine virtually lacks affinity for most receptor types involved in neurotransmission (for review see [67]). Fluvoxamine is the trans-isomer. The cis analogue is significantly less potent.

Litoxetine shares with noxiptiline and fluvoxamine the aromatic A-ring and a nitrogen atom at a distance of five atoms (Tab. 6). Litoxetine inhibits the rat SERT with a pIC_{50} = 7.7. The selectivity ratio for SERT over NET is 89.

Table 6.
Selective SERT inhibitors; miscellaneous structures.

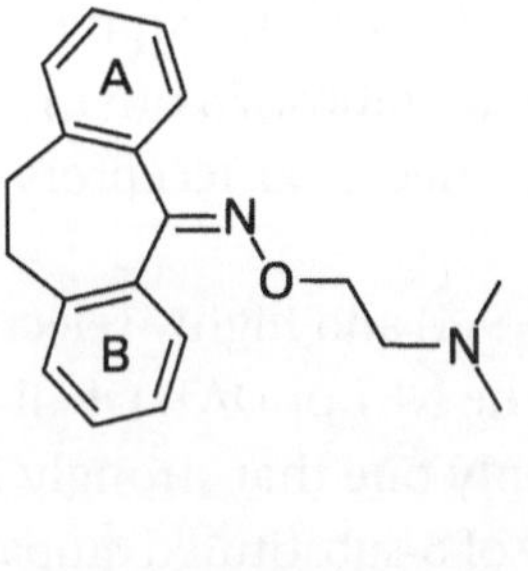

Noxiptiline

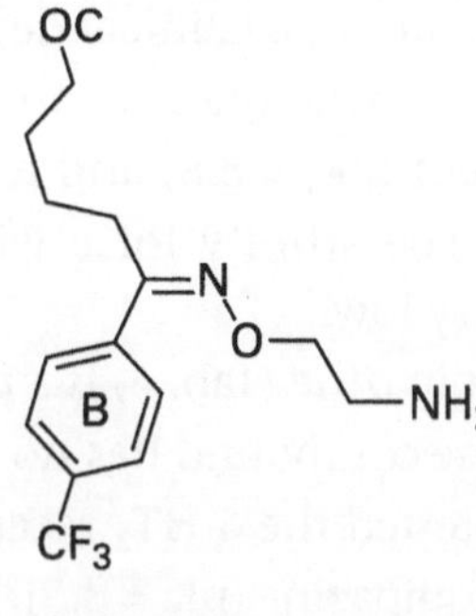

Fluvoxamine $pK_i = 8.3$

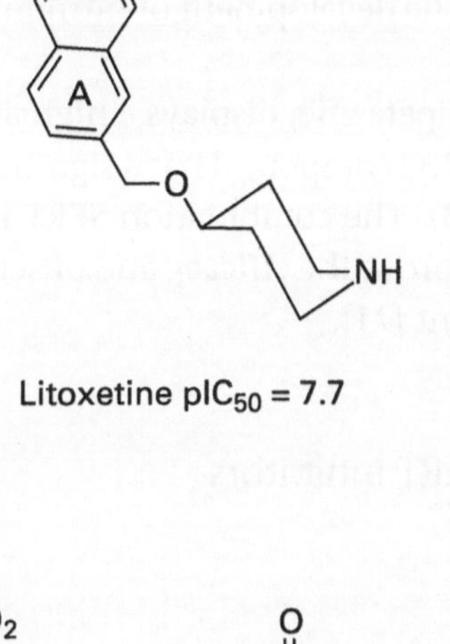

Litoxetine $pIC_{50} = 7.7$

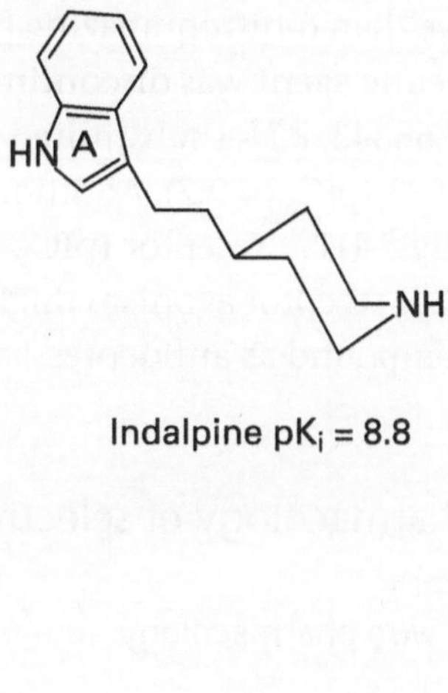

Indalpine $pK_i = 8.8$

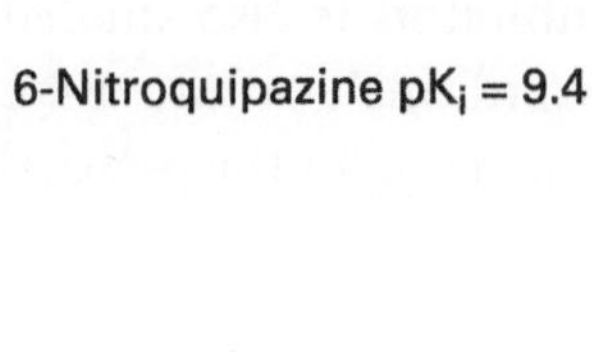

6-Nitroquipazine $pK_i = 9.4$

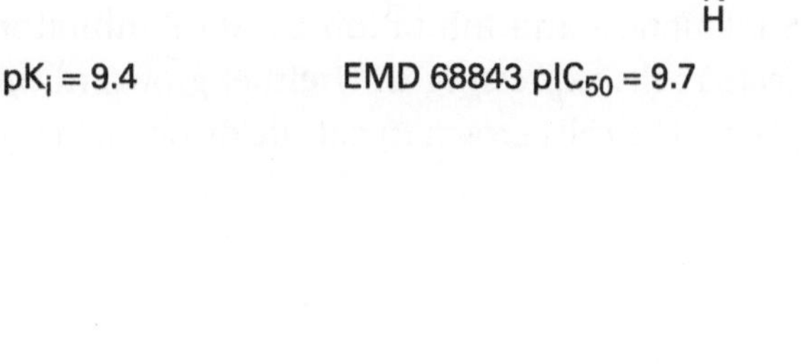

EMD 68843 $pIC_{50} = 9.7$

The affinity for neuroreceptors is negligible except for 5-HT_3 receptors ($pIC_{50} = 6.7$) [68, 69]. The concomitant 5-HT_3 antagonism of litoxetine may limit the gastrointestinal side-effects (nausea or vomiting) induced by the pure SERT inhibitors. Clinical development, however, was halted.

Indalpine is structurally related to litoxetine (Tab. 6). Indalpine, however, is more potent ($pK_i = 8.8$) and more selective (Si ratios: 784 (NET) and 580 (DAT) [52]. The affinity for a wide variety of neuronal receptors is either absent or very low.

6-Nitroquipazine (Tab. 6) is a potent ($pK_i = 9.4$) and highly selective SERT inhibitor. The compound has no affinity for the NET or DAT. Of all the neuroreceptors tested the 5-HT_3 receptor is the only one that strongly interacts with 6-nitroquipazine ($pK_i = 8.5$). The potency of 6-substituted quipazines for the SERT decreases gradually: $NO_2 \geq MeO > Cl > Br = CF_3$. All compounds remain selective for SERT. The unsubstituted quipazine analogue is moderately potent and nonselective versus NET. Substitution of the 4-position of 6-nitroquipazine is well tolerated. The 4-bromo-6-nitroquipazine is only two-fold less active than 6-nitroquipazine [70]. The development of nitroquipazine as a therapeutic agent was discontinued.

EMD 68843, a N-4 substituted arylpiperazine, displays a high affinity for the rat SERT ($pIC_{50} = 9.7$). Additionally the compound has a significant affinity for the 5-HT_{1A} receptor ($pIC_{50} = 9.3$). The combination SERT inhibition and 5-HT_{1A} receptor agonism might improve the efficacy and onset of action of the compound as antidepressive agent [71].

2.7 Pharmacology of selective SERT inhibitors

2.7.1 *In vitro* pharmacology

The uptake of $[^3H]\text{-}5\text{-HT}$ by synaptosomes prepared from the rat frontal cortex and its inhibition by a series of SERT inhibitors was reported by Cheetham et al. [72]. The binding of $[^3H]$ paroxetine to membranes prepared from rat frontal cortex was used to assay its affinity (K_d) and the density of binding sites (B_{max}). This preparation was also used in the assay of the potency of ligands (K_i) competing with $[^3H]$ paroxetine for its binding site. $[^3H]\text{-}5\text{-HT}$ uptake and inhibition by SERT inhibitors is also studied using transfected cells expressing SERT either grown in small culture dishes or in well plates. The cells grown in culture dishes are used for the preparation of

SERT containing membranes, see for instance [24, 27]. The plated cells are used *in situ* for the assay of [³H]-5-HT uptake and inhibition of uptake by incubation with or without added inhibitors in varying concentrations. The uptake is terminated by several washes and after solubilisation of the cells [³H]-5-HT is determined by liquid scintillation counting [20, 29, 31]. Qualitative and quantitative binding of [³H] labelled SERT inhibitors to SERTs in rat- and human slide-mounted brain slices was reported in several publications (e.g. [1, 3, 73]).

2.7.2 *In vivo* pharmacology

In the 5-HTP test the behavioural effects induced by 5-hydroxytryptophan in mice (headtwitches) and rats (wet dog shakes and serotonin syndrome such as forepaw treading, tremor, hindlimb abduction, atactic gait, lordosis) are potentiated by selective SERT inhibitors and much less so by tricyclic antidepressants [52, 62, 74].

A large number of behavioural tests in animal models of depression have been described. In most of the tests the animal is brought into a stress-inducing situation from which a potential antidepressant may allow the animal to escape. In depression tests such as the forced swim test, fluoxetine, paroxetine and sertraline decrease immobility and increase swimming indicative of antidepressant efficacy [75, 76].

In another test, tail suspension, antidepressants like the selective 5-HT reuptake inhibitors reduce the time of immobility of mice suspended by the tail. Antidepressants also increase escape behaviour in animals exposed for a longer period of time to inescapable stress (learned helplessness).

Repeated administration of selective 5-HT uptake inhibitors to olfactory bulbectomized rats reduce hyperactivity in the open field test in which a rat is placed in the centre of the apparatus and the number of crossings of times on the surface are scored [77]. For reviews on animal models of depression see [78, 79].

2.8 Therapeutic applications of selective SERT inhibitors

Various selective SERT inhibitors, such as citalopram, fluoxetine, fluvoxamine, paroxetine and sertraline, are clinically effective in the treatment of major depressive illness (for reviews see [61, 34, 80, 44, 49]). The clinical effect is comparable to that of the tricyclic antidepressants.

The selective SERT inhibitors are well tolerated. The most commonly reported side-effect is nausea. Unlike the TCAs, the selective SERT inhibitors are not cardiotoxic (tachycardia) and devoid of cardiovascular side-effects (orthostatic hypotension). Anticholinergic effects (dry mouth) are minimal or absent. The onset of action of the SERT inhibitors like the TCAs starts after 2–3 weeks of treatment. This delay is probably due to a negative feedback mechanism induced by the 5-HT released. After about 2 weeks of treatment this feedback is downregulated [81]. By that time clinical improvement starts. During long-term maintenance therapy the SERT inhibitors remain effective. The clinical profile of the SERT inhibitors is very similar to each other [82]. A number of selective SERT inhibitors have been studied in obsessive-compulsive disorder (OCD) and/or panic disorder. Fluoxetine, fluvoxamine, paroxetine and sertraline were as effective as the reference compound clomipramine. The compounds were better tolerated than clomipramine (for reviews see [83, 44, 49, 84]). Preliminary results show that paroxetine is more effective than placebo in the treatment of social phobia.

3   The dopamine transporter (DAT)

3.1   Distribution in the CNS

The distribution of DATs in rat brain assessed by immunohistochemical methods was reported by Freed et al. [85]. Dense DAT-like immunoreactivity was found in the striatum, nucleus accumbens, olfactory tubercle, nigrostriatal bundle and lateral habenula. Moderate staining was found in the cell bodies of the substantia nigra pars compacta. Staining was also found in neuronal processes with axonal and dendritic morphologies in the substantia nigra, in laminae I, II and III of the cingulate cortex and in the medial prefrontal cortex.

Another approach to transporter distribution studies of DAT in the CNS is the use of radioactive inhibitors. Incubation of rat brain slices with [^{125}I] RTI121 (3β-(4-iodophenyl)tropane-2β-carboxylic acid isopropylester) selectively labelled striatum, nucleus accumbens, olfactory tubercle and substantia nigra [86].

[^{125}I]RTI55 (3β-(4-iodophenyl)-2β-carboxylic acid methylester), in addition to labelling DAT-rich regions, also labelled SERT-rich areas such as cerebral cortex, hippocampus, brainstem, hypothalamus and thalamus [86].

N-omega-fluoropropyl-2β-carbomethoxy-3-β-(4-iodophenyl) tropane ([^{123}I]FP-CIT) was used for the *in vivo* labelling of DATs in the CNS of rats and monkeys [87]. After intravenous injection in rats a high signal of radioactivity was found in the striatum and a lower signal in brain regions with high densities of SERTs. In monkeys with a unilateral lesion of striatal DA neurons, SPECT showed a severe loss of uptake of radioligand at the lesioned side.

Another radioligand suitable for SPECT or PET imaging of DATs in the CNS is N-(1-iodoprop-1-en-3-yl)-2β-carbomethoxy-3β-(4-fluorophenyl)propane (= [^{125}I] altropane). The CNS distribution of [^{125}I]-altropane was determined *in vitro* or *ex vivo* by quantitative autoradiography of coronal brain sections of the squirrel monkey [88]. *In vitro*, [^{125}I]-altropane was detected primarily in putamen, nucleus caudatus and nucleus accumbens. The putamen/cerebellum ratio exceeded 120. *Ex vivo*, the highest concentrations in putamen, caudate and nucleus accumbens were detected 30 min after i.v. injection and the lowest in cerebellum and cortex. SPECT imaging confirmed the rapid and selective uptake in the striatum. The distribution of [^{125}I]-altropane in postmortem tissue from normal and Parkinson's brains was described by Madras et al. [89]. In tissue sections of normal brains high levels of [^{125}I]-altropane binding were found in caudate and putamen, but 27% lower levels in the nucleus accumbens. In Parkinson's brains the binding levels of [^{125}I]-altropane in putamen, caudate and nucleus accumbens were only 13%, 17% and 25% of the normal values. [^{123}I]-altropane was used for the rapid detection by SPECT of Parkinson's disease [90]. Results from eight male patients were compared to results from seven healthy volunteers. Within 1 h excellent quality images of the accumulation of altropane in the striatum were obtained. In all Parkinson patients the accumulation was markedly reduced and most profound in the posterior putamen while the caudate nuclei were relatively spared. Similar results were obtained by Tissingh et al. [91] using [^{123}I]-FP-CIT in early stage, drug naïve Parkinson patients (n = 21) at 3 h postinjection. The ratio of specific to nonspecific striatal binding of the radioligand was used as the outcome measure. In all Parkinson patients the ratios were significantly lower than in the control group (n = 14). The mean reduction in the putamen was 57%, while the mean reduction in the caudate nucleus was 29% compared to the control group (N = 14).

3.2   Structure of the dopamine transporter

The putative structure of the DAT is shown in Figure 1. The primary structure of DAT was found by isolating a complementary DNA encoding the amino acid sequence of the transporter protein while hydropathicity analysis suggested the tertiary structure. Cloning and expression of the cDNA in different cell systems resulted in the characterization of rat, bovine and human DATs [92–96]. The gene corresponding to hDAT is located on the distal end of chromosome 5 (5p15.3) [96].

The DAT protein consists of 620 amino acids. The bovine DAT protein was reported to consist of 693 amino acids [95]. However, the apparent longer C terminal might be due to a sequencing error giving rise to a frame shift at residue 634 [96]. The hDAT has two PKA and one PKC consensus phosphorylation sites on the N-terminus and one PKA site on the C-terminus. There is also one PKC phosphorylation site on the internal second loop [96]. On the large external second loop there are three glycosylation sites. Conspicuous is the presence of a leucine zipper motif in TM2 and 9 of the hDAT protein [96]. (At least four leucine residues spaced by six amino acids in a helix.) One methionine residue is an alternative to leucine [97]. The presence of one or two leucine zippers suggests the possibility of intramolecular bonding between TM2 and 9 or intermolecular bonding between transporter molecules. Leucine zippers are also present in rat and bovine DATs.

The amino acid sequence in hDAT is 93% identical to the sequence in rDAT and 84% to the sequence in bDAT. The sequence in hDAT is 75% identical to the sequence in the norepinephrine transporter NET, if conservative substituents are taken into account, if not, the homology is 66% [96]. The sequence homology of DAT compared with SERT is only 49%.

3.3   Dopamine transport mechanism

The mechanism of dopamine uptake by DATs is comparable to the mechanism of 5-HT uptake by SERTs with the exception that the stoiochiometry of the cotransporter Na^+- and Cl^--ions is different and that the outward transport of K^+ is not involved in the reorientation step of the transporter. Whereas the stoiochiometry of transport of $5\text{-}HT^+$, Na^+ and $Cl^- = 1:1:1$, the stoiochiometry of transport of DA^+, Na^+ and Cl^- probably is 1:2:1 [98, 99].

3.4 Ligand binding domains

The effect of site-directed mutations in rDAT on the binding of the cocaine analogue $(-)$-2β-carbomethoxy-3β-(4-fluorophenyl) tropane (CFT) and uptake of dopamine and of the neurotoxin 1-methyl-4-pyridinium (MPP$^+$) was investigated by Kitayama et al. [100]. Wild-type DAT and mutants were expressed in COS cells. Aspartate 79 in TM1 was replaced by alanine, glycine or glutamate. The binding (K_D) of [^{3}H]-CFT was substantially reduced compared to the wild-type by all three mutants whereas the B_{max} did not change significantly. This could indicate that the structure of the mutants is comparable to that of the wild-type DAT. The uptake of dopamine and of MPP$^+$ was also severely reduced by the mutants. From these experiments it is obvious that Asp79 in TM1 is essential for the functioning of DAT. Both serine residues 356 and 359 in TM7 were replaced by alanine or glycine. The K_D's of [^{3}H]-CFT binding to the mutants were about twice that of binding to the wild-type whereas the B_{max}'s were similar. The uptake of dopamine and MPP$^+$ was also significantly reduced by both mutants. The serine residues in TM7 may play a role in the binding of catecholamines such as dopamine and norepinephrine by hydrogen bridge formation but that does not account for the MPP$^+$ binding. Both serine residues 403 and 404 in TM8 were replaced by glycine. Binding parameters of [^{3}H]-CFT and uptake parameters of dopamine and MPP$^+$ are similar for both mutants and wild-type DAT indicating that both serine residues in TM8 are not involved in ligand binding. Replacement of serine 527 and 538 and tyrosine 533 in TM11 by alanine resulted in an increased affinity for MPP$^+$-uptake and a slight effect on dopamine uptake in COS cells expressing the rat wild-type DAT and the mutants [101]. In another mutant of rDAT, tyrosine 533 is replaced by phenylalanine, which is the corresponding amino acid residue in hDAT. This mutant showed an increased velocity of MPP$^+$-uptake and decreased affinity compared to the wild-type rDAT. The K_m and V_{max} of dopamine uptake were comparable to those of the wild-type DAT, and so were the binding parameters of CFT [102]. It is possible that tyrosine 533 is important for the functioning of rDAT.

Recently an endogenous Zn^{2+} binding site was found in the hDAT that was absent in the closely related hNET [103]. hDAT, hNET and their mutants were expressed in COS-7 cells. Zn^{2+} was shown to be a non-competitive blocker of dopamine uptake in micromolar concentrations. The effect was reversible. The binding of the dopamine uptake blocker WIN 35.428 (= CFT) increased by 50% in the presence of 10 μM Zn^{2+}. The inhibition of dopamine uptake was caused by a blockade of the translocation step while the increase in binding of WIN 35.428 was the result of an apparent increase in B_{max}. The effects were not observed in the norepinephrine transporter hNET. It was found that a single histidine residue (His 193) in hDAT located in the second extracellular loop of the transporter was responsible for the difference. The corresponding amino acid residue in hNET is lysine. Replacing lysine in hNET by histidine resulted in the same effect of Zn^{2+} on dopamine uptake as in hDAT indicating that His193 in hDAT is important for the binding and functioning of Zn^{2+}. The effect of Zn^{2+} on the transport of dopamine by hDAT is similar to that of hNET when the conserved histidine residue 375 in the fourth extracellular loop of hDAT is replaced by alanine. The data suggest that Zn^{2+} is bound to the hDAT in a coordination complex involving histidine 193 and 375, thereby constraining the transporter in a conformation unfavourable for translocation of the substrate.

Despite the huge efforts to try and unravel the molecular basis of substrate transport by DATs and the mechanism of uptake inhibitors the exact molecular mechanisms are still not known.

3.5 Transporter regulation

Phosphorylation and dephosphorylation of DAT is probably an important regulatory pathway in the intracellular transport and surface membrane expression of the transporter. Endogenous phosphorylation of DAT in rat striatal synaptosomes was enhanced by various activators of phosphokinase C (PKC) but not by PKA activators [104]. The enhancement was also induced by the phosphatase inhibitor okadaic acid. The phosphate incorporation was accompanied by a reduction in DA transport. This reduction caused by the PKC activator phorbol 12-myristate-13-acetate (PMA) was blocked by the PKC inhibitor staurosporine. The transport reduction was caused by a reduced V_{max} with no significant change in K_m. The same effects on DA uptake reduction after activation of PKC by PMA were found when hDAT was expressed in *Xenopus laevis* oocytes [105]. The PMA effects on specific [³H]-mazindol binding to intact oocytes was a 77% decrease in B_{max}, whereas the specific binding to oocyte homogenates in fmol/oocyte was not significantly different from control. PMA also inhibited the hDAT transport-associated current, the substrate-independent leak current, and decreased the membrane capacitance C_m. The results suggest that PMA regulates the membrane surface trafficking of hDAT in *Xenopus laevis* oocytes [105].

Activation of PKC by PMA also reduced DA uptake by hDAT expressed in insect Sf9 and mammalian COS7 cells. The V_{max} was reduced by approx. 40%. The effect was blocked by staurosporine. Pretreatment of the cells with staurosporine alone raised V_{max} by about 30%. The same rise was effected by pretreatment with the potent PKA inhibitor Rp-cAMPS. Activation of PKA by Sp-cAMPS had no significant effect. The decrease of DA uptake induced by PKC activation was correlated with a rapid sequestration/internalization of hDATs from the cell surface membrane whereas the increase of DA uptake resulted from translocation of intracellular hDATs to the surface membrane as was demonstrated by immunofluorescent microscopy [106].

The effects of endogenous arachidonic acid (AA) on the DA uptake and on the binding of the DAT inhibitor WIN34.428 was studied by Zhang and Reith [107] in rat C_6 glioma cells stably expressing hDAT.

Enhancement of the intracellular AA level was attempted in three different ways:

- Stimulation of the production of AA by the phospholipase A_2 activator melittin.
- Blocking of the re-esterification of AA by the re-acylation inhibitor thimerosal.
- Inhibition of the breakdown of AA by the lipooxygenase inhibitor nordihydroguaiaretic acid.

In all three experimental approaches both DA uptake (V_{max}) and binding of WIN34.428 were decreased. The same results were obtained when AA or PMA were applied exogenously. However, the effects of either exogenously applied AA or of AA endogenously raised by melittin were not blocked by the PKC inhibitor staurosporine. This is in contrast to the similar effects by PMA that are blocked by staurosporine. The results indicate that the molecular mechanism of regulation of DATs in the surface membrane by AA or PMA is not identical.

N-glycosylation of DATs and other monoamine transporters could be another conceivable pathway in the regulation of transporter activity. Lenhard et al. reported that DA uptake by hDATs expressed in hamster BHK-21 cells was decreased when N-glycosylation was inhibited by N-tunicamycin. Electronmicroscopic immunogold staining showed that glycosylated DATs were localized in the plasma membrane while translocation of unglycolysated DAT to the plasma membrane was blocked in cells treated with tunicamycin [108].

3.6 Selective DAT inhibitors

(R)-cocaine (Tab. 7), a weak and nonselective inhibitor of DAT, was used as lead compound for the design of potent and selective DAT inhibitors. Numerous analogues were synthetised and tested to elucidate the structural requirements of binding to DAT (for review see [109]). A breakthrough was the observation that the β-benzoyl group at C-3 could be replaced by a β-benzene ring (WIN 35,065-2). This compound is three times more potent than (R)-cocaine (Tab. 7). WIN 35,065-2 was reported as selective with respect to SERT (Si = 87) and NET (Si = 40) [110]. However, the selectivity ratios were calculated from IC_{50} values determined in binding experiments. As the IC_{50} is dependent on the concentration of the radioligand used, erroneous results may be obtained. Using K_i values to calculate selectivity ratios avoids this problem. Note the drop in selectivity ratio from 87 (IC_{50} values) to 3.46 (K_i values) for WIN 35,065-2 [111]. Substitution of the benzene ring at the 4-position is well tolerated (Tab. 7). The rank order of potency based on pIC_{50} values is Cl (RTI-31) ≥ I (RTI-55) > C > OC ~ NO_2 ~ F (WIN 35,428) = CF_3 > NH_2 = H [110, 112, 113]. The compounds are not selective (based on K_i values) [111, 114]. For comparison the selectivity ratios based on IC_{50} values (between brackets) are included (Tab. 7) [110].

There is a significant drop in selectivity ratios. The corresponding 3α-(substituted phenyl) tropane-2β-carboxylic acid methyl esters are slightly less potent than the 2β,2β isomers. This relatively high affinity of these 2β,3α isomers is in sharp contrast to the low affinity of the 2β,3α isomer of cocaine (pIC_{50} = 5.2). Structure analysis showed that the tropane ring of cocaine possesses the chair conformation, whereas the tropane ring of the 2β ester, 3α-phenyl analogues possesses the twist-boat conformation. In the twist-boat conformation the nitrogen atom, the ester group and the benzene ring are located in a similar position as the corresponding groups in the 2β,3β-isomer. These results explain the similar affinities of both stereoisomers [110]. The α-ester, β-phenyl analogue (WIN 35410) is a weak inhibitor of DAT (pIC_{50} = 5.5). The methyl of the carbomethoxy group of the 2β-ester, 3β-phenyltropane analogues, such as RTI-31, can be exchanged for isopropyl or phenyl with

Table 7.
SAR of cocaine analogues for the rat DAT.

	R	pK_i	pIC_{50}	SERT/DAT	NET/DAT
Cocaine		6.4	7.1	0.37 (12)[a]	(12)[a]
Win35,065-2	H	7.0	7.6	3.46 (87)	
Win35,428	F	7.8	7.9	12.3 (58)	43.2 (60)
RTI - 31	Cl		9.0	(40)	(33)
RTI - 55	I	8.9	8.9	0.32 (3.3)	2.0 (29)
	C	8.2	8,8	3.36 (140)	(35)
	OC		8.1		
	CF_3		7.9		
	NO_2		8.0		
	NH_2		7.6		

[a]Note: Between brackets Si rations based on IC_{50} values.

very little loss in affinity (pIC_{50} values: 8.9 and 8.7, resp.) [115]. These results indicate that the transporter for dopamine can accommodate relatively large substituents at C-2. These lipophylic esters, displaying a rather weak affinity for SERT and NET, are more selective for DAT than the parent compound RTI-31. The 2β-ester group can be replaced by various heterocyclic rings such as 1,2-isoxazole, 1,2,4-oxadiazole or 1,3-thiazole [116, 117]. The most potent and selective compound of the 2β-heterocyclic, 3β-phenyltropanes is 3β-(4'-chlorophenyl)-2β-(3'-phenylisoxazol-5-yl)tropane (pIC_{50} = 8.9; Si = 1891 (SERT/DAT); Si = 393 (NET/DAT) based on IC_{50} values). Incorporation of the phenyl ring of 1,3-thiazole into benzthiazole is well tolerated (pIC_{50} values 8.2 and 8.9, respectively). Based on QSAR studies a predominantly electro-static (H-bond) interaction between the 2β-substituents of these ligands and the binding site at DAT is postulated [117]. A different type of interaction at C-2 is proposed by the group of Kozikowski [118]. They showed that relatively large lipophylic substituents at C-2 are tolerated by DAT (Tab. 8). The most potent compound of this series is the cis isomer of the 2β-styrene containing

Table 8.
SAR of 2β-alkyl-3β-phenyltropanes for the rat DAT.

	R	pK_i
RTI - 31	COOC	9.1
	C_2	8.7
	C_3	9.0
	C_4	8.9
	C_5	6.8
	C_6	8.8
	C_2-Phe	8.8
	C = C	9.3
	(E) – C = – Phe	9.5
	(Z) – C = – Phe	9.9

derivative (pK_i = 9.9). This compound is six-fold more potent than the 2β-ester analogue RTI-31. The trans 2β-styrene isomer displays a two-fold lower affinity for DAT than its cis counterpart. The phenethyl analogue inhibits DAT 5–10 times less than its styrene congeners. The affinity of the 2β-alkyl (C2-C4) substituted derivatives is close to that of RTI-31 (Tab. 8).

None of these compounds is capable to interact with DAT via H-bonding. These results indicate the presence of a hydrophobic pocket at DAT in the vicinity of the 2β-substituent [118]. Similar results were obtained by Xu who extended the series with substituents of different lipophylicity (Tab. 9) [119].

Despite the diversity in lipophylicity all compounds bound equally well. No correlation was found between clog P and the pK_i. Recent SAR studies show that DAT can even accommodate 2,3-diphenyltropanes. The 2β,3α-isomers are one to four times more potent and about twice as selective as the corresponding 2β,3β-isomers (Tab. 10). The high affinity of both isomers is due to a difference in the conformation of the tropane ring: chair (2β,3β) or boat (2β,3α). The result is a similar spatial position of the substituents on the tropane ring for both isomers. The 2β-alkyl, 3β-phenyltropanes display a four- to six-fold higher affinity for DAT than the 2β,3α-isomers. The 2β-alkyl substituted 3β- and 3α-phenyltropanes are more selective for DAT than the 2β-ester, 3β-phenyl derivatives (Tab. 10) [111].

3α-(4-fluorophenyl)-2α-[[3,4-(methylenedioxy) phenoxy] methyl] nortropane, a tropane analogue of paroxetine, is a potent inhibitor of DAT (pIC_{50} =

Table 9.
SAR of 2β-substituted-3β-phenyltropanes for the rat DAT.

	R	pK_i	clogP
Win 35,065 - 2	COOC	7.5	2.07
	C = C – COOC	7.7	3.22
	C = C – COOC	7.6	3.13
	C = C – C – OH	7.6	2.23
	C = C – C – OH	8.0	2.71
	C_2 – C – COOC	7.7	4.27
	C_4 – COOC	7.5	4.19
	C_2 – (C = O) – Phe	7.6	4.53
	C_3 – Phe	7.8	6.12

Table 10.
SAR of 2β-substituted, 3β- and 3α-phenyltropanes for the rat DAT.

R_1	R_2	pK_i	SERT/DAT	pK_i	pIC_{50}	SERT/DAT
COOC	H	7.0	3.46			
	C	8.2	3.36			
C_3	H	7.9	12.6	7.1		12.9
	C	8.8	9.35	8.1		4.25
	F	8.3	10.9	7.7		8.2
C_4	C	8.7	11.5	7.9		5.1
Phe	H	7.3	38.1	7.9		64.3
	C	8.6	25.7	8.5		68.9
	F			8.2		26.6
CO – Phe (3,4-O_2C)	F				8.5	(140)

8.5) (Tab. 10) [46]. The selectivity based on IC_{50} values (Si = 140) will be too high [111]. It is obvious that DAT tolerates a variety of structures at the 2β-position of the tropane ring without loss in affinity. Exchanging the N-methyl group by N-alkenyl, N-alkynyl or N-benzyl of for example RTI-55 (β-CIT) enhances the selectivity for DAT, with retention of the affinity. The N-benzyl and the N-3-iodoprop-(2E)-enyl derivatives are 21- and 290-fold more selective than RTI-55 for DAT versus SERT (Si ratios: 2.3, 32 and 0.1, respectively). [^{123}I]-N-(3-iodoprop-(2E)-enyl)-2β-carbomethoxy-3β-(4'-iodo-phenyl) nortropane will be a better SPECT marker for DA neurones than [^{123}I]-RTI-55 [120]. Extension of the tropane ring to granatane reduces the affinity significantly. The 2β-(methoxycarbonyl)-9-methyl-3α-phenyl-9-azabicyclo [3.3.1] nonane derivative is more than two decades less potent than the corresponding tropane analogue (pK_i values: 5.3 and 7.5, resp.) [121]. Contraction of the tropane ring into a 7-azabicyclo [2.2.1] heptane is detrimental for activity at DAT. The 2β-(methoxycarbonyl)-7-methyl-3β-phenyl-7-azabicyclo [2.2.1] heptane is hardly active (pK_i = 4.2). Molecular modelling shows that the spatial position of the substituents on the 7-azabicyclo [2.2.1] heptane are totally different from that of the corresponding tropane analogues [122].

It is obvious that the binding site at DAT is very sensitive towards structural modifications of the tropane ring. However, recent SAR studies show that the presence of the two-carbon bridge of the tropane ring is not a prerequisite for binding to DAT. The piperidines display a lower affinity than the corresponding tropanes. The most potent compound of the series is (–)-4β-(4-chlorophenyl)-3β-(n-propyl)-1-methylpiperidine (pIC_{50} = 8.5). This piperidine analogue is about three times less potent than the tropane derivative (pK_i = 9.0). The difference in affinity for the β-ester is larger (pIC_{50} values: 7.6 (piperidine) and 9.0 (tropane) [123].

Of interest are the results of Meltzer et al., who provided evidence that the presence of a nitrogen atom in the tropane analogues is not essential for binding to DAT [124]. The 8-oxa analogues of 2β-carbomethoxy-3-β-(3,4-dichlorophenyl) tropane and its 2β,3α-isomer are potent inhibitors of the monkey DAT (pIC_{50} values: 8.5 and 8.6, respectively). These 8-oxa containing compounds are only three to six times weaker than the corresponding 8-aza analogues (Tab. 11).

The activity resides mainly in the (R)-enantiomers. The 2β,3α-8-oxa isomer is ten times more selective than its 2β,3β counterpart (Si ratios: 13 and 1.4, respectively). Both compounds are less selective than their 8-aza congeners. In contrast to the 8-azatropanes, substitution with halogen such as

Table 11.
SAR of 8-oxatropanes and 8-azatropanes for the monkey DAT.

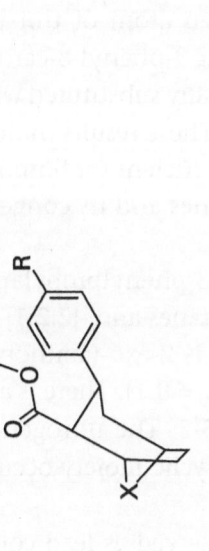

R		X = O	X = N – C		X = O		X = N · C	
		pIC$_{50}$	SERT/DAT	pIC$_{50}$	SERT/DAT	SERT/DAT	pIC$_{50}$	SERT/DAT
RS/R*	H	<6.0	10	(7.6*)	(87)	5.7	6	(7.0*)	(57)
RS/R*	F	6.3	5	8.0*	15	<6.0	10	(7.7*)	(241)
RS/R*	Cl	8.0	11	8.9*	4	7.5	29	(8.6*)	(415)
RS/R*	I	8.2	1.7	(8.9*)	(3)	7.4	2	(8.5*)	(23)
RS	3,4Cl$_2$	8.5	2.0			8.5	21		
R	3,4Cl$_2$	8.5	1.4	9.0	2	8.6	13	9.4	68
S	3,4Cl$_2$	7.3	1.2			7.3	51		

Note: Rat data between brackets. Selectivity ratios too high (cf. Tab. 7)

chlorine, bromine or iodine at the C-4 position of phenyl ring of the 8-oxa-tropanes is necessary for binding to DAT. The unsubstituted and 4-fluo-rophenyl analogues are hardly active. This difference in SAR between the 8-oxa and 8-aza compounds is not due to differences in topology. Both structures are superimposable. Both structures can form a nonionic hydrogen bond between the 8-hetero atom and the aspartic acid residue (Asp 79) in the transmembrane 1 of the transporter. However, the hydrogen bond formed to oxygen is stronger than to nitrogen. Consequently, the length of the hydrogen bond of 8-oxa to Asp 79 is shorter than in the 8-aza analogue. This difference in length affects the position of the 3-phenyl ring relative to the corresponding acceptor site on the transporter. The 3-phenyl ring of the 8-aza analogues can be placed deeper into the acceptor site than the 8-oxa derivatives. The result is a higher potency for the 8-aza compounds. A deeper placement of the 3-phenyl ring of the 8-oxatropanes is obtained by substitution of the phenyl ring at C-4 with appropriate substituents such as chlorine. The result is a significant increase in affinity for DAT [124]. Recently the same group showed that the nitrogen atom of tropane can also be replaced by carbon [125, 159]. The resulting 3-phenyl-8-carbobicyclo [3.2.1] octanes, in which the phenyl ring is optimally substituted with 3,4-dichloro display a relatively high affinity for DAT. These results indicate that a good fit of the 8-carbon atom into a pocket is sufficient for binding. It is obvious that the mode of interaction of the tropanes and its congeners is far from clear.

Differently constrained analogues of 3-phenylpropylamine are the 2-(aminomethyl)-3-phenylbicyclo [2.2.2]-octanes and -[2.2.1] heptanes [126]. The most potent compound of the series is 2-exo-(aminomethyl)-3-exo-4-chlorophenylbicyclo [2.2.1] heptane (pIC_{50} = 8.1). There is a certain overlap between this compound and WIN 35,065-2. The nitrogen atoms and the phenyl rings are in the same area. The bicyclic moiety occupies the area of the 2β-ester of WIN 35,065-2.

The anticholinergic drug benztropine served as lead compound for the design of potent inhibitors of DAT. Benztropine, a 3α-(diphenylmethoxy)-tropane analogue of cocaine, is a weak inhibitor of DAT (pIC_{50} = 6.5). In benz-tropine, however, the structural requirements for binding of cocaine and analogues at DAT are lacking. The compound has no 2β-substituent and the substituent at C-3 has the α-configuration instead of the preferred β-orientation. In order to enhance the affinity of benztropine, a carbomethoxy group was introduced at the C-2 position of the tropane ring. Only one of the eight iso-

Table 12.
SAR of diphenylmethoxytropane analogues for the rat DAT.

	configur	pIC_{50}	SERT/DAT
Difluoropine	(S) 2β 3α	8.0	324
	(S) 2β 3α	5.5	0.5
	(S) 2β 3α	5.1	0.5
	(S) 2β 3α	5.8	2.8
	(R) 2β 3α	5.7	1.0
	(R) 2β 3α	4.9	0.1
	(R) 2β 3α	4.7	0.25
	(R) 2β 3α	5.4	2.4

mers (difluoropine) displays high affinity (pIC_{50} = 8.0) and selectivity (Si = 324) for DAT (Tab. 12).

In contrast to what is expected, this isomer has the (S)-2β-3α-configuration. The isomer with the appropriate (R)-2β-3β orientation hardly binds (pIC_{50} = 4.9) [127]. Unlike the 3-phenyltropanes, the presence of a nitrogen atom at the 8-position of the tropane ring is essential for high affinity. Oxadifluoropine is only a weak inhibitor of DAT (pIC_{50} = 6.3) [124]. These results indicate that the benztropine analogues and the cocaine analogues bind in a different way to DAT. Removal of the 2β-carbomethoxy group of difluoropine has no effect on the affinity for DAT (pK_i = 7.9). The 4,4'-difluoro-substituents can be replaced by 4,4'-dichloro (pK_i = 7.7), but not by 4,4'-dimethoxy (pK_i = 5.7). Monosubstitution with chlorine at the 2-position or trifluoromethyl at the 4-position are less well tolerated (pK_i values: 6.6 and 6.2, respectively) (Tab. 13).

All compounds are selective for DAT with respect to NET and SERT but not for the muscarinic M_1 receptor. Like the lead compound benztropine the substituted benztropine analogues display a high affinity for the muscarinic M_1 receptor [128, 129]. Replacement of the N-methyl group by other N-alkyl or arylalkyl substituents is unfavourable for binding at the muscarinic M_1 receptor. The most potent and selective compound of the series is the N-(4-phenyl-n-butyl) analogue (pK_i = 8.1, Si = 56.8 (M_1/DAT) (Tab. 14). Even the nortro-

Table 13.
SAR of diphenylmethoxytropane analogues for the rat DAT.

	pK_i		pK_i
H	6.9	3,4 - diF	7.6
2-F	7.3	3,4 - diCl	7.7
3-F	7.2	3,4 - diCl,4^1 -F	7.7
4-F	7.5	3,3^1 - diF	7.3
2-Cl	6.6	4,4^1 - diF	7.9
3-Cl	7.7	4,4^1 - diCl	7.7
4-Cl	7.5		
4-OC	7.1	4,4^1 - diOC	5.7
4-CF$_3$	6.2		

Table 14.
SAR of diphenylmethoxytropane analogues for the rat DAT.

R	pK_i	M_1/DAT
H	8.0	13.9
C$_1$	7.9	0.7
C$_4$	7.6	10.2
Phe-C$_1$	7.1	9.4
Phe-C$_3$	7.4	3.2
Phe-C$_4$	8.1	56.8
C-C=O	5.6	

pane analogue is 20 times more selective than the parent compound. A basic nitrogen atom is a prerequisite for high binding to DAT (Tab. 14) [130].

Structurally related to the N-arylalkyl 3α-diphenylmethoxytropane analogues is GBR 12909 (Tab. 15). GBR 12909, a disubstituted piperazine, is a potent and rather selective inhibitor of DAT (pIC$_{50}$ = 8.4). The compound is more selective with respect to NET (Si = 110) than to SERT (Si = 34). GBR 12909 has no affinity for muscarinic M_1, α_2 and $\beta_{1,2}$-adrenoceptors and little affinity for dopamine (D_1, D_2), serotonin (5-HT$_{1A}$, 5-HT$_2$) and α_1-adrenoceptors. The compound, however is not selective with respect to histamine H_1

Table 15.
SAR of diphenylmethoxyalkylpiperazines for the rat DAT.

	R_1	R_2	pIC_{50}	SERT/DAT
GBR12935	Phe	H	8.4	168
GBR12909	Phe	F	8.4	34
	2-Thio	H	8.3	162
	2-Thio	F	8.5	32
	2-Fur	H	8.2	234
	2-Fur	F	8.2	35
	3-Pyr	H	7.1	31
	3-Pyr	F	7.8	175

(pIC_{50} = 7.7) and σ_1 receptors (pIC_{50} = 7.7) [131, 132]. Removal of both fluoro atoms (GBR 12935) enhances the selectivity with respect to SERT (Si = 168) without affecting the potency (pIC_{50} = 8.4). The phenylpropyl side-chain of GBR 12935 and GBR 12909 can be exchanged for a variety of heteroarylalkyl substituents (Tab. 15).

The thiophene and furan analogues for example, are as potent and selective as their parent compounds. The pyridine containing derivatives bind less strong to DAT. In contrast to the lead compounds the bis-(4-fluoro)-substituted pyridine analogue is more selective than the desfluoro analogue (Tab. 15). Introduction of a double bond in the 2- and 3-positions of the phenylpropyl side-chain is well tolerated. The fluoro-containing unsaturated derivatives are about one to four times more potent than their saturated analogues. The desfluoro unsaturated furan-containing compound displays the highest selectivity for DAT versus SERT (Si = 367) (Tab. 16).

Restriction of the conformation of GBR12783 and GBR13069 by incorporation of the benzene ring and the double bond into a benzthiophene, benzfuran or indole ring hardly influences the affinity and selectivity for

Table 16.
SAR of diphenylmethoxyalkylpiperazines for the rat DAT.

	R_1	R_2	pIC_{50}	SERT/DAT
GBR12783	Phe	H	7.9	
GBR13069	Phe	F	9.0	158
	2-Thio	H	8.2	184
	2-Thio	F	8.7	40
	2-Fur	H	8.3	367
	2-Fur	F	8.7	62
	3-Pyr	F	7.4	61
	3-Pyr	F	7.9	25

DAT. The indole-containing derivatives are the most potent and selective compounds of this series. Interestingly the corresponding 2-quinoline analogues are rather weak and non-selective inhibitors of DAT (Tab. 17) [132].

Exchanging the piperazine ring of GBR12935 for homopiperazine (LR-1111) enhances the selectivity for DAT significantly (Si = 4736), whereas the potency for DAT is only slightly affected (pIC_{50} = 8.1). Expansion of the homopiperazine ring to an eight-membered ring is unfavourable for affinity (pIC_{50} = 7.0) as well as for selectivity (Si = 17). Ring opening of the piperazine ring into the corresponding ethylenediamine congener is tolerated (pIC_{50} = 7.7; Si = 136). Replacement of the piperazine ring of GBR12935 by pyrrolidineamine results in a racemic compound. The (S)-enantiomer is a potent (pIC_{50} = 9.2) and selective inhibitor of DAT (Si = 1409). Its antipode is 181 times weaker and much less selective (Si = 25). Similar to GBR 12935, the compounds retain affinity for the σ_1-receptor [133, 134].

The piperidine analogues of GBR12935 and GBR12909 are about half as potent as the parent compounds but significantly less selective (Tab. 18). The

Table 17.
SAR of diphenylmethoxyalkylpiperazines for the rat DAT.

X	R_2	pIC_{50}	SERT/DAT
S	H	7.7	131
S	F	8.4	121
O	H	7.8	110
O	F	8.2	45
NH	H	9.0	619
NH	F	9.2	163
N = C	H	6.7	10
N = C	F	7.3	1

N-phenylpropyl side chain can be replaced by phenethyl or benzyl without reducing the affinity for DAT. The selectivity decreased for the N-phenethyl derivatives but increased for the N-benzyl analogues (Tab. 18). Shortening the diphenylmethoxyethyl substituent with one carbon atom is tolerated for the N-phenylpropyl and the N-phenethyl compounds but not for the N-benzyl analogues. The latter compounds are weak nonselective inhibitors of DAT [135].

Substitution at C-4 of the N-benzyl moiety with a fluoro atom or a nitro group is favourable for DAT selectivity (Tab. 19). Derivatives with a 4-chloro, 4-bromo, 4-methoxy or 4-methyl substituent are about as potent and selective as the unsubstituted N-benzyl analogue. Selectivity drops by substitution with a four-amino group (Tab. 19). The phenyl ring of the N-benzyl side-chain cannot be replaced bioisosterically by 2-thienyl (pIC_{50} = 7.2; Si = 21.2) or by 3-pyridyl (pIC_{50} = 7.3; Si = 13.9). However, thiophene does substitute for one of the phenyl rings in the diphenylmethoxy moiety. The N-4-fluorobenzyl compound displays a good affinity (pIC_{50} = 7.9) and selectivity (Si

Table 18.
SAR of diphenylmethoxyalkylpiperazines for the rat DAT.

		R = H		R = H	
n	m	pIC_{50}	SERT/DAT	pIC_{50}	SERT/DAT
3	2	7.9	19.3	7.8	3.3
2	2	8.0	9.7	7.7	1.6
1	2	7.8	48.9	8.0	20.4
3	1	7.8	4.0	7.9	8.6
2	1	7.0	4.2	7.9	17.5
1	1	6.1	0.7	6.9	6.0

Table 19.
SAR of diphenylmethoxyalkylpiperazines for the rat DAT.

R	X	pIC_{50}	SERT/DAT
H	O	7.8	48.9
F	O	7.8	111.6
Cl	O	7.6	65.1
Br	O	7.5	47.9
OC	O	7.6	44.6
C	O	7.6	60.4
NO_2	O	7.8	107.9
NH_2	O	7.0	15.6
F	NH	8.0	62.2

= 100) for DAT [136]. Similar results are observed for the N-phenylpropyl substituted derivative (pIC_{50} = 8.2; Si = 30) [137].

Interestingly the presence of a benzhydrylic oxygen atom is not a prerequisite for high affinity and selectivity. The oxygen atom can be replaced by nitrogen. The latter is as potent and slightly less selective as its oxygen-containing counterpart (Tab. 19) [138].

3.7 Pharmacology of selective DAT inhibitors

3.7.1 *In vitro* pharmacology

An example of the procedures used in assaying binding affinity and potency in uptake inhibition by DAT inhibitors in rat caudate-putamen membranes and tissue slices was reported by Katz et al. [139] and references therein. General methods of assaying the apparent affinity of radiolabelled DAT inhibitors are illustrated for instance in the paper of Aloyo et al. [140]. In the saturation experiment increasing concentrations of radiolabelled uptake inhibitor were incubated with a fixed amount of membrane preparation until equilibrium is reached and no more radioligand is specifically bound.

In the homotopic displacement experiment a fixed amount of radiolabelled inhibitor is bound to a fixed amount of membrane preparation and the bound radioligand is displaced by increasing concentrations of the unlabelled inhibitor.

From Scatchard plots generated from data of both experiments the affinity of the inhibitor and the density of binding sites are obtained. Both methods should lead to similar results.

3.7.2 *In vivo* pharmacology

In order to study potential stimulant properties of DA uptake inhibitors several behavioural tests can be used such as the forced swimming test in which immobility, swimming and climbing are scored [76] and the locomotor test in which the increase in horizontal ambulation is scored and compared with the effect on locomotor increase induced by cocaine [139]. Whether rats are able to discriminate between cocaine and a DA uptake inhibitor or not is tested in the cueing or discrimination test (see for instance [139]).

3.8   Potential therapeutic applications of selective DAT inhibitors

GBR-12909 was in phase II clinical studies for the indication Parkinson disease. However, further development is suspended. It is possible that GBR-12909 will be replaced by the longer acting decanoate ester of GBR-12909 [141].

A number of DAT inhibitors such as GBR-12909, GBR-12935 and WIN-35065-2 analogues are under development as potential treatment of substance dependence such as cocaine abuse. So far no clinical data have been published. GBR-12909 and GBR-12935 will probably be replaced by the more selective homopiperazine analogue LR 1111 or the long-acting decanoate ester of GBR-12909 [141].

Dopascan (iometopane) is RTI-55 labelled with iodine-123. The compound is in phase II clinical trial as a dopamine imaging agent for the diagnosis of Parkinson's disease. Dopascan fully distinguished patients with Parkinson's disease from those without. Serious side-effects were not observed. Phase III trials are running [141].

GBR-12909, GBR-12935 and the decanoate ester of GBR-12909 have a suppressant effect on appetite in primates. A therapeutic application as anti-obesity agent has to be explored.

4   The norepinephrine transporter (NET)

4.1   Distribution in the CNS

The distribution of NETs in rat brain was investigated by quantitative autoradiography of [³H]-nisoxetine binding to coronal sections of the brain [142]. The highest specific binding (fmol/mg protein) was found in the locus coeruleus (1526 ± 39), anteroventral nucleus of the thalamus (1444 ± 147), ventral portion of the bed nucleus of the stria terminalis (1348 ± 57) and the dorsomedial nucleus of the hypothalamus (1062 ± 37). The binding density was also high (ranging from 847 ± 81 to 672 ± 50) in the paraventricular nucleus of the hypothalamus, paraventricular nucleus of the thalamus, dentate gyrus of the hippocampus and medial zona incerta. Moderate densities were found in the dorsal raphe nucleus, mammilothalamic tract, dorsal area of the bed nucleus of stria terminalis, median raphe nucleus and basolateral nucleus of the amygdala (range 639 ± 27 to 497 ± 30). The other brain regions investigated showed lower densities (about 300–180). The density in the caudate putamen was the lowest (54 ± 11).

NET distribution in human locus coeruleus and raphe nuclei was studied by Ordway et al. [143] using quantitative autoradiography of [^{3}H]-nisoxetine in *post mortem* brain sections. It was found that the density of specific binding of the selective NET inhibitor [^{3}H]-nisoxetine was unevenly distributed along the rostral-caudal axis of the locus coeruleus. The binding correlated well with the number of neuromelanin-containing cells along the axis. The density of binding site was also uneven along the rostral-caudal axis of the dorsal raphe nucleus. The highest density was found in the ventral subnucleus, the ventrolateral subnucleus and the interfascicular subnucleus. In some regions of the dorsal raphe the density of [^{3}H]-nisoxetine binding sites was as high or even higher than in the locus coeruleus. The results of the investigations make it plausible that NETs in the dorsal raphe reside on norepinephrine fibers terminating near or at serotonergic cell bodies.

4.2   Structure of the norepinephrine transporter

The putative general structure of NET is shown in Figure 1. The primary structure of NET was found by isolating a complementary DNA encoding the amino acid sequence of the transporter protein while hydropathicity analysis suggested the tertiary structure.

Cloning and expression of the cDNA in different cell systems resulted in the characterization of human, bovine and rat NETs [144–146]. The NET protein consists of 617 amino acids. hNET and bNET have three glycosylation sites situated on the second external loop whereas rNET has only two. All three NETs have one PKC phosphorylation site on the second internal loop. bNET has an additional two phosphorylation sites on the internal C-terminal whereas rNET has one PKC phosphorylation site and one casein kinase II phosphorylation site on the internal C-terminal. There is a very high degree of amino acid conservation in the aligned amino acid sequences of the three NETs (human vs. bovine 93.5%, rat vs. human 93% and rat vs. bovine NET 91%). A leucine zipper motif is present in TM2 of all three NETs suggesting the possibility of intermolecular oligomer formation.

The chromosomal localization of the gene responsible for the production of NETs is 16q12.2.

4.3 Norepinephrine transport mechanism

The stoichiometry of NE translocation by NETs ($NE^+:Na^+:Cl^- = 1:1:1$) is different from translocation of serotonin by SERTs ($5\text{-}HT^+:Na^+:Cl^- = 1:1:1$ and coupled to the efflux of one K^+ ion) and from translocation of dopamine by DATs ($DA^+:Na^+:Cl^- = 1:2:1$) (see [98]).

Recently, sophisticated experiments using voltage clamp and amperometric recordings in patches of HEK 293 cells stably transfected with hNETs revealed that a voltage-dependent inward NE flux correlated temporally with NE transporter currents in the same path [147]. The experiments further showed that NE transport occurs in bursts distinct from stoichiometric transport. It seems more likely that NETs transport NE via channels especially in the first stage of transport, when relatively large amounts of NE have to be cleared from the synaptic cleft (see also Kavanaugh's commentary [148]).

4.4 Ligand binding domains

From the analysis of a large series of chimeric rDAT/hNETs it was concluded that transmembrane spanning domains 5–7 of NET are important for high affinity binding of the selective NE uptake inhibitors desipramine and nisoxetine. The region including TM1-3 of NET is also involved in the binding of desipramine and nisoxetine [149]. The apparent affinity of NE and DA for their transporters reside in membrane spanning regions TM1-3 and TM10-11 suggesting that residues in both regions may interact. The domain possibly involved in translocation of the substrates includes the regions TM4-8 [149, 150].

The experiments by Giros et al. [151] using a series of functionally expressed rNET/hDAT chimera suggest a different pattern of binding and translocation domains. Regions from the N-terminal through TM1-5 are considered responsible for translocation and ionic dependence. Regions comprising TM6-8 are involved in the binding of tricyclic translocation inhibitors and the regions from TM9 through the C-terminal tail are involved in high affinity binding of substrates. It is clear that further research is needed before the interaction between transporter and ligand on the molecular level is more precisely known.

4.5 Transporter regulation

Regulation of the functioning of NETs in the surface membrane of noradrenergic neurons by phosphorylation and dephosphorylation is probably only one factor in a complex regulatory system. It was shown by Apparsundaram et al. [152] that activation of PKC by the phorbolesters β-PMA and β-PDBu (phorbol-12,13-dibutyrate) resulted in a significantly diminished NE uptake capacity by hNETs in stably transfected HEK293 and LLC-PK1 cells as also in transiently transfected COS-7 cells. The affinity of NE for the hNETs did not change. Neither the mRNA synthesis inhibitor actomycin D nor the translation inhibitor cycloheximide had any impact on the effects of β-PMA on the NE uptake capacity. Binding of the selective NET inhibitor [^{3}H]-nisoxetine to hNETs expressed in HEK293 cells showed that its K_d in β-PMA treated cells is similar to that in untreated cells, whereas the B_{max} is significantly reduced. When the binding studies of [^{3}H]-nisoxetine were repeated with total membranes of lysed β-PMA-treated cells or vehicle-treated control cells, both K_d and B_{max} in both systems were identical. The results indicate that the reduction in B_{max} in whole cells treated with β-PMA is caused by internalization of part of the hNETs in the surface membrane. The redistribution of hNETs in the surface membrane was visualized in LLC-PK$_1$ cells by using confocal microscopy after immunofluorescent labelling of hNETs with N430 antibody. Using this technique it was clearly demonstrated that hNETs are internalized from the surface membrane after treatment with β-PMA and that this process was blocked by treatment with staurosporine.

The effect of glycosylation on surface expression and transport activity of NETs was investigated by Nguyen et al. [153] and Melikian et al. [154]. The canonical N-glycosylation sites in hNET situated in the second extracellular loop between TM3 and 4 (Asn184, Asn192 and Asn198) were all mutated to Gln (QQQ mutant). In the other mutant only Asn192 and Asn198 were mutated to Gln (NQQ mutant). hNET and mutants were transiently expressed in HeLa cells or stably expressed in Madin-Darby canine kidney cells (MDCK cells) [153]. Expressed in HeLa cells the NQQ mutant showed a two-fold diminution in transport velocity compared with hNET while the diminution was 20-fold in the QQQ mutant. The affinity of NE for the mutants was similar to that for the wild type hNET. The apparent affinity K_i of the mutants for the NE uptake inhibitors mazindol, desipramine and (–)cocaine was also similar to that of the wildtype hNET. Quantitation of biotinylated NE transporters in HeLa cells showed that the density of hNETs is two-fold higher than that of the NQQ mutant and about ten-fold higher than that of the QQQ mutant, suggesting that the difference in surface expression explains the difference in transport efficiency. Also in MDCK cells the fully glycosylated hNET is preferentially directed to the cell surface membrane whereas the unglycosylated QQQ mutant was barely detectable. Melikian et al. [154] reported that hNETs stably expressed in LLC-PK1 cells and treated with the glycosylation inhibitor tunicamycin depletes the surface membrane of hNET glycoproteins. Transiently expressed QQQ mutants in HeLa or COS_1 cells suffered severe losses in uptake capacity, 96 and 70% respectively. Expressed in HeLa cells the affinity of the QQQ mutant for the substrate and for the uptake inhibitors desipramine and nomifensine was the same as that of the wild-type hNET. Further experiments suggested that the reduction in uptake capacity of the QQQ mutant is caused by a decrease in the efficiency of the uptake mechanism.

4.6   Selective NET inhibitors

Nisoxetine belongs to the class of substituted 3-phenoxy-3-phenyl-propanamines (Tab. 20). In contrast to its structural analogue fluoxetine, a selective inhibitor for SERT, nisoxetine is selective for NET. Nisoxetine displays a high affinity for the rat NET ($pK_i = 8.9$) and human NET ($pK_D = 9.0$) [66, 152]. The selectivity ratios with respect to SERT are 238 (rat) and with respect to DAT 392 (rat). Similar to fluoxetine, nisoxetine has little or no affinity for various neurotransmitter receptors [155, 156]. Nisoxetine is a racemate and the activity for NET resides mainly in the (R)-isomer. The development of nisoxetine was halted in the clinical phase.

Replacement of the 2-methoxy group of nisoxetine by 2-methyl (tomoxetine) increases the affinity for NET (pK_i values: 9.2 (rat); 8.7 (human)). Tomoxetine is less selective with respect to SERT (Si = 6.1 (rat); 4.5 (human)). The affinity for DAT is weak (pK_i values: 5.9 (rat); 6.0 (human)) [36, 53]. Tomoxetine hardly binds to other receptor subtypes. Almost all activity resides in the (R)-enantiomer [155]. Tomoxetine is in development for the indication attention deficit/hyperactivity disorder (cf. section 4.8).

Exchanging the 2-methyl group of tomoxetine by halogen is well tolerated. The rank order of potency is bromine ~ iodine ($pK_i = 9.5$) ≥ chlorine ($pK_i = 9.3$) > fluorine ($pK_i = 8.8$). The 2-fluorine substituted analogue displays the highest selectivity with respect to SERT (Si = 200). The 2-iodine analogue

Table 20.
Selective NET inhibitors of the aryloxypropanamine type.

Nisoxetine pK$_i$ = 8.9   Tomoxetine pK$_i$ = 9.2   289306 pK$_i$ = 9.4

Reboxetine pK$_i$ = 7.1   Viloxazine pK$_i$ = 6.8

is three-fold less selective. Resolving the 2-iodine compound (289306) (Tab. 20) results in a potent and selective (R)-enantiomer (303926: pK$_i$ = 9.5; Si = 128) and a non-selective (S)-enantiomer (303884: pK$_i$ = 8.0; Si = 5.1). [^{123}I]-303926 may be a useful tool for SPECT. The 2-fluorine and 2-bromine analogues may provide ligands for PET [157].

In reboxetine the sidechain of the 2-ethoxy analogue of nisoxetine is incorporated into a morpholine ring (Tab. 20). Reboxetine, possessing the (RR,SS)-configuration, is selective for NET. The activity resides mainly in the (SS)-enantiomer (pIC$_{50}$ = 8.4) Its (RR)-counterpart is about 24 times weaker (pIC$_{50}$ = 7.1) [158]. Reboxetine does not bind or hardly binds to various neuron receptors. Recently reboxetine has been launched worldwide as an antidepressant (cf. section 4.8).

Table 21.
Selective NET inhibitors derived from constrained benzylamines.

Nomifensine $pK_i = 8.3$ Mazindol $pK_i = 9.3$

Viloxazine is structurally related to reboxetine (Tab. 20). Viloxazine, a racemate, displays a moderate affinity for the rat and human NET ($pK_i = 6.8$). The compound is selective with respect to SERT (Si ~ 100 (rat, human)), and to DAT (Si = 300 (rat), Si > 645 (human)) [66, 53]. Viloxazine does not bind to various other receptors [156].

Viloxazine has been on the market as an antidepressant since 1976.

Nomifensine (Tab. 21) is a constrained benzylamine derivative, structurally related to Mc-N-5652-Z (cf. Tab. 3). In contrast to Mc-N-5652-Z, a potent SERT inhibitor, nomifensine binds to NET with high affinity (pK_i values: 8.3 (rat); 7.8 (human)). Nomifensine is highly selective with regard to SERT (Si ratios: 256 (rat); 65 (human)). The degree of selectivity for NET over DAT is only ten-fold [66, 53]. Nomifensine was on the market as a stimulatory antidepressant. Due to the high incidence of induction of acute haemolytic anemia, nomifensine was withdrawn from the market.

A differently constrained benzylamine is mazindol (Tab. 21). Mazindol displays a high affinity for the rat NET ($pK_i = 9.3$). The compound is selective with respect to human SERT (Si = 224). The degree of selectivity for NET with respect to DAT is less [39, 29]. Due to the relatively high affinity for DAT ($pK_i = 7.8$), [^{3}H]-mazindol was frequently used to label DAT in the striatum. However, [^{3}H]-nisoxetine and [^{3}H]-tomoxetine are significantly more selective for NET. These radioligands are more suitable tools to label NET than [^{3}H]-mazindol. As DAT inhibitors have a suppressant effect on appetite, mazindol is developed as anti-obesity agent and is launched in many countries.

Table 22.
Selective NET inhibitors derived from TCA.

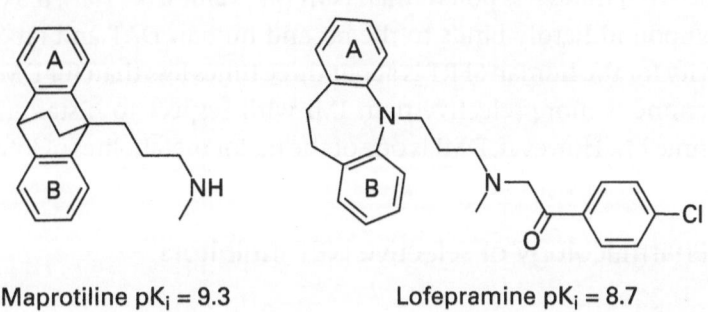

Talsupram pK$_i$ = 9.3   R=H DMI   pK$_i$ = 9.5   Nortriptyline pK$_i$ = 9.0
=H CLODMI pK$_i$ = 9.5

Maprotiline pK$_i$ = 9.3   Lofepramine pK$_i$ = 8.7

Talsupram (Tab. 22) is a structure analogue of citalopram (cf. Tab. 5). In contrast to citalopram, a selective inhibitor of SERT, talsupram is selective for NET. The compound binds with high affinity to NET (pK$_i$ = 9.3). The affinity for SERT is weak (pK$_i$ = 6.1) and for DAT nihil (pK$_i$ = 5.1) [52].

A representative number of selective inhibitors of NET, derived from the first generation of tricyclic antidepressants (TCAs) is illustrated in Table 22.

Desipramine (DMI), desmethylclomipramine (cloDMI) and nortriptyline display nanomolar affinities for the rat as well as for the human NET. The rank order of potency for the rat NET is DMI = cloDMI (pK$_i$ = 9.5) > nortriptyline (pK$_i$ = 9.0). The compounds bind about two-fold weaker to the human NET. In rats the degree of selectivity for NET over SERT is greater for DMI (Si = 416) than for cloDMI (Si = 113) and nortriptyline (Si = 60). The compounds are significantly less selective for the human NET (Si ratios: 35 (DMI);

21 (cloDMI); 8 (nortriptyline) [39, 62, 53]). The affinity for DAT is nihil [36, 53, 62]. Selectivity with respect to various neurotransmitter receptors is lacking. DMI and nortriptyline have pronounced antagonistic effects on α_1-adrenoceptors, histamine H_1 and muscarinic M_1 receptors. CloDMI acts as a histamine H_1 antagonist. However, the desmethyl derivatives are more selective than their corresponding parent compounds [39, 156, 62].

Maprotiline (Tab. 22) is a tetracyclic antidepressant. The compound is a selective inhibitor of NET, both in rat (pK_i = 8.1) and human (pK_i = 8.0). Maprotiline hardly binds to SERT (pK_i = 5.5 (rat); pK_i = 5.2 (human). The degree of selectivity for NET over DAT is greater for rat (Si = 391) than for human (Si = 90) [66, 39]. Like the TCAs, maprotiline is not selective with respect to a number of neurotransmitter receptors, such as histamine H_1 and α_1-adrenoceptors [156].

Lofepramine (Tab. 22) is an N-substituted DMI derivative. Lofepramine is only six to ten times less potent than DMI (pK_i values: 8.7 (rat); 8.3 (human)). The compound hardly binds to the rat and human DAT and rat SERT. The selectivity for the human SERT is about three times less than for DMI [36, 53]. Lofepramine is more selective than IMI with respect to histamine H_1 and muscarinic M_1. However, DMI is one of the major metabolites of lofepramine.

4.7   Pharmacology of selective NET inhibitors

4.7.1   In vitro pharmacology

The affinity of NE re-uptake inhibitors for NETs and their potency in inhibiting NE uptake is often assayed using synaptosomes prepared from rat hypothalamus or cerebral cortex (see for instance [157, 142]).

An example of ex vivo assays for the determination of the effective dose (ED_{50}) of NE uptake inhibitors in rats is reported by Andersen [131] and by Gehlert et al. [160]. Different dose levels of the drug under investigation were administered to rats. After decapitation and isolation of the cerebral cortex, slices of the tissue were cross-chopped and assayed in suspension for [^{3}H]-NE uptake.

Quantitative autoradiography of rat brain slices incubated with [^{3}H]-NE in the presence or absence of a high concentration of competitor is a useful technique to detect brain regions rich in NETs as shown for instance by Tejani-Butt [142].

An example for the binding assay of NE uptake inhibitors using membranes of transfected HEK 293 cells expressing hNETs was described by Tatsumi et al. [53]. An example of antagonist binding assay on intact transfected HEK 293 cells expressing hNETs was shown by Apparsundaram et al. [152]. The parameters K_m and V_{max} of NE transport are assayed by incubation of intact cells expressing NETs with buffers containing either [^{3}H]-NE or [^{3}H]-DA (see for example [152, 154, 98]). In order to enhance the metabolic stability of [^{3}H]-NE in the cell the incubation buffer has to contain 3-4-dihydroxy-methyl propiophenone (U-0521) to inhibit catechol-O-methyl transferase and pargyline to inhibit monoamine oxidase. As dopamine is more stable than NE the addition of the enzyme inhibitors is not necessary. More important probably is the fact that DA is at least as good a substrate for NETs as NE, if not better [98].

4.7.2 *In vivo* pharmacology

Several tests for potential antidepressant properties of NET inhibitors have been reported such as prevention of tetrabenazine induced ptosis, muscle rigidity and decreased exploratory activity in rats [74], the forced swim test and the open field behavioural test using olfactory bulbectomized rats [161, 77].

4.8 Therapeutic applications of selective NET inhibitors

Recently (January 1999) reboxetine was launched worldwide for the indication depression. Reboxetine was proven to be clinically effective in patients with major depressive disorder and dysthymia (for review see [162]). The efficacy is maintained for at least up to one year. Reboxetine is superior to the selective SERT inhibitor fluoxetine in severely ill patients and in improving social functioning [163]. Reboxetine is well tolerated. The most frequently reported side-effect (urinary resistancy) is different from that of fluoxetine (nausea). Similar to the selective SERT inhibitors reboxetine is not cardiotoxic and is devoid of orthostatic hypotension.

Tomoxetine was undergoing expanded phase III trials for the treatment of major depressive illness. Although effective in depressed patients, the development of tomoxetine as an antidepressant has been discontinued. At present tomoxetine is in phase II trial for the treatment of attention deficit/hyperactivity disorder [141]. Preliminary results show that tomoxetine is effective in attention deficit/hyperactivity disorder and well tolerated [164].

Acknowledgement

The excellent technical support of Marijke Mulder is gratefully acknowledged.

References

1   P.D. Hrdina, B. Foy, A. Hepner and R.J. Summers: J. Pharmacol. Exp. Therap. 252, 410–418 (1990).

2   R. Cortés, E. Soriano, A. Pazos, A. Probst and J.M. Palacios: Neuroscience 27, 473–496 (1988).

3   G.E. Duncan, K.Y. Little, J.A. Kirkman, R.S. Kaldas, W.E. Stumpf and G.R. Breese: Brain Res 591, 181–197 (1992).

4   M.C. Austin, Ch.C. Bradley, J.J. Mann and R.D. Blakely: J. Neurochem. 62, 2362–2367 (1994).

5   D. Bengel, O. Jöhren, A.M. Andrews, A. Heils, P. Mössner, G.L. Sanvitto, J.M. Saavedra, K.-P. Lesch and D.L. Murphy: Brain Res 778, 338–345 (1997).

6   M. Fujita, H.M. Shimada, T. Nishimura and M. Tohyama: Neurosci. Lett. 162, 59–62 (1993).

7   D.P. McLaughlin, K.Y. Little, J.F. Lopez and S.J. Watson: Neuropsychopharmacology 15, 523–529 (1996).

8   Y. Qian, H.E. Melikian, D.B. Rye, A.I. Levry and R.D. Blakely: J. Neurosci. 15, 1261–1274 (1995).

9   F.C. Zhou, Y. Xu, S. Bledsoe, R. Lin and M.R. Kelley: Mol. Brain. Res. 43, 267–278 (1996).

10 F.C. Zhou, J.-H. Tao-Cheng, L. Segu, T. Patel and Y. Wang: Brain. Res. 805, 241–254 (1998).

11 M.A. Bunin and R.M. Wightman: J. Neurosci. 18, 4854–4860 (1998).

12 R.D. Blakely, H.E. Berson, R.T. Fremeau, M.G. Caron, M.M. Peek, H.K. Prince and Ch.C. Bradley: Nature 354, 66–70 (1991).

13 B.J. Hoffman, E. Mezey and M.J. Brownstein: Science 254, 579–580 (1991).

14 W. Mayser, H. Betz and P. Schloss: FEBS Lett. 295, 203–206 (1991).

15 S. Ramamoorthy, A.L. Bauman, K.R. Moore, H. Han, T. Yang-Feng, A.S. Chang, V. Ganapathy and R.D. Blakely: Proc. Natl. Acad. Sci. 90, 2542–2546 (1993).

16 K.P. Lesch, B.L. Wolozin, H.C. Estler, D.L. Murphy and P.J. Riederer: J. Neural. Transm. [Gen. Sect.] 91, 67–72 (1993).

17 A.S. Chang, S.M. Chang, D.M. Starnes, S. Schroeter, A.L. Bauman and R.D. Blakely: Mol. Brain. Res. 43, 185–192 (1996).

18 G. Rudnick and J. Clark: Biochem. Biophys. Acta Bio-Energetics 1144, 249–263 (1993).

19 A.S. Chang and D.M. Lam: J. Physiol. London 510 (Pt3), 903–913 (1998).

20   E.L. Barker, H.L. Kimmel and R.D. Blakely: Mol. Pharmacol. 46, 799–807 (1994).

21   E.L. Barker and R.D. Blakely: Mol. Pharmacol. 50, 957–965 (1996).

22   J-G Chen, A. Sachpatzidis and G.Rudnick: J. Biol. Chem. 272, 28321–28327 (1997).

23   C. Sur, P. Schloss and H. Betz: Biochem. Biophys. Res. Comm. 241, 68–72 (1997).

24   J.-G. Chen, S. Liu-Chen and G. Rudnick: Biochemistry 36, 1479–1486 (1997).

25   M.M. Stephan, M.A. Chen, K.M.Y. Penado and G. Rudnick: Biochemistry 36, 1322–1328 (1997).

26   C. Sur, H. Betz and P. Schloss: Proc. Natl. Acad. Sci. 94, 7639–7644 (1997).

27   P. Schloss and H. Betz: Biochemistry 34, 12590–12595 (1995).

28   C.J. Humphreys, S.C. Wall and G. Rudnick: Biochemistry 33, 9118–9125 (1994).

29   E.L. Barker, M.A. Perlman, E.M. Adkins, W.J. Houlihan, Z.B. Pristupa, H.B. Niznik and R.D. Blakely: J. Biol. Chem. 273, 19459–19468 (1998).

30   Y. Qian, A. Galli, S. Ramamoorthy, S. Risso, J.L. DeFelice and R.D. Blakely: J. Neurosci. 17, 45–47 (1997).

31   S. Ramamoorthy, E. Giovanetti, Y. Qian and R.D. Blakely: J. Biol. Chem. 273, 2458–2466 (1998).

32   K.J. Miller and B.J. Hoffman: J. Biol. Chem. 44, 27351–27356 (1994).

33   Ch.G. Tate and R.D. Blakely: J. Biol. Chem. 269, 26303–26310 (1994).

34   D.T. Wong, F.P. Bymaster and E.A. Engelman: Life Sci. 57, 411–441 (1995).

35   D.T. Wong, F.P. Bymaster, L.R. Reid, D.A. Mayle, J.H. Krushinski and D.W. Robertson: Neuropsychopharmacol 8, 337–344 (1993).

36   C. Bolden-Watson and E. Richelson: Life Sci. 52, 1023–1029 (1993).

37   D.T. Wong, F.P. Bymaster, L.R. Reid and P.G. Threlkeld: Biochem. Pharmacol. 32, 1287–1293 (1983).

38   D.T. Wong, P.G. Threlkeld and D.W. Robertson: Neuropsychopharmacol 5, 43–47 (1991).

39   M.J. Owens, W.N. Morgan, S.J. Plott and C.B. Nemeroff: J. Pharmacol. Exp. Therap. 283, 1305–1322 (1997).

40   S. Chumpradit, M.P. Kung, Ch. Panyachotipun, V. Prapansiri, C. Foulon, B.P. Brooks, S.A. Szabo, S. Tejani-Butt, A. Frazer and H.F. Kung: J. Med. Chem. 35, 4492–4497 (1992).

41   D.R. Michals and H.E. Smith: Chirality 5, 20–23 (1993).

42   R.J. Cregge, E.R. Wagner, J. Freedman and A.L. Margolin: J. Org. Chem. 55, 4237–4238 (1990).

43   P. Plenge, E.T. Mellerup, T. Honoré and P. Lefèvre Honoré: J. Pharm. Pharmacol. 39, 877–882 (1987).

44   N.S. Gunasekara, S. Noble and P. Benfield: Drugs 55, 85–120 (1998).

45   Ch.A. Mathis, J.M. Gerdes and J.D. Enas: J. Pharm. Pharmacol. 44, 801–805 (1992).

46   K.I. Keverline-Frantz, J.W. Boja, M.J. Kuhar, P. Abraham, J.P. Burgess, A.H. Lewin and F.I. Caroll: J. Med. Chem. 41, 247–257 (1998).

47   H. Takeuchi, H. Yatsugi, K. Hatanaka, K. Nakato, H. Hattori, R. Sonoda, K. Koshiya, M. Fujii and T. Yamaguchi: Eur. J. Pharmacol. 329, 27–35 (1997).

48   D.W. Robertson, D.C. Thompson, L.R. Reid and D.T. Wong: FASEB J 4, A988 (1990).

49   C.M. Perry and P. Benfield. CNS Drugs 6, 480–500 (1997).

50   W.M. Welch, A.R. Kraska, R. Sarges and B.K. Koe: J. Med. Chem. 27, 1508–1515 (1984).

51   K.P. Bøgesø, A.V. Christensen, J. Hyttel and T. Liljefors: J. Med. Chem. 28, 1817–1828 (1985).

52   J. Hyttel: Prog. Neuro. Psychopharmacol. Biol. Psychiat. 6, 277–295 (1982).

53   M. Tatsumi, K. Groshan, R.D. Blakely and E. Richelson: Eur. J. Pharmacol. 340, 249–258 (1997).

54   J.O. Marcusson, U. Norinder, T. Högberg and S.B. Ross: Eur. J. Pharmacol. *215*, 191–198 (1992).

55   B.E. Maryanoff, J.L. Vaught, R.P. Shank, D.F. McComsey, M.J. Constanzo and S.O. Nortey: J. Med. Chem. *33*, 2793–2797 (1990).

56   M. Holliday and P. Benfield: Drugs *49*, 280–294 (1995).

57   J.P. Yardley, G.E.M. Husbands, G. Stack, J. Butch, J. Bicksler, J.A. Moyer, E.A. Muth, T. Andree, H. Fletcher, M.N.G. James et al.: J. Med. Chem. *33*, 2899–2905 (1990).

58   E.A. Muth, J.A. Moyer, J.T. Haskins, T.H. Andree and G.E.M. Husbands: Drug Dev. Res. *23*, 191–199 (1991).

59   J.-C. Béïque, N. Lavoie, C. de Montigny and G. Debonnel: Eur. J. Pharmacol. *349*, 129–132 (1998).

60   P.R. Carlier, M.M.C. Lo, P.C.K. Lo, E. Richelson, M. Tatsumi, I.J. Reynolds and T.A. Sharma: Bioorg. Med. Chem. Ltt. *8*, 487–492 (1998).

61   S. Noble and P. Benfield: CNS Drugs *8*, 410–431 (1997).

62   J. Hyttel: Int. Clin. Psychopharmacol. *9* (Suppl. 1), 19–26 (1994).

63   J. Bigler, K.P. Bøgesø, A. Toft, W. Hansen: Eur. J. Med. Chem. *12*, 289–295 (1977).

64   G.P. Luscombe, W.R. Buckett: Drug Dev. Res. *29*, 235–248 (1993).

65   J. Hyttel and J.J. Larssen: Acta Pharmacol. Toxicol. *56* (Suppl. 1), 146–153 (1985).

66   E. Richelson, M. Pfenning: Eur. J. Pharmacol. *104*, 277–286 (1984a).

67   K.J. Palmer and P. Benfield: CNS Drugs *1*, 57–87 (1994).

68   B. Scatton, Y. Claustre, D. Graham, T. Dennis, A. Serrano, S. Arbilla, C. Pimoule, H. Schoemaker, D. Bigg and S.Z. Langer: Drug Dev. Res. *12*, 29–40 (1988).

69   I. Angel, H. Schoemaker, M. Prouteau, M. Garreau and S.Z. Langer: Eur. J. Pharmacol. *232*, 139–145 (1993).

70   K. Hashimoto and T. Goromaru: Neuropharmacology *31*, 869–874 (1990).

71   G.D. Bartoszyk, R. Hegenbart and H. Ziegler: Eur. J. Pharmacol. *322*, 147–153 (1997).

72   S.C. Cheetham, J.A. Viggers, N.A. Slater, D.J. Heal and W.R. Buckett: Neuropharmacology *32*, 737–743 (1993).

73   C.A. Stockmeier, L.A. Shapiro, J.W. Haycock, P.A. Thompson and M.T. Lowy: Brain Res. *727*, 1–12 (1996).

74   R.M. Ferris, L. Brieaddy, N. Mehta, E. Hollingsworth, G. Rigdon, C. Wang, F. Soroko, W. Wastila and B. Cooper: J. Pharm. Pharmacol. *47*, 775–781 (1995).

75   M.J. Detke, M. Rickels and I. Lucki: Psychopharmacology *119*, 47–54 (1995).

76   S.E. Hemby, I. Lucki, G. Gatto, A. Singh, C. Thornley, J. Matasi, N. Kong, J.E. Smith, H.M.L. Davies and S.I. Dworkin: J. Pharmacol. Exp. Therap. *282*, 727–733 (1997).

77   A. Harkin, J.P. Kelly, M. McNamara, T.J. Connor, K. Dredge, A. Redmond and B.E. Leonard: Eur. J. Pharmacol. *364*, 123–132 (1999).

78   R.D. Porsolt, A. Lenègre and R.A. Mc Arthus, in: B. Olivier, J. Mos and J.L. Slangen (eds.): Animal models in psychopharmacology. Birkhäuser Verlag, Basel 1991, 137–159.

79   P. Willner, in: P. Willner (ed.): Behavioural models in psychopharmacology: theoretical, industrial and clinical perspectives. Cambridge University Press, Cambridge UK 1991, 91–125.

80   M.R. Ware: J. Clin. Psychiatry *58* (Suppl. 5), 15–23 (1997).

81   F. Artigas, L. Romero, C. De Montigny and P. Blier: TINS *19*, 378–383 (1996).

82   F. De Jonghe and J. Swinkels: CNS Drugs *7*, 452–467 (1997).

83   T.A. Pigott and S.M. Seay: J. Clin. Psychiatry *60*, 101–106 (1999).

84   B. Fulton and D. Mc Tavish: CNS Drugs *3*, 305–322 (1995).

85   C. Freed, R. Revay, R.A. Vaughan, E. Kriek, S. Grant, G.R. Uhl and M.J. Kuhar: J. Com-

parative Neurol. *359*, 340–349 (1995).

86   J.W. Boja, J.L. Cadet, T.A. Kopajtic, J. Lever, H.H. Seltzman, C.D. Wyrick, A.H. Lewin, P.Abraham and F.I. Carroll: Mol. Pharmacol. *47*, 779–786 (1995).

87   J. Booy, G. Andringa, L.J.M. Rijks, R.J. Vermeulen, K. de Bruin, G.J. Boer, A.G. Janssen and E.A. van Royen: Synapse *27*, 183–190 (1997).

88   B.K. Madras, L.M. Gracz, M.A. Fahey, D.R. Elmaleh, P.C. Meltzer, A.Y. Liang, E.G. Stopa, J. Babich and A.J. Fischman: Synapse *29*, 116–127 (1998).

89   B.K. Madras, L.M. Gracz, P.C. Meltzer, A.Y. Liang, D.R. Elmaleh, M.J. Kaufman and A.J. Fischman: Synapse *29*, 102–115 (1998).

90   A.J. Fischman, A.A. Bonab, J.W. Babich, E.P. Palmer, N.M. Alpert, D.R. Elmaleh, R.J. Callahan, S.A. Barrow, W. Graham, P.C. Meltzer, R.N. Hanson and B.K. Madras: Synapse *29*, 128–141 (1998).

91   G. Tissingh, J. Booij, P. Bergmans, A. Winogrodzka, A.G. Janssen, E.A. van Royen, J.C. Stoof and E.C. Wolters: J. Nucl. Med. *39*, 1143–1148 (1998).

92   S. Shimada, S. Kitayama, C.-L. Lin, A. Patel, E. Nanthakumar, P. Gregor, M. Kuhar and G. Uhl: Science *254*, 576–578 (1991).

93   J.E. Kilty, D. Lorand and S.G. Amara: Science *254*, 578–579 (1991).

94   B. Giros, S. El Mestikawy, L. Bertrand and M.G. Caron: FEBS Lett *295*, 149–154 (1991).

95   T.B. Usdin, E.Mezey, C. Chen, M.J. Brownstein and B.J. Hoffman: Proc. Natl. Acad. Sci. *88*, 11168–11171 (1991).

96   B. Giros, S. El Mestikawy, N. Godinot, K. Zheng, H. Han, T. Yang-Feng and M.G. Caron: Mol. Pharmacol. *42*, 383–390 (1992).

97   W.H. Landschulz, P.F. Johnson and S.L. McKnight: Science *240*, 1759–1764 (1988).

98   H. Gu, S.C. Wall and G. Rudnick: J. Biol. Chem. *269*, 7124–7130 (1994).

99   H. Gu and G. Rudnick: Soc. Neurosci. Abstr. *22*, 370 (1996).

100   S. Kitayama, S. Shimada, H. Xu, L. Markham, D.M. Donovan and G.R. Uhl: Proc. Natl. Acad. Sci. USA *89*, 7782–7785 (1992).

101   S. Kitayama, J.B. Wang and G.R. Uhl: Synapse *15*, 58–62 (1993).

102   C. Mitsuhata, S. Kitayama, K. Morita, D. Vandenbergh, G.R. Uhl and T. Dohi: Mol. Brain Res. *56*, 85–88 (1998).

103   L. Norregaard, D. Frederiksen. E.Ø. Nielsen and U. Gether: EMBO J *17*, 4266–4273 (1998).

104   R.A. Vaughan, R.A. Huff, G.R. Uhl and M.J. Kuhar: J. Biol. Chem. *272*, 15541–15546 (1997).

105   S.-J. Zhu, M.P. Kavanaugh, M.S. Sonders, S.G. Amara and N.R. Zahniser: J. Pharmacol. Exp. Therap. *282*, 1358–1365 (1997).

106   Z.B. Pristupa, F. McConkey, F.Liu, H.Y.Man, F.J.S. Lee, Y.T. Wang and H.B. Niznik: Synapse *30*, 79–87 (1998).

107   L. Zhang and M.E.A. Reith: Eur. J. Pharmacol. *315*, 345–354 (1996).

108   T. Lenhard, K. Marheineke, B. Lingen, W. Haase, R. Hammermann, H. Michel and H. Reilander: Cell Mol. Neurobiol. *18*, 347–360 (1998).

109   F.I. Carroll, A.H. Lewin, J.W. Boja and M.J. Kuhar: J. Med. Chem. *35*, 969–981 (1992).

110   C.R. Holmquist, K.I. Keverline-Frantz, P. Abraham, J.W. Boja, M.C. Kuhar and F.I. Carroll: J. Med. Chem. *39*, 4139–4141 (1996).

111   A.P. Kozikowski, G.L. Araldi, K.R.C. Prakash, M. Zhang and K.M. Johnson: J. Med. Chem. *41*, 4973–4982 (1998).

112   F.I. Carroll, Y. Gao, M.A. Rahman, P. Abraham, K. Parham. A.H. Lewin, J.W. Boja and M.J. Kuhar: J. Med. Chem. *34*, 2719–2725 (1991).

113   J.W. Boja, F.I. Carroll, M.A. Rahman, A. Philip, A.H. Lewin and M.J. Kuhar: Eur. J. Pharmacol. *184*, 329–332 (1990).

114   J.L. Neumeyer, G. Tamagnan, S. Wang, Y. Gao, R.A. Milius, N.S. Kula and R.J. Baldessarini: J. Med. Chem. *39*, 543–548 (1996).

115   F.I.Carroll, P.Abraham, A.H.Lewin, K.A.Parham, J.W. Boja and M.J. Kuhar: J. Med. Chem. *35*, 2497–2500 (1992).

116   F.I. Carroll, J.L. Gray, P. Abraham, M.A. Kuzemko, A.H. Lewin, J.W. Boja and M.J. Kuhar: J. Med. Chem. *36*, 2886–2890 (1993).

117   P. Kotian, S.W. Mascarella, P. Abraham, A.H. Lewin, J.W. Boja, M.J. Kuhar and F.I. Carroll: J. Med. Chem. *39*, 2753–2763 (1996).

118   A.P. Kozikowski, M.K. Eddine Saiah, K.M. Johnson and J.S. Bergmann: J. Med. Chem. *38*, 3086–3093 (1995).

119   L. Xu, S.V. Kelkar, S.A. Lomenzo, S. Izenwasser. J.H. Katz, R.K. Kline and M.L. Trudell: J. Med. Chem. *40*, 858–863 (1997).

120   P. Emond, L. Garreau, S. Chalon, M. Boazi, M. Caillet, J. Bricard, Y. Frangin, L. Mauclaire, J-C. Besnard and D. Guilloteau: J. Med. Chem. *40*, 1366–1372 (1997).

121   Z. Chen, S. Izenwasser, J.L. Katz, N. Zhu, C.L. Klein and M.L. Trudell: J. Med. Chem. *39*, 4744–4749 (1996).

122   C. Zhang, S. Izenwasser, J.L. Katz, P.D. Terry and M.L. Trudell: J. Med. Chem. *41*, 2430–2435 (1998).

123   A.P. Kozikoswki, G.L. Araldi, J. Boja, W.M. Meil, K.M. Johnson, J.L. Flippen-Andersen, C. George and E. Saiah: J. Med. Chem. *41*, 1962–1968 (1998).

124   P.C. Meltzer, A.Y. Liang, P. Blundell, M.D. Gonzalez, Z. Chen, C. George and B.K. Madras: J. Med. Chem. *40*, 2661–2673 (1997).

125   P.C. Meltzer, P. Blundell and B.K. Madras: Med. Chem. Res. *8*, 12–34 (1998).

126   H.M. Deutsch, D.M. Collard, L. Zhang, K.S. Burnham, A.K. Deshpande, S.G. Holtzman and M.M. Schweri: J. Med. Chem. *42*, 882–895 (1999).

127   P.C. Meltzer, A.Y. Liang and B.K. Madras: J. Med. Chem. *37*, 2001–2010 (1994).

128   A.H. Newman, R.H. Kline, A.C. Allen, S. Izenwasser, C. George and J.L. Katz: J. Med. Chem. *38*, 3933–3940 (1995).

129   R.H. Kline, S. Izenwasser, J.L. Katz, D.B. Joseph, W.D. Bowen and A.H. Newman: J. Med. Chem. *40*, 851–857 (1997).

130   G.E. Agoston, J.H. Wu, S. Izenwasser, C. George, J. Katz, R.H. Kline and A.H. Newman: J. Med. Chem. *40*, 4329–4339 (1997).

131   P.H. Andersen: Eur. J. Pharmacol. *166*, 493–504 (1989).

132   D. Matecka, D. Lewis, R.B. Rothman, C.M. Dersch, F.H.E. Wojnicki, J.R. Glowa, A. Courtney De Vries, A. Pert and K.C. Rice: J. Med. Chem. *40*, 705–716 (1997).

133   D. Matecka, R.B. Rothman, L. Radesca, B.R. de Costa, C.M. Dersch, J.S. Partilla, A. Pert, J.R. Glowa, F.H.E. Wojnicki and K.C. Rice: J. Med. Chem. *39*, 4704–4716 (1996).

134.   R.N. Hanson, S-W Choi, D.R. Elmaleh and A.J. Fischman: Bioorg. Med. Chem. Lett. *7*, 2559–2564 (1997).

135   A.K. Dutta, C. Xu and M.E.A. Reith: J. Med. Chem. *39*, 749–756 (1996).

136   A.K. Dutta, L.L. Coffey and M.E.A. Reith: J. Med. Chem. *40*, 35–43 (1997).

137   A.K. Dutta, L.L. Coffey and M.E.A. Reith: J. Med. Chem. *41*, 699–705 (1998).

138   A.K. Dutta, C. Xu and M.E.A. Reith: J. Med. Chem. *41*, 3293–3297 (1998).

139   J.L. Katz, S. Izenwasser, R.H. Kline, A.C. Allen and A.H. Newman: J. Pharmacol. Exp. Therap. *288*, 302–315 (1999).

140   V.J. Aloyo, J.S. Ruffin, P.S. Pazdalski, A.L. Kirifides and J.A. Hatrvey: J. Pharmacol. Exp. Therap. *273*, 435–444 (1995).

141   Pharmaprojects CD v 2.0 (1999).

142   S.M. Tejani-Butt: J. Pharmacol. Exp. Ther. *260*, 427–436 (1992).

143   G.A. Ordway, C.A. Stockmeier, G.W. Cason and V. Klimek: J. Neurosci. *17*, 1710–1719 (1997).

144   T. Pacholczyk, R.D. Blakely and S.G.Amara: Nature *350*, 350–354 (1991).

145   B. Lingen, M. Brüss and H. Bönisch: FEBS Lett. *342*, 235–238 (1994).

146   M. Brüss, P. Pörzgen, L.J. Bryan-Lluka and H.Bönisch: Mol. Brain Res. *52*, 257–262 (1997).

147   A. Galli, R.D. Blakely and L.J. DeFelice: Proc. Natl. Acad. Sci. USA *95*, 13260–13265 (1998).

148   M.P. Kavanaugh: Proc. Natl. Acad. Sci. USA *95*, 12737–12738 (1998).

149   K.J. Buck and S.G. Amara: Mol. Pharmacol. *48*, 1030–1037 (1995).

150   K.J. Buck and S.G. Amara: Proc. Natl. Acad. Sci. USA *91*, 12584–12588 (1994).

151   B. Giros, Y.-M. Wang, S. Suter, S.B. McLeskey, Ch. Pifi and M.G. Caron: J. Biol. Chem. *269*, 15985–15988 (1994).

152   S. Apparsundaram, S. Schroeter, E. Giovanetti and R.D. Blakely: J. Pharmacol. Exp. Ther. *287*, 744–751 (1998).

153   T.T. Nguyen and S.G. Amara: J. Neurochem. *67*, 645–655 (1996).

154   H.E. Melikian, S. Ramamoorthy, Ch.G. Tate and R.D. Blakely: Mol. Pharmacol. *50*, 266–276 (1996).

155   D.T. Wong, P.G. Threlkeld, K.L. Best, F.P. Bymaster: J. Pharmacol. Exp. Ther. *222*, 61–65 (1982).

156   E. Richelson and A. Nelson: J. Pharmacol. Exp. Therap. *230*, 94–102 (1984).

157   D.R. Gehlert, D.A. Schober, S.K. Hemrick-Luecke, J. Krushinski, J.J. Hobert, D.W. Robertson, R.W. Fuller and D.T. Wong: Neurochem. Int. *26*, 47–52 (1995).

158   M. Strolin-Benedetti, E. Frigerio, P. Tocchetti, G. Brianceschi, M.G. Castelli, C. Pellizzoni and P. Dostert: Chirality *7*, 285–289 (1995).

159   P.C. Meltzer, P. Blundell, Z. Chen, Y.F. Yong and B.K. Madras: Bioorg. Med. Chem. Lett. *9*, 857–862 (1999).

160   D.R. Gehlert, L. Dreshfield, F. Tinsley, M.J. Benvenga, S. Gleason, R.W. Fuller, D.T. Wong and S.K. Hemrick-Luecke: J. Pharmacol. Exp. Therap. *287*, 122–127 (1998).

161   B.E. Leonard: Eur. Neuropsychopharmacol. *7* (Suppl. 1), S11–16 (1997).

162   G.D. Burrows, K.P. Maguire and T.R. Norman: J. Clin. Psychiatry *59* (Suppl. 14), 4–7 (1998).

163   J. Massana: J. Clin. Psychiatry *59* (Suppl. 14), 8–10 (1998).

164   T. Spencer, J. Biederman, T. Wilens, J. Prince, M. Hatch, J. Jones, M. Harding, S.V. Faraone and L. Seidman: Am. J. Psychiatry *115*, 693–695 (1998).

Progress in Drug Research, Vol. 54 (E. Jucker, Ed.)
©2000 Birkhäuser Verlag, Basel (Switzerland)

Neuropeptides in drug research

By David Poyner[1], Helen Cox[2], Mark Bushfield[3], J. Mark Treherne[3] and Melissa K. Demetrikopoulos[3]

[1]Aston University, Pharmaceutical and Biological Sciences, Aston Triangle, Birmingham B4 7ET, UK;
[2]Centre for Neuroscience, King's College London, GKT School of Biomedical Sciences, St Thomas' Campus, Lamberth Palace Road, London SE1 7EH, UK;
[3]Cambridge Drug Discovery Ltd., Cambridge Science Park, Milton Road, Cambridge CB4 0FG, UK

David Poyner

is currently a lecturer in the Pharmaceutical Sciences Institute, Aston University, Birmingham, UK. He was previously at the MRC Molecular Neurobiology Unit/Laboratory of Molecular Biology, Cambridge and has worked within the National Institute for Medical Research, London with Drs. E.C. Hulme and N.J.M. Birdsall and at Cambridge University, with Professor Sir Arnold Burgen. His research focuses on CGRP and he was co-organiser of CGRP '98 Meeting and was editor of the conference proceedings.

Helen M. Cox

is currently a Senior Lecturer in Pharmacology at Kings College, London. She was previously a lecturer in Pharmacology at The Royal College of Surgeons and prior to this was a postdoctoral scientist at Cambridge University for 6 years. Her interests include the enteric neuropeptides, particularly NPY and she co-organised the NPY '93 Meeting in Cambridge, UK and the NPY '99 meeting in Grand Cayman.

Mark Bushfield

is currently Chief Scientific Officer at Cambridge Drug Discovery Ltd, UK. He was previously Senior Principal Scientist, Gastrointestinal Diseases, at Pfizer Central Research, UK. Before that, he spent 5 years working on cellular signalling at the State University of New York, Stony Brook and at Glasgow University. His interests include signal transduction and ion channel research.

J. Mark Treherne

is currently Chief Executive at Cambridge Drug Discovery Ltd., UK. He was previously Senior Principle Scientist, Neurodegenerative Diseases at Pfizer Central Research in the UK for 5 years. Before that, he was a Research Fellow at the Biozentrum in Basel, where he moved after completing his Ph.D and first post-doctorate in Cambridge. His interests include ion channel research and the pathology of neurodegenerative disease.

Melissa K. Demetrikopoulos

is currently Director of Scientific Communication at the Institute for Biomedical Philosophy, USA. She was previously at the Department of Psychiatry and Behavioural Sciences at Emory University, and completed her training at the University of Medicine and Dentistry of New Jersey. Her interests include understanding the neural substrates important in immune functioning and issues involving scientific literacy.

Summary

Neuropeptides have been a subject of considerable interest in the pharmaceutical industry over the last 20 years or more. Many drug discovery teams have contributed to our understanding of neuropeptide biology but no significant drugs that act selectively upon neuropeptide receptors have yet emerged from the clinic. There are, however, a plethora of clinically useful drugs that act at other classes of neurotransmitter and neuromodulator receptors, many of them discovered over the last 20 years. Nevertheless, we think that the future for the discovery of novel drugs acting at neuropeptide receptors looks bright for two reasons: (1) there has been a substantial increase in our understanding of the function of neuropeptides; and (2) high-throughput screening (HTS) against neuropeptide receptors has now begun to yield many interesting drug-like molecules, rather than peptides, that have the potential to become clinically useful drugs.

The objective of this review is to summarise our current understanding of specific areas of neuropeptide biology and pharmacology in the CNS as well as the PNS. We will also speculate on where we think the new generation of neuropeptide agonists and antagonists could emerge from the clinic.

Contents

Keywords

Neuropeptides, peripheral nervous system, central nervous system, neuropeptide Y, opioid peptides, cholecystokinin, substance P, galanin, calcitonin gene-related peptide (CGRP)

Glossary of abbreviations

HTS, high-throughput screening; CNS, central nervous system; NPY neuropeptide Y; CCK, cholecystokinin; CGRP, calcitonin gene-related peptide; PNS, peripheral nervous system; VIP, vasoactive intestinal polypeptide; alpha-MSH, alpha melanocyte stimulating hormone; HPA hypothalmic pituitary adrenal axis; SubP, substance P; NK, neurokinin; CRF, corticotropin releasing factor; NA, noradrenaline; VTA, ventral tegmental area; LC, locus coeruleus; CRLP, calcitonin receptor-like protein; RAMP, receptor activity modifying protein; ENS, enteric nervous system; PYY, peptide YY; PP, pancreatic polypeptide.

1   Introduction

The discovery of neuropeptides as a class of novel bioactive molecules is of considerable importance to our understanding of neurobiology [1]. Neuropeptides can act as neurotransmitters, neuromodulators and hormones. They control or influence many varied types of behaviour (e.g. mating, feeding, exploration, memory, learning, and pain perception) via actions on the central nervous system (CNS). In addition, they also regulate many systemic functions via their central role in the functioning of the peripheral nervous system (PNS).

The term "neuropeptides" was first coined in 1971 to refer to fragments of peptide hormones lacking the activity of the intact hormone but capable of producing behavioural changes [1]. Subsequently, peptide hormones and their fragments, endogenous opioids (morphine-like peptides) and other biogenic peptides came to be classified as neuropeptides. The key features that united these different peptides were that they originated from the nervous system and other specialised peptide-secreting cells, their biosynthesis, secretion, metabolism and their bioactivity at very low concentrations [1]. In 1978, it was reported in the first issue of "Trends in Neuroscience" that there were 18 different peptides that could be listed [2]. Seventeen years after that period of post-enkephalin euphoria, the same author reported the number to exceed 50 [3]. That rapid increase in the number of neuropeptides came from the recognition that evolution has yielded families of structurally related peptides. Consequently, the enkephalins were joined by the endorphins and dynorphins, substance P (SP) by the tachykinins and vasoactive intestinal peptide (VIP) by other members of the secretin family. Rapidly following the discovery of these novel peptides was the discovery of the neuropeptide receptors by which they exerted their actions.

It soon became clear that the diversity of neuropeptide signalling resulted from the existence of neuropeptides very early in evolution, since they appear to be ubiquitous signalling molecules in all metazoan species possessing a nervous system [4]. This diversity of neuropeptides and their receptors has provided a huge impetus to identify novel drug targets, modulators of which have the potential for selectively modifying behavioural as well as systemic disorders. A key problem, however, has been to turn peptides, which are useful as pharmacological tools, into drug-like molecules suitable for clinical evaluation. Although significant advances have been made in "designing" non-peptide, small molecule agonists and antagonists of neuropeptides [5], high-throughput screening (HTS) against human neuropeptide receptors cloned and expressed in all lines offers real potential for rapidly discovering novel drug-like molecules [6].

2   Neuropeptides of the central nervous system (CNS)

The conclusions that a variety of neuropeptides are involved in normal neuronal functioning and in the pathogenesis of (CNS) disease are well established. However, the large molecular weight and chemical composition of these neuropeptides has limited their pharmaceutical usefulness in the past due to the difficulties involved in their administration. Prokai [7] recently reviewed the challenges of delivering peptide drugs across the blood brain barrier and presented several possible avenues for drug delivery such as disruption of the blood brain barrier, manipulations of the transported peptides, and the use of biological carriers. The potential utilisation of these various neuropeptide delivery options will allow the further development of clinically useful compounds for combating CNS disease.

While it is beyond the scope of this review to catalogue thoroughly all of the neuropeptides and their various functions, the following sections survey a variety of neuropeptides and give illustrative examples of selected functions in order to explore their relevance to drug research. The papers reviewed address several issues important for drug design including the development of agonist and antagonist compounds, the delineation of receptor subtypes and their anatomical distribution, the delivery of peptide compounds to the CNS, and an understanding of the issues involved in the development of potentially clinically useful compounds.

2.1 Neuropeptide Y (NPY)

Neuropeptide Y (NPY), a member of the pancreatic polypeptide family, has at least five pharmacologically distinct receptor subtypes that are all members of the G-protein-coupled receptor superfamily [91]. NPY receptor subtypes differ in both their anatomical and chemical specificity [91] as outlined in detail in Table 1 and section 3.2.3. Beyond its widely studied effects in the peripheral nervous system, NPY has been shown to have important CNS effects such as stimulating feeding behaviour through ventromedial arcuate nucleus innervation of the hypothalamus [8]. It has been suggested that this system may be disregulated in anorexia since a mouse model of genetic anorexia involves impaired release of hypothalamic NPY [10]. The effects of NPY on feeding most likely involve several NPY receptor subtypes and the interaction of other neuropeptides within the hypothalamus since the orexigenic effects of NPY are blocked by glucagon-like peptide (GLP) but not by α-melanocyte-stimulating hormone (α-MSH) or neurotensin [11]. In addition to regulating feeding, NPY is important for the central regulation of a variety of physiologically important phenomena such as blood pressure, learning and memory, thermoregulation, and hypothalamic-pituitary-adrenal (HPA) axis regulation [9]. Since it is likely that the mechanisms controlling these biological systems display NPY receptor subtype specificity, the development of compounds that can selectively target the various NPY receptor subtypes represents an important avenue for drug discovery. The use of molecular modelling has allowed investigators to examine the structure of NPY and propose NPY analogues. Since it is thought that both the N and C termini of NPY are important to receptor binding, analogues have been designed which have the central turn region removed while retaining the same orientation of the termini. For example, Krstenansky and colleagues suggest that residues 7–17 are not directly involved in receptor binding but serve a structural purpose by stabilising a conformation that allows receptor binding [12]. In addition to designing various peptide analogues that can be used to study NPY systems, non-peptide antagonists have been developed as tools for differentiating the various NPY receptor subtypes [13]. Jacques and colleagues have demonstrated that BIBP3226, a nonpeptide NPY receptor antagonist, is selective for the Y_1 receptor but not on the Y_2 or Y_3 subtypes. The design of such selective antagonists is critical for determining the functional significance of the receptor subtypes and thus for the development of clinically useful compounds.

2.2 Opioid peptides

Opioid peptides, including the enkephalins, endorphins and dynorphins, have been shown to produce a variety of physiological effects such as analgesia, respiratory depression, immune suppression, dependence, and gut motility. It is thought that they have a high degree of conformational flexibility that may be reflected in the complexity of the physiological response to opiates [14]. This flexibility may allow a specific ligand to bind to several receptor subtypes depending on the particular conformation it has assumed. Therefore, drug discovery has concentrated on the design of highly receptor-selective agonists and antagonists to differentiate the various opioid receptor subtypes. Conformationally constrained opioid peptides have been designed using binding assays and *in vitro* bioassays with various spectroscopic methods [14]. For example, Kawasaki and colleagues designed several dynorphin A analogues that are conformationally constrained in the "address" sequence of the peptide [14]. They demonstrated additional subtype specificity such that Cys5, Cys11 and Cys8, Cys13 differed in their affinity for central versus peripheral κ and μ receptors. This same group of investigators further characterised the centrally acting Cys5, Cys11 peptides by synthesising a series of cyclic peptides and thus demonstrated that the conformation at residue 5 is important in aligning the message segment to the address segment [15]. In addition to the design of conformationally constrained opioid peptides, another approach to central analgesic drug design has involved the development of compounds formulated to inhibit peptidases that normally inactivate the enkephalins. Chen and colleagues designed a dual inhibitor to the membrane-bound zinc metallopeptidases, aminopeptidase N and neutral endopeptidase-24, 11, which inactivate enkephalins [16]. They developed aminophosphinic compounds that acted as dual inhibitors with nanomolar affinities and produced antinociceptive responses similar to those produced by morphine. This suggests the potential for developing analgesic agents that are clinically superior to morphine in terms of their lack of opioid side-effects. An additional approach to analgesic drug design incorporates a brain-targeted chemical delivery system that allows the delivery of an analgesic agent across the blood-brain barrier and protects the compound from inactivating peptidases. Prokai-Tatrai and colleagues utilised a retro-metabolic drug design to deliver a leu-enkephalin analogue centrally [17]. The brain-targeting delivery system utilised a biologically inert molecule that was then converted to the active peptide in the CNS. These systems have the advantage of producing the analgesia centrally and thus avoid peripheral side-effects. Furthermore, additional refinement of the system should allow optimal clinical therapeutic effects by providing a mechanism for controlling the rate of central peptide release.

2.3   Cholecystokinin (CCK)

Cholecystokinin (CCK) has been shown to have CNS effects on satiety, analgesia, dopamine modulation (important for schizophrenia and Parkinson's disease) and GABA modulation (important for anxiety) through the CCK-B receptor subtype [18]. Additionally, experimental models of hypovolemia and hypotension have demonstrated that CCK in the lateral parabrachial nuclei is involved in thirst and salt appetite [19]. Furthermore, CCK regulates burst firing of thalamic reticular neurons by suppression of K^+ conductance in the dendrites [20]. Since it has been shown that CCK has numerous CNS affects of potential clinical importance, the development of selective agonist and antagonist agents is crucial. Horwell [18] used a multi stepped process to design potentially therapeutically useful CCK-related compounds that began with the examination of the contiguous and non-contiguous fragments of the target neuropeptide and then proceeded to identification of the "minimum fragment" in binding assays. After the "minimum fragment" was identified, the N and C termini and other functional groups were chemically modified to optimise the bioavailability of the fragment. Finally, the agonist/ antagonist profiles of the compounds were determined by bio- and pharmacological assays as well as by behavioural testing. Using this methodology, Horwell was able to synthesise an orally active antagonist agent capable of crossing the blood-brain barrier to produce potent anxiolytic effects. Another approach to antagonist development involves the modification of the potent CCK-B antagonist spiroglumide [21]. Makovec and colleagues utilised a mixed anhydride method by which the spiroglumide was reacted in THF with a mixed amino acid aqueous solution. This method yielded compounds that exhibited activity 70-170 times greater than the original antagonist. Similarly, Freidinger et al. took as their starting point the key structural feature of asperlicin, the 1,4 benzodiazepine, to design devazepide or L-364,718. This ligand was a CCK-A receptor antagonist with extremely high affinity. Further chemical modification yielded a range of CCK-B receptor specific antagonists exemplified by L-365,260 [22] and L-368,395 [23]. Taken together, these investigators demonstrated that new therapeutic agents can be derived from either endogenously occurring substrates or further refinement of previously synthesised compounds.

2.4 The tachykinins

Substance P (SP) is a small, 11 amino acid peptide that has extensive CNS and PNS effects partly due to its distribution to a variety of brain regions including the hypothalamus, brain stem and pontine laterodorsal nuclei, and its regulation of the HPA axis [24]. SP, along with neurokinins A and B, forms part of a family of neuropeptides called tachykinins that share a common C terminal sequence. The tachykinins are subdivided into two groups with SP in the aromatic subgroup. Four receptors have been described for the tachykinins: NK_1, NK_2, NK_3 and NK_4. Typically, activation of these G-protein-linked receptors leads to a cascade of events that ultimately results in opening of Ca^{2+} channels and a rise in intracellular Ca^{2+} [24]. SP-containing terminals are widely distributed in brain regions known to be important in pressor responses including the nucleus amygdaloideus centralis, nucleus paraventricularis, nucleus ventromedialis, lateral hypothalamus-perifornical region, periaqueductal gray matter, nucleus parabrachialis, locus coeruleus, and rostral ventrolateral medulla [25]. Ku and colleagues [25] demonstrated a hypertensive response when either SP or corticotropin-releasing factor (CRF) was injected into these regions. Beyond producing a hypertensive response, SP has anxiolytic effects when micro-injected into the nucleus basalis magnocellularis region [26]. Hasenohrol et al. [26] found that rats injected with SP into the nucleus basalis spent more time in the open arms of the plus-maze and increased their social interaction times. Obviously, it is critically important to the discovery of a SP agent for the clinical treatment of anxiety to target the system specifically so that the hypertensive response does not occur as an unwanted side-effect of the compound.

SP produces many of its effects in conjunction with other neurotransmitter systems. For example, SP has been shown to regulate dopamine activity in the striatum [27]. This effect was shown to be mediated through NK_1 but not NK_3 receptors and thus demonstrated receptor subtype specificity. Similarly, SP depolarizes cholinergic interneurons in the striatum using the NK_1 receptor subtype [28]. It has been suggested that this occurs through a phosphoinositide signalling pathway. In addition to the various systems that SP effects through changes in Ca^{2+} channels, SP has also been shown to produce its physiological effects through other channel systems. For example, SP produced an inward current in auditory efferent neurons that occurred in the absence of Ca^{2+} in solution [29]. In this model, Wang and Robertson suggest that SP's effect was due to the opening of a relatively non-selective unknown cation channel and closure of the inward rectifier K^+ channels. In the locus coeruleus, Shen and North [30] showed SP acted by opening a non-selective cation channel and closing an inwardly rectifying potassium channel. The results were confirmed and extended by Koyano et al., who showed that only the potassium channel effect was mediated by a G-protein [31]. Similarly, Ca^{2+} influx was not required for SP enhancement of N-methyl-D-aspartate (NMDA) channel function in hippocampal dentate gyrus granule cells [32]. Lieberman and Mody suggested that SP may gate the activation of hippocampal network activity by increasing the duration of NMDA channel openings. While a thorough review of the physiological effects of SP is beyond the scope of this review, the above examples were chosen to illustrate the complexity of this system. Potential SP drug design must consider all these factors to develop site and receptor specific compounds.

2.5 Galanin

The 29 amino acid peptide galanin is evident in widespread regions of the CNS [33]. Galanin has been shown to hyperpolarise monoaminergic neurons [34] and inhibit dopaminergic neurons [35]. Although galanin is often co-localised with noradrenaline (NA), the release of galanin from NA terminals is dependent on the rate of NA terminal depolarisation. It has been suggested that galanin release occurs during burst firing of NA neurons but not during slow regular rates of depolarisation [33]. This differential release of galanin may be important in the production of stress-induced behavioural depression [36]. This hypothesis suggests that, under basal conditions, locus coeruleus (LC) neurons undergo slow, regular rates of depolarisation thus releasing NA, but not galanin, leading to the stimulation of dopaminergic cells within the ventral tegmental area (VTA) by interaction with excitatory α_1 adrenoceptors. However, under stressful conditions, NA becomes depleted in the LC resulting in a functional blockade of α_2 receptors and subsequent burst firing of LC neurons. This LC neuronal burst firing causes the release of galanin into the VTA that will hyperpolarize the cells and inhibit dopamine release. Decreased dopamine release will result in the behavioural manifestations generally observed in stress-induced depression such as inactivity and anhedonia. Support for this hypothesis demonstrated that VTA administration of exogenous galanin produced a dose-dependent behavioural depression that showed antagonism by galantide [37]. Therefore, galanin appears to be involved in stress-induced depression through its interaction with a variety of other neurotransmitter systems. However, other investigators have examined the release of galanin from the hypothalamic paraventricular nucleus and the median eminence and found no change in response to 120 min of immobilisation stress [38]. Taken together, these studies show that galanin release during stress is site specific and suggest new avenues of drug discovery for depression. In addition to its effects on depression, galanin may play an important role in memory by stimulating the NMDA receptor/nitric oxide synthase/cyclic GMP pathway in the ventral hippocampus [39]. Consolo and colleagues demonstrated that galanin raises cyclic GMP in the ventral hippocampus in a dose-dependent and site-specific manner. This phenomenon could be blocked by the galanin antagonist M40, NMDA receptor antagonists, or nitric oxide synthase inhibitors. Similarly, Sobreviela and colleagues demonstrated co-localisation of nitric oxide synthase and galanin within the cholinergic basal forebrain [40]. The galanin positive neurones were primarily localised within the septal-diagonal band complex and some of these neurones within the horizontal limb of the diagonal band displayed nitric oxide synthase reactivity. The authors proposed that the co-localisation of these compounds within the cholinergic basal forebrain neurons indicates a complex chemical signal and possible novel pharmacological means for preventing neurodegenerative processes. Galanin may also affect neurodegenerative processes by modulating the cholinergic vasodilatatory basalocortical system [41]. Cholinergic stimulation of the substantia innominata by carbachol increased cerebral blood flow that was blocked by co-administration of galanin. Thus, it may be possible to exploit the potential protective role of galanin in cerebrovascular reactivity in order to develop a drug treatment for neurodegeneration.

2.6 Neurotrophic factors

It is widely accepted that neurotrophic factors serve a neuro-protective role during neuronal development [42]. They are thought to be necessary for the maintenance of neurons by suppressing the activation of suicide genes that lead to apoptosis. However, the role of neurotrophic factors in the maintenance of the adult nervous system is less well established. It has been suggested that neurotrophic factors are important in maintaining normal neuronal functioning and that loss of these factors may be responsible for age-related neuronal atrophy and a variety of neurodegenerative diseases. Thus, neurotrophic factors have tremendous therapeutic potential since they may protect diseased and injured neurons, induce neuronal sprouting, and increase neuronal functioning. A variety of neurotrophic agents including nerve growth factor, brain-derived neurotrophic factor, neurotrophin-3, glial cell line-derived neurotrophic factor, transforming growth factor α, and insulin-like growth factor-I serve numerous neuro-protective functions. For example, nerve growth factor is believed to be important in the maintenance of cholinergic neurons and clinically important for Alzheimer's disease and alcohol induced neurotoxicity. Similarly, glial cell line-derived neurotrophic factor has clinical implications for Parkinson's disease, Alzheimer's disease and Huntington's disease; and neurotrophin-3 may be important for neuronal survival following injury. In addition to their neuro-protective effects, there is increasing evidence that neurotrophic agents may be able to correct age-related impairments. For example, Markowska and colleagues demonstrated that insulin-like growth factor-I was able to improve working and reference memory in aged rats [43].

The systemic administration of these proteins is often ineffective in alleviating adverse CNS symptomatology due to the impermeability of the blood-brain barrier, consequently delivery of potentially therapeutic neurotrophic agents to the brain is a critical component of drug discovery. Several methodologies for CNS delivery of neurotrophic factors have been explored including the use of polymeric implants, continuous infusion pumps, and the transplantation of protein-secreting cells [44]. The differences in these methodologies translate into their various strengths such that polymeric implants allow the administration of the highest possible local concentration of the peptide agent, while infusion pumps provide greater control, and the transplantation of cell "factories" may offer lifelong treatment. However, in each case, the penetration into tissues is quite low, resulting in a small treatment region. Recently, design issues have tried to address this problem by exploring the distribution, diffusion and elimination of neurotrophic factors in the brain. Several biophysical techniques including quantitative autoradiography, fluorescence microscopy, and magnetic resonance imaging can be used to measure the fate of centrally administered neurotrophic factors. An understanding of these basic phenomena has facilitated the development of customised methods for the local administration of agents such as nerve growth factor. This has been accomplished by stabilisation of the protein in order to reduce its elimination [44]. Taken together, these technologies provide new avenues of drug design for the clinically relevant neurotrophic factors.

2.7 Calcitonin gene-related peptide (CGRP)

Although more widely studied in the periphery, calcitonin gene-related peptide (CGRP) has a wide range of potential CNS effects due to its broad distribution in the hypothalamus, medial forebrain area, medial amygdaloid nucleus, hippocampus, thalamus, medial lemniscus, ventral tegmentum, lateral lemniscus, superior olive, and many other structures [45]. At least 2 CGRP receptors have been described pharmacologically, as outlined in section 3.1.1. These receptors display G protein-coupling and regulation of K^+ channels and Ca^{2+} currents. CGRP has a role in sensory (olfaction, audition, and vision); motor; and integrative systems (learning, and feeding). Despite its prevalence in a variety of CNS systems, there is little data supporting pathology associated with CGRP. However, CGRP may be clinically important in pain since it has been shown to be elevated in the cerebral circulation during migraine [45] and increased in the nucleus gracilis of rats with injured sciatic nerves [46]. Wimalawansa recently reviewed CGRP's receptor physiology and therapeutic potential [47] and has suggested that crystallographic and NMR-based imaging of CGRP and its receptors will enhance the understanding of this peptide by suggesting the design of nonpeptide mimetic agents.

2.8   Other CNS neuropeptides

The above sections discussed drug discovery issues relating to selected neuropeptides. Although the list of neuropeptides is quite extensive, the neuropeptides were chosen from the recent literature to illustrate various concerns and opportunities in drug development. The issues raised by these examples have relevance to the other neuropeptides not discussed, including angiotensin II, vasopressin, atrial natriuretic peptide, bombesin, corticotropin, gastrin, glucagon, inhibin, melanocortin, motilin, neurotensin, oxytocin, secretin, vasoactive intestinal polypeptide, and the hypothalamic regulating hormones. Many of these agents were first described in the periphery where they serve as hormones.

These examples provide evidence that various neuropeptides produce their effect through their interaction with other neuropeptides and various neurotransmitter systems. The suprachiasmatic nucleus, which generates circadian rhythmicity and contains at least 25 neurotransmitters and neuropeptides, is an excellent neuro-anatomical site for examining the potential interactions of these compounds [48]. Circadian entrainment is partially due to the glutamate and SP retinal projections, the NPY and GABA thalamic projections, and the serotonergic midbrain projections. Furthermore, the terminal field of these afferent fibres contains vasoactive intestinal peptide, histidine, isoleucine, and gastrin-releasing peptide. Along with these agents, somatostatin and vasopressin have been shown to have endogenous rhythms within the suprachiasmatic nucleus. Huhman and colleagues [48] have shown that various neuropeptides interact synergistically to affect suprachiasmatic function and that there is further interaction with the neuropeptides and classical neurotransmitters. Although the chemical complexity in this neuro-anatomical region is particularly intricate, it serves as an illustrative example of the types of interactions that may be involved in physiological functioning and thus must be addressed in drug development. Ultimately, clinically useful compounds must be able to produce their effects in the whole organism where a variety of complicated neurochemical interactions are occurring in a site-specific manner.

3   Neuropeptides in the PNS

Rather than provide a comprehensive list of all neuropeptides present in the PNS, this section reviews two key neuropeptide families that represent important areas of drug discovery research. In each of these areas, CGRP and NPY, we give an overview of the current status of research and discuss opportunities for the discovery of new therapeutic agents. This is followed by a discussion of the prospects for the discovery of new neuropeptides and neuropeptide receptors.

3.1 CGRP and related peptides

CGRP is a 37 amino acid neuropeptide with an extensive distribution including sensory and some motor nerves and within the CNS.

It shows homology with amylin (46% amino acid identity) and adrenomedullin (24%) and also has a more distant relationship with calcitonin. CGRP, amylin and adrenomedullin show a complex pattern of cross-reactivity at each other's receptors [49, 50].

3.1.1 CGRP pharmacology

CGRP pharmacology is a complicated area; the nature and extent of CGRP receptor heterogeneity is still unclear and interactions between other peptides adds further problems. The concept of CGRP receptor heterogeneity was first established with the discovery that CGRP fragments such as $CGRP_{12-37}$ and $CGRP_{8-37}$ were able to antagonise the actions of CGRP with high affinity in tissues such as the guinea pig atrium ($pA_2 \geq 7$) but not others such as the vas deferens. Conversely the linear CGRP analogue CysACM-CGRP was an agonist at the vas deferens but not the atrium. On this basis two subtypes were proposed: $CGRP_1$ (high affinity for $CGRP_{8-37}$) and $CGRP_2$ (low affinity for $CGRP_{8-37}$, activated by CysACM-CGRP) [51, 52]. This classification represents a good working framework, but is likely to be an oversimplification of the real situation. A wide variety of pA_2 values for $CGRP_{8-37}$ have been reported, from below 6 to above 8 [53]. Some of the variation may reflect species or experimental variation, but the spread remains uncomfortably wide. It is difficult to be certain that CGRP is really the endogenous ligand for all of these receptors. An additional problem is that it has never been possible to match the heterogeneity seen in functional assays with the results from radioligand binding assays [51,52]. CGRP interacts with members of the G-protein coupled receptors. Recently the orphan receptor calcitonin receptor-like receptor (CRLR) was identified as a CGRP receptor [54]. However for this to exhibit responsiveness to CGRP it must be co-expressed with members of a family of smaller single transmembrane proteins termed receptor activity modifying proteins (RAMPs) [55]. CRLR co-expressed with RAMP1 produces a CGRP receptor, whereas expression with RAMP2 is said to produce an adrenomedullin receptor [55]. The mechanism of RAMP action is unclear although it effects CRLR glycosylation. The CRLR receptor behaves as a $CGRP_1$ subtype. The distribution of CRLR suggests that it probably does not account for all CGRP receptors or binding sites; thus tissues with high CGRP binding activity such as liver or cerebellum have little or no detectable CRLR mRNA. The current data relating to the molecular biology of CGRP receptors thus points to heterogeneity.

As noted previously, there is significant cross-reactivity between members of the CGRP family of peptides. A simple summary of the situation is that adrenomedullin, at modest concentrations, and amylin, at high (100 nM) concentrations, can activate the CGRP receptor; high concentrations of CGRP can activate amylin but not adrenomedullin receptors [50]. The clinical significance of the above data is that CGRP can interact with a variety of receptors both for itself and for other peptides. Within the category of genuine CGRP receptors there is almost certainly heterogeneity. This may be of importance in the design of selective agonists and antagonists. At the moment, the only widely available CGRP receptor antagonist is the peptide fragment $CGRP_{8-37}$, a poor tool for *in vivo* or clinical studies. There are, however, initial reports of non-peptide antagonists [56] which should greatly facilitate studies on CGRP.

3.1.2 Cardiovascular actions of CGRP

CGRP receptors are found throughout the cardiovascular system and CGRP is an extremely potent vasodilator. This has numerous potential clinical applications. In Raynaud's disease CGRP has been shown to produce a longer-lasting increase in hand skin blood flow than prostsacyclin [57]. Other peripheral vascular diseases might also benefit from CGRP administration; for example there is evidence that there is loss of CGRP-containing nerve fibres in diabetic neuropathy causing circulatory complications [58]. The vasodilatory properties of CGRP could be useful in treatment of impotence [47]. In subarachnoid haemorrhage there is a reflex vasospasm that can lead to ischaemia and this can be reversed in animal models by CGRP; however clinical trials in humans have shown at best mixed results [59, 60]. CGRP has been reported to improve coronary circulation and to delay the onset of myocardial ischaemia, suggesting a role for the treatment of angina [61]. CGRP acts as a powerful renal vasodilator whilst also increasing glomerular filtration rate and may be suitable for treatment of acute renal failure [47]. The roles and possible benefits of CGRP in hypertension are complicated. Although administration may be useful in some circumstances, the stimulatory actions on the heart may cause problems. Furthermore, its effectiveness as a vasodilator may be reduced where there is damage to the endothelium [62].

3.1.3 Inhibition of CGRP-mediated vasodilatation

Cranial blood vessels have an extensive CGRP-containing innervation originating from the trigeminal nucleus, and these vessels are known to be sensitive to excessive dilation. There is good evidence for excessive CGRP release in many forms of neuro-vascular headaches such as migraine, cluster headache etc. Agents that decrease CGRP release can reduce headache severity and there is obvious potential here for the use of selective CGRP receptor antagonists for treatment of vascular headaches [63].

There are other conditions where excessive CGRP-mediated vasodilation may be undesirable; chronic pelvic pain in women is associated with pelvic venodilation and these patients may show greater sensitivity to CGRP [64]. In septic or other forms of shock, CGRP antagonists may work both to inhibit vasodilation and to prevent release of other vasorelaxants.

3.1.4 CGRP in heart failure

CGRP has positive chronotropic and inotropic effects, and together with its other cardiovascular actions it has attracted attention as a possible treatment for heart failure. Clinical trials have shown mixed results [65, 66].

3.1.5 CGRP in inflammatory disease

CGRP has well documented pro-inflammatory effects and as neurogenic inflammation underlies conditions from arthritis to asthma, this is of great significance. A large part of its actions are due to its properties as a vasodilator, increasing blood flow and hence oedema in affected areas. It can synergise with other inflammatory mediators such as SP. However CGRP receptors have been observed on many types of lymphocytes and leucocytes. These receptors can inhibit T cell proliferation, B cell and monocyte differentiation and the antigen-presenting function of human Langerhans cells. It is also reported to enhance the chemotactic response to leukotrienes in eosinophils from allergic but not normal subjects [67]. There are numerous reports of increased CGRP levels in inflammatory exudates. Consequently, beneficial effects of CGRP antagonists might be expected in many conditions involving neurogenic inflammation. However little clinical data is available, and given the multitude of other mediators that might be released in these conditions CGRP antagonists, at best, may have to be used in combination with other therapies.

3.1.6 Trophic and mitogenic actions of CGRP

There is considerable evidence that CGRP can act as a mitogen on numerous cell types including endothelial and epithelial cells. This may mean that the agent is useful in promoting wound healing [68]. CGRP has been shown to improve survival of surgical flaps. In the short term this is probably due to local vasodilation improving blood flow, but the mitogenic and trophic effects may be significant if it is used for chronic treatment.

3.2 Neuropeptide Y and the pancreatic polypeptides

This section focusses on the pancreatic polypeptides whose differential localisation within the enteric nervous system (ENS) indicates their role(s) in the control of mucosal ion and fluid transport. The pharmacology of antisecretory actions induced by the pancreatic polypeptides (NPY, PYY and PP) are discussed in the light of recent advances in our knowledge of Y receptor heterogeneity.

3.2.1 Enteric neuropeptides: co-localisation and plasticity

The presence of different families of neuropeptide precursors and their cleaved products within discrete enteric neurone populations that innervate mammalian gastrointestinal (GI) mucosa, has stimulated numerous studies investigating their potential functional significance. The last decade has seen the emergence of a number of prominent neuropeptides with major effects upon mucosal ion transport (either stimulating or inhibiting fluid and electrolyte secretion) and the aims of this section are to highlight some trends focussing on the pancreatic polypeptides.

Secretory neuropeptides such as SP, VIP or CGRP, and antisecretory neuropeptides, e.g. NPY, galanin and somatostatin have been identified within intrinsic cholinergic, and non-cholinergic enteric neurones in different mammalian species. The combinations of co-localised, unrelated neuropeptides can vary vastly between species and most importantly, between intestinal areas in the same species (for comprehensive descriptions see [69–73]). The permutations of neuropeptide co-localisations within the enteric nervous system (ENS) has provided a chemical basis for coding in parallel with morphological and electrophysiological coding methods. Assessing the potential role(s) subserved by specific peptide-containing neuronal networks has produced some unexpected findings. For example, submucous neurones immunohistochemically positive for VIP/peptide histidine isoleucine (PHI) and NPY account for one-third or more of the total number of neurones innervating the rat small intestine mucosa [71, 73]. The co-packaging of VIP and NPY [74] and co-release of these neuropeptides in the mucosa where they exert physiologically antagonistic effects upon epithelial function, is one example of the violation of Dale's Law that has frequently been observed within the ENS.

The consequences of neuropeptide release may be to stimulate responses indirectly (via neurogenic or other non-neuronal mechanisms) or directly by interacting with selective receptor populations in basolateral epithelial membranes. It is also becoming increasingly evident that neuropeptide receptor expression and localisation can alter significantly along the length of the intestine, e.g. neurokinin-2 (NK_2) receptor expression changes in the guinea-pig intestine [75]. In addition, neuropeptide expression also alters during development [76] and major changes in both the patterns and levels of peptide expression occur in animal models of disease, e.g. diabetes ([77], see also review [78]). Such plasticity and differential distribution of neuropeptides and their receptors continues to provide a challenging prospect for the functional characterisation of prominent peptidergic innervation within the intestinal mucosa, the manipulation of which may provide novel therapeutic targets in the future.

139

3.2.2 Pancreatic polypeptides

The pancreatic polypeptides include NPY, peptide YY (PYY) and pancreatic polypeptide (PP), together with their C-terminal metabolites, e.g. (3–36) PYY which is functionally significant [79]. To varying degrees each of these peptides has been shown to exert an antisecretory effect upon gastrointestinal mucosae dependent upon the Y receptor type (s) expressed (Tab. 1). Of the three mature members of the PP family NPY is the established neurotransmitter, being extensively expressed in intrinsic myenteric and submucous neurones, and in extrinsic sympathetic neurones. NPY is located throughout the mammalian ENS in virtually every species studied thus far, including guinea-pig, rat, and man [70, 71, 80]. In the rat, a near constant 98% of submucous NPY-positive neurones also express VIP along the small intestine, while in the descending colon variations in both the number and proportion of these double-labelled neurones is observed [81]. PYY, a 36 amino acid analogue with 70% homology to NPY, is located in endocrine cells particularly in the distal small intestine and colon in rat, pig and man [82] and has a similar spectrum of GI actions as NPY, presumably because the same Y receptor populations are activated by both peptides [83]. Infusion of PYY intravenously into humans has been shown to cause a long-lasting reduction in intestinal secretion induced by VIP [84] and a similar antisecretory effect has been demonstrated following NPY infusion when hypersecretion was prestimulated with prostaglandin E_2 [85]. In man the release of PYY into the circulation in response to ingestion of a mixed meal, but particularly of fat, indicated over a decade ago that PYY might play a significant hormonal role facilitating absorption and be involved in the phenomenon "ileal break" (see review [86]).

The third major member of this peptide group is PP, initially identified in pancreatic acini and GI endocrine cells distinct from those expressing insulin, glucagon or somatostatin. PP is also released into the circulation following ingestion of a meal, but the time-course is significantly different from the postprandial PYY response. Although PP appears to be effective in fewer GI targets compared with NPY or PYY, its status as a circulating hormone involved in digestion is assured (for reviews see [86, 87]). One area of particular interest currently is the role played by all three PP's in food intake. Centrally administered NPY, PYY [88] and PP are potent orexigenic agents, increasing the rate and duration of feeding in satiated rats. The Y receptor type(s) responsible for these effects continues to be a subject of considerable controversy [89], the resolution of which will provide a new therapeutic target for the management of obesity. The obesity protein leptin inhibits NPY release [90] and this mechanism contributes to leptin's potent inhibition of feeding.

3.2.3 Y receptor pharmacology

The functional significance of each pancreatic polypeptide exhibits yet further complexity as a consequence of the characterisation of at least six mammalian Y receptor types, five of which have been cloned to date (Y_1, Y_2, Y_4, Y_5, and Y_6) and a sixth (Y_3) which exhibits an atypical NPY-preferring pharmacology, but has yet to be characterised at the molecular level (see review [91]). The orders of potency exhibited by the most commonly used Y agonists are shown in Table 1, which includes a summary of the current pharmacological characteristics for each Y receptor type. The lack of specificity exhibited by most, if not all available Y receptor agonists (see Tab. 1), has in the past resulted in frequent erroneous conclusions concerning receptor identity. The recent availability however, of selective antagonists (e.g. for the Y_1 receptor, BIBP3226, SR120107A) and specific antibodies raised to epitopes of the different Y receptor types now finally allows a definitive characterisation of Y receptor expression in different target tissues.

3.2.4 Y receptors in the GI tract

Both NPY and PYY exert numerous inhibitory effects in the GI tract [86, 92] for example both peptides attenuate epithelial anion and fluid secretion in the small intestine [93, 94] and descending colon *in vitro* [95, 96] and they are similarly inhibitory upon gastrointestinal motility [97, 98]. In epithelial preparations from the rat jejunum independent functional and binding studies have shown the presence of Y_2-like receptors with sensitivity to a series of C-terminal NPY and PYY fragments and truncated analogues [99–101]. This pharmacology appears however to be subtly different from that of Y_2 receptors cloned from the CNS and northern analysis of Y_2 mRNA levels in peripheral tissues including the small intestine indicates low levels of expression of this receptor type compared with that in the CNS [102]. The possibility that another Y_2 subtype exists, predominantly in peripheral targets, has been suggested [103] but remains unproven to date.

Table 1.
The basic pharmacology of different Y receptor types

Receptor	Agonist order	Defining characteristics
Y_1	PYY/NPY/Pro^{34}NPY>>(13–36)NPY>PP	PYY-preferring, Pro^{34}-analogues are potent, BIBP3226, GR231118 (also known as 1229U91) inhibit.
Y_2	PYY>NPY>(3–36)PYY>>>Pro^{34}NPY=PP	PYY-preferring, C-terminal fragments are effective, no antagonism with BIBP3226 or GR231118.
Y_3	NPY>Pro^{34}NPY>(13–36)NPY>PP>PYY	NPY-preferring, PYY poor, (3–36)PYY inactive, no antagonism by BIBP3226.
Y_4	hPP Pro^{34}NPY>>>PYY=NPY	hPP-preferring, PYY/NPY and C-terminal fragments little/no effect, no antagonism with BIBP3226 but GR231118 has affinity (agonist?).
Y_5	NPY=PYY Pro^{34}PYY=hPP>(13–36)NPY	A nonselective receptor, expressed in CNS antagonists pending as novel anti-obesity drugs.
Y_6	NPY=PYY Pro^{34}NPY>>(13–36)NPY>>>hPP	Relatively nonselective, limited K_i data only.

BIBP3226: ((R)-N^2-(diphenylacetyl)-N-[(4-hydroxyphenyl)methyl]-argininamide), a nonpeptide Y_1 selective antagonist.
BIBO3304: latest nonpeptide Y_1 selective antagonist (Wieland et al.: BJP 125, 549–555, 1998)
GR231118 (1229U91): Ile Glu Pro Dpr Tyr Arg Leu Arg Tyr-NH$_2$
Dpr = 2,3-diaminopropionic acid
H$_2$N-Tyr Arg Leu Arg Tyr Dpr Pro Glu Ile
a peptide (equal mixture of parallel and antiparallel isomers) Y_1 antagonist, but also with affinity for Y_4 receptors.

There is clear evidence of Y receptor heterogeneity along the length of the GI tract within the same species. Whilst in rat jejunum mucosa only Y_2-like receptors are expressed, in the rat descending colon a combination of Y_1 (BIBP3226-sensitive) and Y_2-like receptors are found [96]. *In situ* hybridisation studies show that human colon also expresses Y_1 receptor mRNA in the mucosa, in basal glands and in submucous and myenteric ganglia [104], while Northern analysis also indicates Y_4 receptor expression in colonic tissue with lower mRNA levels in human small intestine [105]. Few human epithelial cell lines constitutively express Y receptors but we [96, 106] have identified Y_1 receptors in an untreated adenocarcinoma cell line while others have stimulated Y_1 expression following butyrate treatment of HT-29 cells [106]. Recently we have also discovered the presence of Y_4-like receptors in a further adenocarcinoma cell line (Cox et al., unpublished) and the antisecretory responses stimulated by human and bovine PP (but not rat PP) are reminiscent of the PP competition binding isotherms described by Gingerich et al. (1991) in canine intestine basolateral membranes [108].

The lack of selective agonists and the availability (until recently) of only a few selective Y_1 receptor antagonists has resulted in frequent confusion and misinterpretation of functional data. A further potential problem, all too often overlooked in functional studies (though of obvious significance in GI preparations) is the differential stability of agonist peptides, the consequence of which will provide additional variation in the relative orders of agonist potency. For example, we have described an impressive PYY preference (of native and Pro^{34}-substituted analogues) for Y_1 receptors stably transfected into HT-29 cells [109] and this PYY preference was still evident (although not as pronounced) in binding assays with HT-29 membranes in the presence of protease inhibitors [110]. It is most likely that preferential degradation of NPY and its Pro^{34} analogue by dipeptidyl peptidase IV [111] is responsible for this apparent difference in potency, as this particular peptidase is expressed by HT-29 epithelia [112]. A Y_1-expressing clone selected from another human adenocarcinoma cell line exhibits a similar functional PYY preference but this was not apparent in competition binding studies in the presence of inhibitors [113]. Difficulty can therefore be experienced in functional characterisations in isolation, even in clonal cell lines where a single known receptor population is expressed.

Notwithstanding these limitations the most commonly observed Y receptor types in mammalian epithelia or mucosae *in vitro* are of the Y_1, Y_2 or Y_4 type. While studies with human mucosal tissue *in vitro* have yet to identify the Y receptor type(s) responsible for the antisecretory effects of NPY or PYY in *in vivo* studies [84, 86] other Y receptor types may also have been described in GI preparations. For example in rabbit distal colon an apparently nonselective Y receptor phenotype has been observed [114] which could either be the Y_5 receptor or a combination of Y_1, Y_2 and Y_4 types. Another apparently nonselective profile was observed by autoradiography in porcine myenteric plexi and, despite its inactivation, abundant Y_6 (not Y_{2b}, as published) transcript has been identified in human small intestine, with low levels of expression in colonic tissue [115]. The functional significance of the latter mammalian pseudogene also remains to be determined. The recent description of a selective Y_2 antagonist, BIIE0246 (116) should certainly assist pharmacological investigations in PNS and CNS and the pharmaceutical focus on Y_5 antagonists as potential anti-obesity drugs has resulted in the description of a novel, selective drug, CGP 71683A [117].

In conclusion, therefore, the next few years should see major advances in the identification of novel, selective Y receptor antagonists as well as stable agonists. In mimicking the potent, broad spectrum inhibitory effects of the PP's upon fluid and electrolyte secretion, an agonist specific for the predominant Y receptor expressed in human colonic mucosa could be therapeutically significant as a novel anti-diarrhoeal drug.

3.3 Other PNS neuropeptides

In addition to the two neuropeptide families considered above, there are a vast array of neuropeptides in the PNS. These include the tachykinins, neurotensin, the opioid related peptides, vasopressin, oxytocin, VIP, somatostatin, endothelin, corticotrophin-releasing factor, gastrin and CCK, bradykinin, angiotensin, the orexins/hypocretins, bombesin and gallanin. Many of these have important physiological functions and have been dealt with in other reviews (see e.g. [66–69, 118]).

Despite the wealth of information on neuropeptides and their receptors, it seems likely that several new members of this wide family will be discovered in the next few years. The discovery of novel neuropeptides and receptors remains a thriving industry [119]. This is exemplified by the reports last year of a biologically active peptide, nocistatin, derived from the nociceptin/orphanin FQ precursor but which does not bind to the ORL-1 receptor [120], and of two peptides called orexin A and orexin B (or hypocretin 1

144

and hypocretin 2), which exhibit substantial sequence homology to secretin [120, 121].

The orexins stimulate food consumption through binding to two previously identified G-protein coupled receptors [121]. Like the hypocretins/orexins, it is likely that some of the newly discovered neuropeptides will be found to be the endogenous ligands for orphan receptors. However, it is also likely that the targets of new neuropeptiddes will turn out to be "old targets", i.e. previously characterised receptors [121].

4 Conclusion and future prospects

In conclusion, this review has demonstrated that neuropeptide receptors are exciting drug targets. A multiplicity of neuropeptide receptors have been identified in both the CNS and PNS. Whilst much attention has been focused on developing drugs for these targets it is clear that the majority of such drug discovery programmes have, to date, yielded excellent biological tools without producing clinically useful drugs. Hopefully, the introduction of technologies such as HTS into the drug discovery process will accelerate the discovery of new drug-like non-peptide agonists and antagonists. This should help to fuel the finding of a new generation of drugs acting on neuropeptide receptors.

References

1   Klaviedva, M.M.: Frontiers Neuroendocrinol. *16*, 293–321 (1995).
2   Iversen, L.L.: Trends Neurosci. *1*, 15–16 (1978).
3   Iversen, L.L.: Trends Neurosci. *18*, 49–50 (1995).
4   Shaw, C.: Parasitol. *113*, S35–45 (1996).
5   Horwell, D.C.: Trends Biotechnol. *13*, 132–134 (1995).
6   Kenny, B.A., Bushfield, M., Parry-Smith, D.J., Fogarty, S. and Treherne, J.M.: Progress in Drug Research *51*, 246–269 (1998)
7   Prokai, L.: Progress in Drug Research *51*, 95–131 (1998).
8   Hokfelt, T., Broberger, C., Zhang, X., Diez, M., Koop, J., Xu, Z., Landry, M., Bao, L., Schalling, M., Koistinaho, J. et al.: Brain Research Reviews *26*, 154–166 (1998).
9   Malendowicz, L., Markowska, A. and Zabel, M.: Histol. Histopathol. *11*, 485–494 (1996).
10   Broberger, C., Johansen, J., Schalling, M. and Hokfelt, T: J. Comp. Neurol. *387*, 124–135 (1997).
11   Tritos, N., Vicent, D., Gillette, J., Ludwig, D., Flier, E. and Maratos-Flier, E.: Diabetes *47*, 1687–1692 (1998).

12   Krstenansky, J., Owens, T., Buck, S., Hagaman, K. and McLean, L.: Proc. Natl. Acad. Sci. *86*, 4377–4381 (1989).
13   Jacques, D., Cadieux, A., Dumont,Y. and Quirion, R.: Eur. J. Pharm. *278*, R3–R5 (1995).
14   Kawasaki, A., Knapp, R., Kramer, T., Wire, W., Vasques, O., Yamamura, H., Burks, T. and Hruby, V.: J. Med. Chem. *33*, 1874–1879 (1990).
15   Meyer, J., Collins, N., Lung, F., Davis, P., Zalewska, T., Porreca, F., Yamamura, H. and Hruby, V.: J. Med. Chem. *37*, 3910–3917 (1994).
16   Chen, H., Nobel, F., Coric, P., Fournie-Zaluski, M. and Roques, B.: Proc. Nat. Acad. Sci. *95*, 12028–12033 (1998).
17   Prokai-Tatrai, K., Prokai, L. and Bodor, N.: J. Med. Chem. *39*, 4775–4782 (1996).
18   Horwell, D.: Neuropeptides *19*, 57–64 (1991).
19   Menani, J. and Johnson, A.: Am J. Physiol. *275*, R1421–R1437 (1998).
20   Sohal, V., Cox, C. and Huguenard, J.: J. Neurophysiol. *79*, 2820–2824 (1998).
21   Makovec, F., Peris, W., Frigerio, S., Giovanetti, R., Letari, O., Mennui, L. and Revel, L.: J. Med. Chem. *39*, 135–142 (1996).
22   Freidinger R.M., Bock M.G., DiPardo R.M., Evans B.E., Rittle K.E., Whitter W.L., Veber D.F. Anderson P.S., Chang R.S.L. and Lotti V.J., in: Hughes, Dockary & Woodruff: The Neuropeptide Cholecystokinin, Ellis Horwood Ltd, 123–132, 1998.
23   Freedman S.B., Patel S., Smith A.J., Chapman K., Fletcher A., Kemp J.A., Marshall G.R., Hargreaves R.J., Scholey K., Mellin E.C.et al., in: Reeve, Eysselein, Solomon and Laing: Cholecystokinin, Ann. Acad. Sci. *713*, 312–330, 1994.
24   Nussdorfer, G. and Malendowicz, L.: Peptides *19*, 949–968 (1998).
25   Ku, Y., Tan, L., Li, L. and Ding, X.: Peptides *19*, 677–682 (1998).
26   Hasenohrol, R., Jentjens O., De Souza-Silva, M., Tomaz, C. and Huston, J.: Eur J. Phamacol. *354*, 123–133 (1998).
27   Tang, F., Chiu, T. and Wang, Y.: Experimental. Neurol. *152*, 41–49 (1998).
28   Bell, M., Richardson, P. and Lee, K.: Neurosci. *87*, 649–658 (1998).
29   Wang, X. and Robertson, D.: J. Neurophysiol. *80*, 218–229 (1998).
30   Shen, K.Z and North, R.A.: Neurosci. *50*, 345, (1992).
31   Koyano, K., Velimirovic, B.M., Grigg, J.J., Nakajima, S. and Nakajima, Y.: Eur. J. Neurosci. *5*, 1189 (1993)
32   Lieberman, D. and Mody, I.: J. Neurophysiol. *80*, 113–119 (1998).
33   Bartfai, T., Iverfeldt, K., Fisone, G. and Serofozo, P.: Ann. Rev. Pharmacol. Toxicol. *28*, 285–310 (1988).
34   Seutin, V., Verbanck, P., Massotte, L. and Dresse, A.: Eur J. Pharmacol. *164*, 373–376 (1989).
35   Gopalan, C., Tian, Y., Moore, D. and Lookingland, K.: Neuroendocrinol. *58*, 287–293 (1993).
36   Weiss, J., Demetrikopoulos, M., West, C. and Bonsall, R.: Depression *3*, 225–245 (1995).
37   Demetrikopoulos, M.K., Kreiss, J.H., Turner, A.J., Koski, P.A., Bonsall, R.W. and Weiss J.M.: Soc. Neurosci. Abstr. *22*, 812–818 (1996).
38   Kiss, A. and Jezova, D.: Histochem. J. *30*, 569–575 (1998).
39   Consolo, S., Uboldi, M., Caltavuturo, C. and Bartfai, T.: Neurosci. *85*, 819–826 (1998).
40   Sobreviela, T., Jaffar, S. and Mufson, E.: Neurosci. *87*, 447–461 (1998).
41   Barbelivien, A., MacKenzie, E. and Dauphin, F.: Brain Res. *789*, 92–100 (1998).
42   Connor, B. and Dragunow, M.: Brain Res. Rev. *27*, 1–39 (1998).
43   Marowska, A., Mooney, M. and Sonntag, W.: Neurosci. *87*, 559–569 (1998).
44   Haller, M. and Saltzman, W.: Pharmaceutical Res. *15*, 377–385 (1998).

45   Van Rossum, D., Hanisch, U. and Quirion, R.: Neurosci and Biobehav. Rev. *21*, 649–678 (1997).
46   Ma, W. and Bisby, M.: Exp. Neurology *152*, 137–149 (1998).
47   Wimalawansa, S.J.: Endocrin Rev. *17*, 533–585 (1996).
48   Huhman, K., Gillespie, C., Marvel, C. and Albers, H.: Ann. N. Y. Acad. Sci. *814*, 300–304 (1997).
49   Quirion, R. and Dumont, Y., in: D.R. Poyner, I. Marshall, I. and S.D. Brain (ed.): The CGRP family: CGRP, amylin and adrenomedullin. Landes Biosciences, Texas 2000.
50   Marshall, I., Poyner, D.R., Sexton, P.M. and Smith, D.M.: Trends Pharmacol. Sci. (Nomenclature supplement), 5th edition, 20–21 (1999).
51   Dennis, T.B., Fournier, A. St. Pierre, S. and Quirion, R.: J. Pharmacol. Exp. Ther. *251*, 718–725 (1989).
52   Quirion, R., Van Rossum, D., Dumont, Y., St. Pierre, S. and Fournier, A.: Ann. N.Y. Acad. Sci. *657*, 88–105 (1992).
53   Poyner, D.R.: Biochem. Soc.Trans. *25*, 1032–1036 (1997).
54   Aiyar, N., Rand, K., Elshourbagy, N.A., Zeng, Z.Z., Adamou, J.E., Bergsma, D.J. and Li, Y.: J. Biol. Chem. *271*, 11325–11329 (1996).
55   McLachtie, L.M., Fraser, N.J., Main, M.J., Wise, A., Brown, J., Thompson, N., Solari, R., Lee, M.G. and Foord, S.M.: Nature *393*, 333–339 (1998).
56   Daines, R.A., Sham, K.K.C., Taggart, J.J., Kingsbury, W.D, Chan, J., Breen, A., Disa, J. and Aiyar, N.: Bioorg. Med. Chem. Lett. *7*, 2673–2676 (1997).
57   Shawket, S., Dickerson C., Hazleman, B and Brown M.J.: Brit. J. Clin. Pharmacol. *32*, 209–213 (1991).
58   Bennett, G.S., Radhika Kajekar, R., Garrett, N.E., Diemel, L.T., Tomlinson, D.R. and Brain, S.D., in: D.R. Poyner, I. Marshall and S.D. Brain (eds.): The CGRP family: CGRP, amylin and adrenomedullin. Landes Biosciences, Texas 2000.
59   Johnston, F.G., Bell, B.A., Robertson, I.J., Miller, J.D., Hailburn, C., O'Shaughnessy, D., Riddell, A.J. and O'Laoire, S.A.: Lancet *335*, 869–872 (1990).
60   Bailey, I.C., Lyttle, J.A., Matthew, B., Braadvedt, G., Nelson, R.J., Stranjalis, G., Castel, J.P., Orgogozo, J.M., Aziz, A.M., Buckley, T.F. et al.: Lancet *339*, 831–834 (1992).
61   Uren, N.G., Seydoux, C. and Davies, G.J.: Cardiovasc. Res. *27*, 1477–1488 (1993).
62   Uren, N.G., Ludman, P.F., Crake, T. and Oakley, C.M.: J. Am. Coll. Cardiol. *19*, 835–841 (1992).
63   Goadsby, P.J., in: D.R. Poyner, I. Marshall and S.D. Brain (eds.): The CGRP family: CGRP, amylin and adrenomedullin. Landes Biosciences, Texas 2000.
64   Stones, R.W., Thomas, D.C. and Beard, R.W.: Clin. Auton. Res. *2*, 343–348 (1992).
65   Dubisrande, J.L., Merlet, P., Benveniste, C., Sediame, S., Macquinmavier, I., Charbier, E., Braquet, P., Castaigne, A. and Adnot, S.: Am. J. Cardiol. *70*, 906–912 (1992).
66   Stevenson, R.N., Roberts, R.H. and Timmis, A.D.: Int. J. Cardiol. *37*, 407–414 (1993).
67   McGillis, J.P. and Figueiredo, H.F., in: J.A. Marsh and MD. Kendall (eds.): The Physiology of Immunity, CRC Press, London 1996, 127–143
68   Brain, S.D.: Immunopharmacol. *37*, 133–152, (1997).
69   Furness, J.B. and Costa, M.: The Enteric Nervous System, ed. 1, Churchill Livingstone, New York 1987.
70   Furness, J.B., Costa, M., Gibbins, I.L., Llewellyn-Smith, I.J. and Oliver, J.R.: Cell Tiss. Res. *241*, 155–163 (1985).
71   Ekblad, E., Winter, C., Ekman, E., Håkanson, R. and Sundler, F.: Neurosci. *20*, 169–188, (1987).

72   Ekblad, E., Ekman, R., Håkanson, R. and Sundler, F.: Neurosci. *27*, 655–674 (1987).
73   Gershon, M.D., Kirchgessner, A.L. and Wade, P.R., in: R. Leonard: Physiology of the Gastrointestinal Tract, Raven Press, New York 1994, vol. 1, 381–414.
74   Cox, H.M., Rudolph, A. and Gschmeissner, S.: Neurosci. *59*: 469–476 (1994).
75   Portbury, A.L., Furness, J.B., Southwell, B.R., Wong, H., Walsh, J.H. and Bunnett, N.W.: Cell & Tissue Res. *286*: 281–292 (1996).
76   Saffrey, M.J. and Burnstock, G.: J. Autonom. Nerv. System. *49*, 183–196 (1994).
77   Belai, A. and Burnstock, G.: Gastroenterol. *98*: 1427–1436 (1990).
78   Goyal, R.K. and Hirano, I.: New Engl. J. Med. *334*, 1106–1115 (1996).
79   Grandt, D., Schimiczek, M., Beglinger, C., Layer, P., Goebell, H., Eysselein, V.E. and Reeve, J.R.: Reg. Peptides *51*, 151–159 (1994).
80   Wattchow, D.A., Furness, J.B., Costa, M., O'Brien, P.E. and Peacock, M.: Gastroenterol. *93*: 1363–1371 (1987).
81   Browning, K.N. and Lees, G.M.: Neurosci. *62*: 1257–1266 (1994).
82   Böttcher, G,, Sjölund, K., Ekblad, E., Håkanson, R., Schwartz, T. and Sundler, F.: Reg. Peptides *8*, 261–266 (1984).
83   Pappas, T.N., Chang, A.M., Debas, H.T. and Taylor, I.L.: Gastroenterol. *91*, 1386–1389 (1986).
84   Playford, R.J., Domin, J., Beacham, J., Parmar, K.B., Tatemoto, K., Bloom, S.R. et al.: Lancet *335*, 1555–1557 (1990).
85   Holzer-Petsche, U., Petritsch, W., Hinterleitner, T., Eherer, A., Sperk, G. and Krejs, G.J.: Gastroenterol. *101*, 325–330 (1991).
86   Playford, R.J. and Cox, H.M.: Trends Pharmacol. Sci. *17*, 436–438 (1996).
87   Walsh, J.H., in: L.R. Johnson (ed.): Physiology of the Gastrointestinal Tract, Raven Press New York 1994, vol. 1, 1–128.
88   Stanley, B.G., Daniel, D.R., Chin, A.S. and Leibowitz, S.F.: Peptides *6*, 1205–1211 (1985).
89   O'Shea, D., Morgan, D.G.A., Meeran, K., Smith, D.M., Ghatei, M.A. and Bloom, S.R.: Endocrinol. *138*, 196–202 (1987).
90   Stephens, T.W., Basinski, M., Bristow, P.K., Zhang, X.-Y. and Heiman, M.: Nature *377*, 530–532 (1995).
91   Michel, M.C., Beck-Sickinger, A., Cox, H.M., Doods, H.N., Herzog, H., Larhammar, D., Quirion, R., Schwartz, T.W. and Westfall, T.: XVI. Pharmacol Rev. *50*, 143–150 (1998).
92   Cox, H.M., in: W. Colmers and C. Wahlestedt (eds): The biology of NPY and related peptides, Humana Press Inc., New Jersey 1993, 273–313
93   Saria, A. and Beubler, E.: Eur. J. Pharmacol. *119*, 47–52 (1995).
94   Cox, H.M., Cuthbert, A.W., Håkanson, R. and Wahlestedt, C.: J. Physiol. *398*, 65–80 (1998).
95   Strabel, D. and Diener, M.: Br. J. Pharmacol. *115*, 1071–1079 (1995).
96   Tough, I.R. and Cox, H.M.: Eur. J. Pharmacol. *310*, 55–60 (1996).
97   Holzer, P., Lippe, I.T., Bartho, L. and Saria, A.: Gastroenterol. *92*, 1944–1950 (1997).
98   Krantis, A., Potvin, W. and Harding, R.K.: Naunyn-Schmeid. Arch. Pharmacol. *338*, 287–292 (1998).
99   Cox, H.M. and Cuthbert, A.W.: Br. J. Pharmacol. *101*, 247–252 (1990).
100   Cox, H.M. and Krstenansky, J.L.: Peptides *12*, 323–327 (1991).
101   Servin, A.L., Rouyer-Fessard, C., Balasubramanian, A., St-Pierre, S. and Laburthe, M.: Endocrinol. *124*, 692–700 (1989).
102   Gehlert, D.R., Beavers, L.S., Johnson, D., Gackenheimer, S.L., Schober, D.A. and Gadski, R.A.: Mol. Pharmacol. *49*, 224–228 (1996).

103 Blomqvist, A. and Herzog, H.: Trends Neurosci. *20*, 294–298 (1997).

104 Wharton, J., Gordon, L., Byrne, J., Herzog, H., Selbie, L.A., Moore, K. et al.: Proc. Natl. Acad. Sci. *90*, 687–691 (1993).

105 Lundell, I., Blomqvist, A., Berglund, M.M., Schober, D.A., Johnson, D., Statnick, M.A., Gadski, R.A., Gehlert, D.R. and Larhammar, D.: J. Biol. Chem. *270*, 29123–29128 (1995).

106 Cox, H.M. and Tough, I.R.: Br. J. Pharmacol. *116*, 2673–2678 (1995).

107 Mannon, P.J., Mervin, S.J. and Sheriff-Carter, K.D.: Am. J. Pharmacol. *267*, G901–G907 (1994).

108 Gingerich, R.L., Akpan, J.O., Gilbert, W.R., Leith, K.M., Hoffman, J.A. and Chance, R.E.: Am. J. Physiol. *261*, E319–324 (1991).

109 Holliday, N.D. and Cox, H.M.: Br. J. Pharmacol. *119*, 321–329 (1996).

110 Holliday, N.D. and Cox, H.M.: Br. J. Pharmacol. *120*, 290P (1997).

111 Mentlein, R., Dahms, P., Grandt, D. and Kruger, R.: Reg. Peptides *49*, 133–144 (1993).

112 Howell, S., Kenny, A.J. and Turner, A.J.: Biochem. J. *284*, 595–601 (1992).

113 Holliday, N.D. and Cox, H.M.: Reg. Peptides *71*, P11 (1997).

114 Ballantyne, G.H., Goldenring, J.R., Fleming, F.X., Rush, S., Flint, J.S., Fielding, L.F., Binder, H.J. and Modlin, I.M.: Am. J. Physiol. *264*, G848–G854 (1993).

115 Walsh, D.A., Wharton, J., Blake, D.R. and Polak, J.M.: Br. J. Pharmacol. *108*, 304–311 (1993).

116 Doods, H., Gaida, W., Wieland, H.A., Dollinger, H., Schnorrenberg, G., Esser, F., Engel, W., Eberlein, W. and Rudolf, K.: Eur. J. Pharmacol. (in press).

117 Criscione, L., Rigollier, P., Batzl-Hartman, C., Rueger, H. et al.: J. Clin. Invest. *102*, 2136–2145 (1998)

118 Darlinson, M.G. and Richter, D.: Trends Neurosci. *22*, 81–88 (1999).

119 Okuda-Ashitaka, E.: Nature *392*, 286–289 (1998).

120 De Lecea, L.: Proc. Nat. Acad. Sci. U.S.A. *95*, 322–327 (1998).

121 Sakurai, T.: Cell *92*, 573–585 (1998).

Progress in Drug Research, Vol. 54 (E. Jucker, Ed.)
©2000 Birkhäuser Verlag, Basel (Switzerland)

Regulation of NMDA receptors by ethanol

By Meena Kumari and
Maharaj K. Ticku

Department of Pharmacology,
University of Texas Health Science
Center, 7703 Floyd Curl Drive,
San Antonio, TX 78229, USA

Meena Kumari

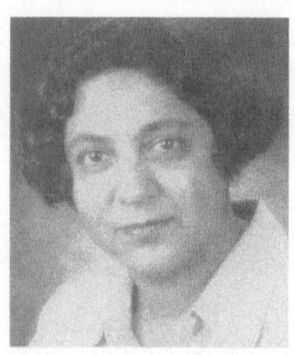

received her Ph.D. from the University of Delhi, India. Thereafter she worked as an Alexander von Humboldt fellow at the University of Marburg, Germany. After post-doctoral training at Northwestern University, Evanston, and the Southwest Foundation for Biomedical Research at San Antonio, she joined the Department of Pharmacology at the University of Texas Health Science Center at San Antonio in 1996. She currently holds the position of assistant professor. Dr. Kumari's primary research interests focus on effects of ethanol on regulation of gene expression of NMDA receptors.

Maharaj K. Ticku

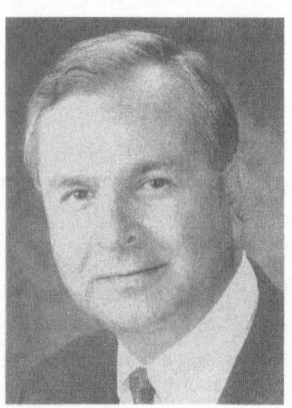

received his Ph.D. in biochemical pharmacology from the State University of New York at Buffalo, N.Y., USA. He joined the University of Texas Health Science Center at San Antonio, TX, USA, as an assistant professor of pharmacology in 1978 and was promoted there to full professor of pharmacology and psychiatry in 1986. He has utilized behavioral, biochemical, pharmacological and molecular biological approaches to understand how drugs modulate and regulate GABA$_A$ and NMDA receptors. His current research is aimed at defining the molecular mechanisms involved in drug (alcohol, benzodiazepines, and neurosteroids)-induced tolerance and physical dependence. He has an extensive publication history in this area of research.

Summary

NMDA receptors are glutamate-gated ion channels, mediating excitatory neurotransmission in the brain. These widely distributed receptors are known to play a role in neuronal development and synaptic plasticity, but over stimulation of these receptors can lead to neurotoxicity. In recent years, NMDA receptors have emerged as an important site of action of ethanol. It is believed that at least some of the deleterious effects of ethanol like alcohol dependence, development of tolerance to alcohol and alcohol withdrawal syndrome are mediated via NMDA receptors. The sensitivity of NMDA receptors to ethanol, however, varies regionally. This diversity of NMDA receptor sensitivity is believed to result, at least in part, from heterogeneity of receptor subunit composition. Ethanol's effects on NMDA receptors, including alteration in receptor function and number, probably result from interplay of multiple mechanisms some of which are discussed here.

Contents

Keywords

NMDA, receptors, ligand-gated ion channel, acute ethanol treatment, chronic ethanol treatment, signal transduction, phosphorylation, brain function, gene expression, excitotoxicity, neurotransmission, ethanol dependence, ethanol withdrawal syndrome.

Glossary of abbreviations

Akt, protein kinase B; AMPA, α-amino-3-hydroxy-5-methyl-4-isoxazole-propionic acid; AP5, amino-5-phosphonopentanoic acid; BDNF, brain-derived neurotrophic factor; Ca^{2+}, calcium ions; $[Ca^{2+}]_i$, intracellular calcium; cGMP, cyclic GMP; CHO cells, Chinese hamster ovary cells; CKII, cam kinase II; CNS, central nervous system; CPP, 3-(($\pm$)-2-carboxypiperazin-4-yl)propyl-1-phosphonic acid; cRNA, antisense ribonucleic acid; DNA, deoxyribonucleic acid; GABA, γ-amino-butyric acid; $GABA_A$, γ-amino-butyric acid receptor subtype A; GluR, glutamate receptors; HEK 293 cells, human embryonic kidney cells; $5-HT_3$, serotonin receptor subtype 3; K^+, potassium ions; LTP, long-term potentiation; Mg^{2+}, magnesium ions; MK-801, (+)-5-methyl-10,11-dihydro-5H-dibenzo[a,d]-cyclo-hepten-5,10-imine hydrogen maleate; mRNA, messenger ribonucleic acid; MS, median septum; Na^+, sodium ions; NANM, (+)-N-allyl-normetazocine; NGF, nerve growth factor; NMDA, N-methyl-D-asparatate; NO, nitric oxide; NOS, nitric oxide synthase; NR1, NMDA R1 receptor subunit in rat (ζ in mouse); NR2, NMDA R2 receptor subunit in rat (ε in mouse) (four subtypes); PCP, phencyclidine; PKA, protein kinase A; PKC, protein kinase C; PMA, phorbol 12-myristate 13-acetate; 5' UTR, 5' untranslated region.

1 Introduction

Alcohol (ethanol) is the most widely used and abused drug by all segments of our society. Ethanol abuse alters the function of almost all parts of the body resulting in a wide range of pathological conditions affecting the brain, liver, cardiovascular system, and can also lead to cancer. It is estimated that ethanol related costs to a country like the USA may total over $125 billion annually (accidents, suicide, alcohol-related health problems, decreased productivity and lost employment). While it is known that ethanol consumption produces brain damage (loss of neurons), the underlying mechanisms are unknown. Since ethanol consumption is generally associated with loss of food intake, at the present time it is not clear whether neuronal damage involves both neuronal excitotoxicity and lack of nutrition. In humans, ethanol consumption produces thiamine deficiency that leads to Korsakoff's syndrome characterized by anterograde amnesia and cognitive deficits [1]. During thiamine deficiency, levels of glutamate in brain tissue increases. Glutamate, being one of the major excitatory neurotransmitters, may produce excitotoxicity resulting in neuronal damage leading to central nervous system (CNS) effects [2, 3].

A low dose of ethanol produces mild motor incoordination, loss of righting reflex and ataxia, while higher doses of ethanol produce effects like euphoria, sedation, loss of righting reflex, confusion, even coma and death. In some cases, chronic ethanol consumption produces cerebral atrophy and sleep apnea. Since different brain regions mediate these behavioral effects, ethanol must act on various neurochemical processes in various regions of the brain.

The molecular basis for ethanol's effects on the brain, and the potential mechanisms involved in ethanol tolerance and physical dependence have yet to be established. In 1986, three independent groups demonstrated that the GABAergic system was affected by ethanol treatment [4–6]. Three years later, several other groups pointed out that the glutaminergic system may also be involved in ethanol's action on brain function [7–10]. In addition, other ligand-gated ion channels such as acetylcholine, adenosine, glycine [11–18], 5-HT$_3$ receptors [19, 20], voltage-gated ion channels and second messenger systems [21–29] may all play a role in ethanol-induced changes in brain function. Most of the ligand-gated ion channels are allosteric proteins and are composed of multiple subunits [25, 29, 30]. The exact site of ethanol's action on these receptors is not known. However, it is known that ethanol affects these receptors at pharmacologically relevant concentrations via signal transduction pathways [25, 28, 31–37]. In neurons, activation of signal transduction pathways can lead to changes at the membrane level such as trafficking of receptor proteins [25, 38] and an increase in channel opening time [39, 40]. Alterations in the cytoplasm such as translocation of proteins [41, 42] and changes in the levels of polypeptides [31, 43–46] have also been reported. At the nuclear level, ethanol has been shown to alter the rate of gene transcription [47, 48] and this may be achieved by interaction of specific proteins, i.e. the transcription factors, with ethanol-responsive *cis*-acting DNA regulatory elements in the respective gene. To date ethanol-responsive regulatory elements have been identified for two genes in *Saccharomyces cerevisiae* [49, 50] and four genes in mammals [51–54].

In this review, we have focused on the effects of ethanol on a subtype of glutamate receptors, the N-methyl-D-aspartate (NMDA) receptor. The NMDA receptors are heteromeric complexes, and they gate a ligand-gated ion channel. The major properties of the NMDA receptor are: (a) sensitivity to neurotransmitter and voltage; (b) requirement of a co-agonist, glycine; (c) high permeability to Ca^{2+} and Na^+; (d) slow kinetics; (e) blockade by physiological concentrations of Mg^{2+}; and (f) allosteric modulation by drugs [55–57]. Like other ligand-gated ion channels, NMDA receptors are expressed throughout the brain and exhibit a differential expression in different brain regions. The general consensus is that chronic agonist treatment results in downregulation of NMDA receptors, whereas chronic antagonist treatment results in upregulation of the receptors. Although ethanol is not referred to as a NMDA receptor antagonist, ethanol treatment does inhibit NMDA receptor responses.

2   NMDA receptors

In the central nervous system, glutamate is one of the major excitatory neurotransmitters. Glutamate activates the glutamate receptors (GluR) resulting in the most rapid excitatory synaptic transmission [58]. The development and use of selective pharmacological tools made it possible to classify these receptors into two families: (a) the ionotropic glutamate receptor family, and (b) the metabotropic glutamate receptor family [59–63]. Activation of metabotropic GluR by L-glutamate results in stimulation of phospholipase C in neurons [64–66]. In contrast, activation of ionotropic GluR results in an increase in cell membrane permeability to mono- and divalent-cations, specifically Na^+, K^+ and Ca^{2+}, and neuronal excitation [67–72]. The ionotropic glutamate receptors comprise a group of ligand-gated ion channels and are further classified into three major types: (i) NMDA receptors which are activated by N-methyl-D-aspartate (NMDA), (ii) Kainate receptors are activated by kainic acid, and (iii) AMPA receptors are activated by α-amino-3-hydroxy-5-methyl-4-isoxazole-propionic acid (AMPA). These three receptors are named after their selective agonists [61, 73, 74].

NMDA receptors have multiple drug binding sites. Binding of a drug at one site influences the binding of another drug at a different site on the receptor (allosteric regulation). Activation of NMDA receptors by glutamate at the NMDA site of the NMDA receptor opens the ion channel allowing the influx of calcium into the cell. However, for full activation of the NMDA receptor, glycine, a co-agonist, is required. At least two molecules of glycine must bind to their site for complete activation of the NMDA receptor [75–77]. Drugs acting at other sites on the receptor such as the polyamine site can lead to allosteric modification of the receptor. NMDA receptors also have a non-competitive phencyclidine (PCP) site that is located within the ion channel itself. The NMDA receptor antagonist, MK-801 ((+)-5-methyl-10, 11-dihydro-5H-dibenzo[a,d]-cyclo-hepten-5,10-imine hydrogen maleate), acts at this site to prevent the influx of calcium into the neuron. At the resting membrane potential, NMDA receptors are blocked by physiological concentrations of magnesium ions that are located in the channel pore. When neurons are depolarized, a voltage-dependent removal of magnesium ions from the channel pore occurs, thus allowing the influx of calcium. A detailed account of various binding sites on the NMDA receptors and the ligands that bind to these sites has recently been published [57].

Two unique properties of NMDA receptors, i.e. their voltage dependence and high permeability to calcium, have made them a target of intensive research [68, 74, 78, 79]. Through these efforts, it is clear that NMDA receptors play a role in neuronal development, neuronal plasticity, maintenance of neuronal excitability and long-term potentiation, a process involved in learning and memory [80–85]. Over-stimulation of NMDA receptors is involved in many neurodegenerative diseases [86].

The NMDA receptor complex has a heteromeric structure as revealed by agonist and antagonist binding studies using neuronal membrane preparations [87]. Quantitative autoradiographic binding studies performed with [³H]-glutamic acid, [³H]-CPP (3-((±)-2-carboxypiperazin-4-yl)propyl-1-phosphonic acid), [³H]-MK-801, D-[³H]-AP5 (D-2-[³H]-amino-5-phosphonopen-tanoic acid) and [³H]-CGP 39653 showed differences in binding patterns of these drugs in brain suggesting regional differences in the subunit compo-sition of NMDA receptors in various parts of the CNS [88–98]. Additional evidence for the presence of multiple polypeptides in the NMDA receptor complex came from molecular cloning and experiments involving *in vitro* expression of NMDA receptor subunits in *Xenopus* oocytes [99–102]. The NR1 subunit which was the first subunit to be cloned [99], has eight isoforms generated by alternative splicing of a single gene named *nmdar1* (Fig. 1) [103, 104]. The NR2 family consists of four subunits: NR2A, NR2B, NR2C and NR2D in rat (or ε 1–4 in mouse or hNR2A-D in human) (Fig. 2) [100–102, 105–107]. The NR2 subunits are highly homologous (50–70%) with one another, but are only 15–20% identical with the NR1 subunit [101, 102]. The NR2 subunits are products of four different genes named, *nmdar2a, nmdar2b, nmdar2c* and *nmdar2d* (Figs. 3, 4) [108–110]. Each of these five genes (ζ1 and ε 1–ε 4) in mouse was mapped to a single chromo-some location [109].

The exact subunit composition of NMDA receptors is not known. How-ever, results from a number of different studies suggest that native NMDA receptors are comprised of combinations of NR1 and NR2 subunits. For instance, (A) the heterogeneity of functional NMDA receptors was deter-mined by employing functional assays using either a *Xenopus* oocyte expres-sion system [97, 101, 102, 105, 111–113] or co-transfected human embryonic kidney (HEK) 293 cells and Chinese hamster ovary (CHO) cells [114–116]. Although the NR1 subunit formed functional homomeric NMDA receptors in *Xenopus* oocytes [106, 112], similar results could not be obtained in trans-fected mammalian tumor cell lines [117, 118]. On the other hand, when members of the NR2 family were combined with the NR1 subunit, NMDA receptors with distinct pharmacological properties were formed [100–102, 105, 106, 114–116, 119–123]. (B) Structural evidence for the presence of both NR1 and NR2 subunits in the NMDA receptor complex came from immuno-cytochemical localization of NR1 and NR2 subunits at the ultrastructural level in the central nervous system of rat. Specifically, it was observed that distribution of NR1 and NR2 polypeptides overlapped in most neurons in the rat CNS [124, 125]. (C) Single-channel current patterns suggested that NMDA receptors are pentamers composed of three NR1 and two NR2 subunits [126]. (D) Radioligand binding results indicated that there is a regional specificity in the stoichiometry of the subunits in rat brain [97, 98]. Lastly, (E) Co-

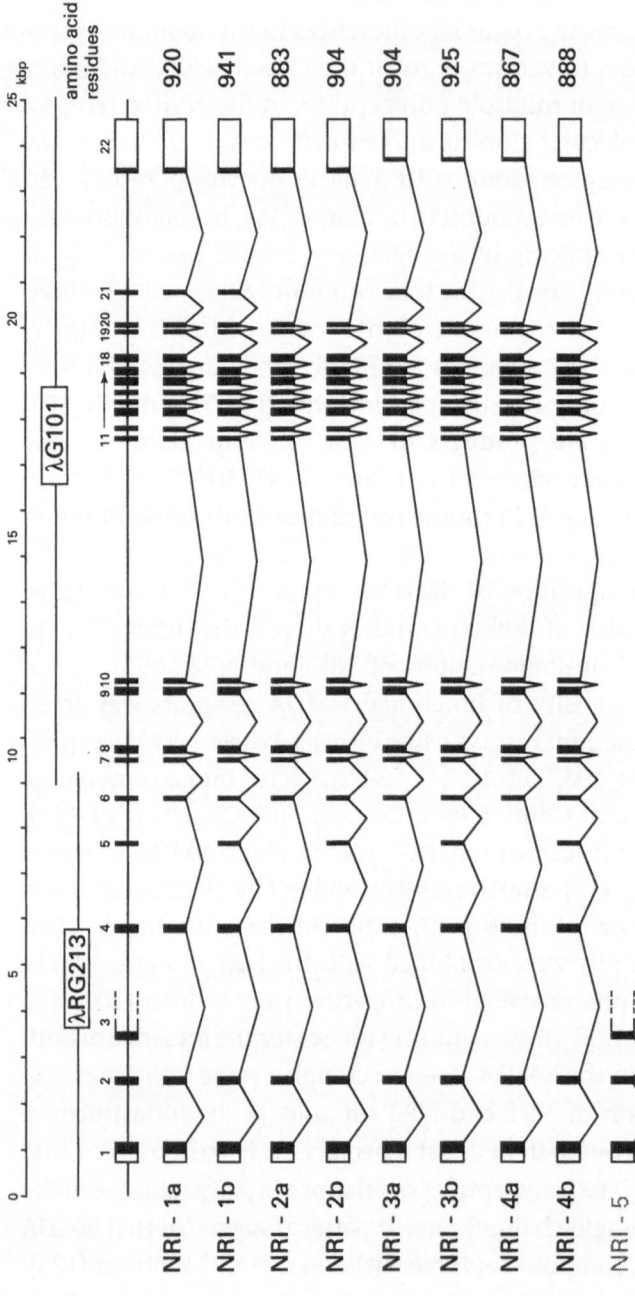

Fig. 1

Genomic structure of the rat NR1 gene and the isoforms generated by alternative splicing

The rat NR1 gene consists of 22 exons shown as numbered solid black boxes. Exons 1, 3 and 22 also contain either 5' or 3' untranslated sequences which are indicated by open boxes. Individual exons have the following lengths (in base pairs) and occur at the indicated positions: exon 1= 473 bp, exon 2= 135 bp, exon 3= ≥ 2700 bp, exon 4= 177 bp, exon 5= 63 bp, exon 6= 101 bp, exon 7= 122 bp, exon 8= 175 bp, exon 9= 145 bp, exon 10= 84 bp, exon 11= 142 bp, exon 12= 128 bp, exon 13= 165 bp, exon 14= 119 bp, exon 15= 113 bp, exon 16= 149 bp, exon 17= 158 bp, exon 18= 162 bp, exon 19= 110 bp, exon 20= 146 bp, exon 21= 111 bp, exon 22= 1248 bp. The NR1 isoforms generated by alternative splicing of exons 5, 21 and 22 are shown below the NR1 gene structure and numbers of the amino acid residues of the proposed mature subunits are indicated on the right. (Modified from Hollmann et al.: Neuron 10, 943–954 (1993)).

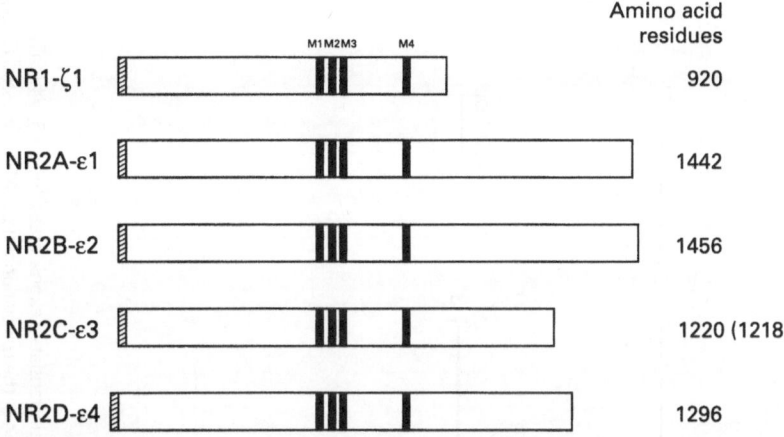

Fig. 2
Schematic representation of the NMDA receptor channel subunits
Putative signal peptides and four internal hydrophobic segments are indicated by hatched and filled boxes respectively. Numbers of amino acids of the proposed mature subunits are indicated on the right; the rat subunit, if different from that of the mouse counterpart, is given in parenthesis. (Modified from Mori and Mishina: Neuropharmocology 34, 1219–1237 (1995)).

immunoprecipitation studies provided direct evidence on the actual composition of the heteromeric NMDA receptor complex in rat cortex [114, 122, 123, 127].

The NR1 subunit (mRNA and polypeptide) is ubiquitously expressed in the brain [106, 119, 128, 129]. The NR2 subunits (mRNAs and their respective polypeptides), however, have a more restrictive pattern of expression in the brain [72, 102, 111, 121, 130–134]. Differential expression of both the NR1 splice variants as well as the NR2 subunits occurs during development [111, 127, 135–138]. The most prominent developmental change in the NR2 subunit is seen with the NR2B subunit. The NR2B subunit is widely expressed in the forebrain and cerebellum up to 2 weeks after birth, but thereafter it is selectively repressed to undetectable levels in the cerebellum. At the same time, expression of NR2C subunit begins in the cerebellum [106, 139, 140]. A similar developmental switch in the expression of NR1-1a/NR1-1b and NR2B/NR2A-NR2C mRNA was observed *in vitro* in cultured cerebellar granule cells [141].

The biological importance of various NMDA receptor subunits was delineated by the gene knock-out/knock-in technology [142]. The targeted disruption of NR2A (NR2A$^{-/-}$) or NR2C (NR2C$^{-/-}$) or NR2A/NR2C (NR2A$^{-/-}$/

Meena Kumari and Maharaj K. Ticku

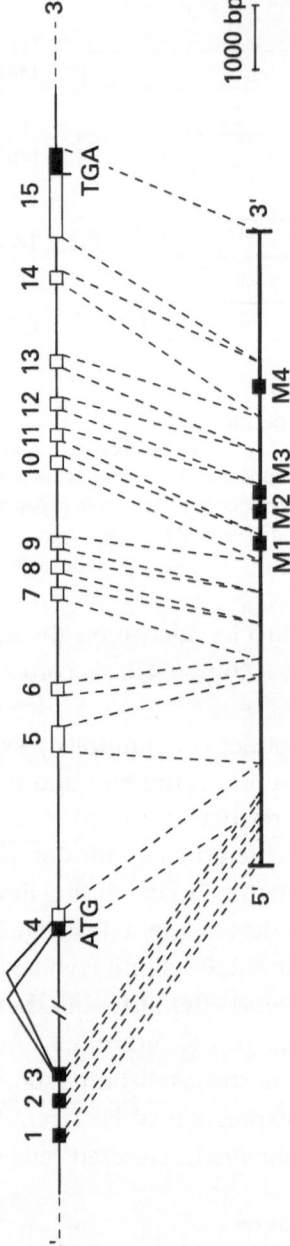

Fig. 3
Schematic drawing of the murine NR2C gene organization
The exon-intron organization is shown in the upper part. Exons 1-15 are boxed and filled boxes represent untranslated exonic areas. Intron 3, which is ~ 6 kb in length, is not drawn to scale. The two alternate splice variants between exons 3 and 4, and the position of the translational start (ATG) and stop (TGA) codons are indicated. The exon alignment of the NR2C cDNA is depicted in the lower part. Coding areas for the four putative transmembrane regions (M1-M4) are shown by filled boxes. (Modified from Suchanek et al.: J. Biol. Chem. 270, 41–44 (1995)).

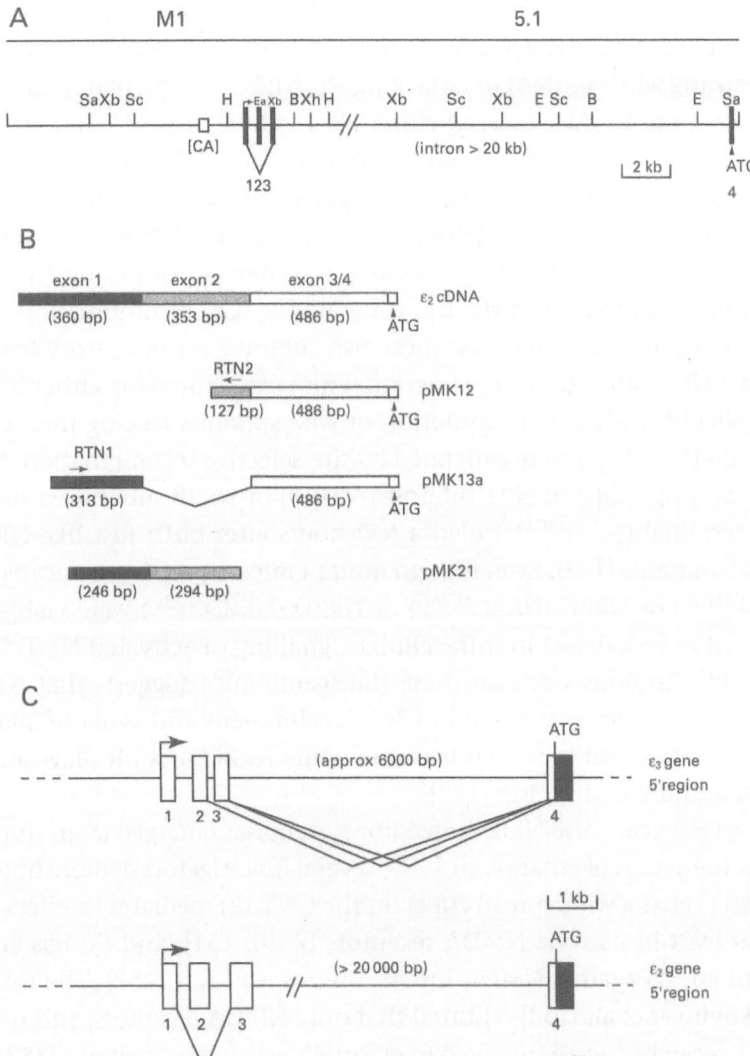

Fig. 4

Sequence and structure of the ε_2 gene promoter and 5' UTR

(A) Genomic structure of the 5' part of the ε_2 gene. The ATG start codon is marked with a triangle, the transcription initiation point is marked by an arrow. Exons are solid boxes, the [CA] repeat is given by an open box. (B) Schematic view of the ε_2 cDNA variants cloned by RACE. (C) Comparison of the 5'-non-coding regions of the ε_3 and the ε_2 genes are shown in the upper part. Untranslated exon sequences are marked as open boxes, translated sequences as solid boxes. Sequence of the promoter region of the ε_2 gene is shown in the lower part. Alternative splice variants of ε_2 and ε_3 are indicated. (Modified from Klein et al.: Gene 208, 259–269 (1998)).

NR2C$^{-/-}$) subunits was not lethal and resulted in viable offspring [143–145]. Mutant mice lacking the NR2A subunit showed a moderate deficiency in spatial learning while mutant mice lacking the NR2C subunit had normal motor co-ordination. In mice lacking either NR2C alone or NR2A and NR2C subunits, NMDA receptor-mediated components of EPSP in cerebellar granule cells were abolished. However, the targeted disruption of NR1 (NR1$^{-/-}$) or NR2B (NR2B$^{-/-}$) subunit was lethal. Mutant mice pups died within a few hours after birth [146–148]. Electrophysiological studies performed on NR1, NR2B, and hippocampal-restricted NR1 (generated by Cre-recombination system) knock-out pups suggested that these two subunits are obligatory for synaptic plasticity [146, 148–150]. Functional mutants expressing either NR1 subunit (NR1$^{q/q}$) with a point mutation or NR2 subunits lacking their carboxy terminus (NR2$^{\Delta C/\Delta C}$) were generated by site-selective recombination. Mutant mice carrying mutated NR1 subunit (NR1$^{q/q}$) or NR2B subunit without carboxy terminal (NR2B$^{\Delta C/\Delta C}$) died a few hours after birth just like NR1$^{-/-}$ or NR2B$^{-/-}$ mutants [142]. Even though mutant mice expressing truncated NR2A (NR2A$^{\Delta C/\Delta C}$) or NR2C (NR2C$^{\Delta C/\Delta C}$) or NR2D (NR2D$^{\Delta C/\Delta C}$) were viable, there appeared to be a defect in intracellular signalling of activated NMDA receptors [142]. Arduous work on these transgenic mice suggests that NR1 and NR2B play an important role in CNS development and synaptic plasticity. NR2A is implicated in spatial learning while NR2C subunit plays an active role in motor coordination [142].

In recent years, the NMDA receptor system has emerged as an important site for the action of ethanol. In 1989, several investigators demonstrated that ethanol (1) has a wide spread effect on the CNS; (2) mediates its effect on the CNS at least in part via NMDA receptors [7–10, 151]; and (3) has anticonvulsant effects against NMDA-induced seizures in rats [152]. The following year, Lovinger et al. [153] reported that only NMDA receptors, and not non-NMDA receptors, were involved in ethanol's action on the brain [153]. Later studies demonstrated that NMDA receptors composed of NR1/NR2B subunits display high ethanol sensitivity in cultured cortical neurons and cerebellar granule cells [154–156]. Recombinant NMDA receptor subunits were expressed in *Xenopus* oocytes to determine the sensitivity of NMDA receptor subunits to ethanol. The heteromeric assemblies of NR1/NR2A and NR1/NR2B were found to be significantly more sensitive to ethanol than NR1/NR2C or NR1/NR2D [157–159]. The sensitivity of NR1 splice variants to acute ethanol is still in debate [72, 160, 161]. The observed differences in ethanol sensitivity of NR1 splice variants may be due to post-translational modifications of the NMDA receptor subunits and/or cellular proteins that interact with NMDA receptor subunits [162]. Recently, it was demonstrated that phosphorylation of NMDA receptor subunits occurred in response to acute ethanol treatment [25, 28, 33, 36]. If phosphorylation of the NMDA receptor is necessary to observe ethanol's effect on NMDA receptor function, then it may not be surprising that contrary results have been reported using different systems [72, 160, 161].

Through intensive research efforts of several laboratories, we now know that acute ethanol treatment *in vivo* inhibits NMDA receptor function [163]. In contrast, chronic ethanol treatment *in vivo* increases NMDA receptor number and function [163]. With recent advances in molecular biology and cloning of NMDA receptor subunits we can now ask: What are the molecular mechanisms that are involved in ethanol's action on brain function? The answer to this question is complex because a number of laboratories have demonstrated that ethanol can modulate gene expression of NMDA receptors by altering (i) the rate of gene transcription in the nucleus, and (ii) post-transcriptional and post-translational events in the cytoplasm. In addition, several reports indicated that ethanol may affect NMDA receptor polpeptides and/or complexes by direct interaction at the cell membrane level or indirectly by modifications of receptor polypeptides via activation of signal transduction pathways [33, 35, 36].

3   Acute effects of ethanol on NMDA receptors

3.1 *In vivo* effects

Acute ethanol ingestion causes several changes in the CNS function leading to behavioral effects such as sedation, anxiolysis and cognitive impairment [44]. Acute ethanol ingestion also impairs memory in humans at concentrations associated with mild intoxication. In rats, severe intoxication including marked ataxia was seen within 30–45 min of systemic administration of ethanol (1.5 g and 2.5 g/kg body weight) [164].

Experimental evidence suggested that the NMDA receptor is not the only candidate that participates in mediating ethanol's effect on the brain. In our laboratory, we have investigated the anticonvulsant effect of ethanol against NMDA and other convulsants in rats [152]. We observed that ethanol was effective against picrotoxin and NMDA, but not against kainate-induced seizures. These results suggest that the anticonvulsant effect of ethanol *in vivo* may involve both $GABA_A$ receptors and NMDA receptors, but not kainate receptors [152]. In another independent *in vivo* study, the effect of systemically administered ethanol on the median septum (MS), a brain region previously shown to be affected by ethanol, was examined. Systemic administration of a pharmacologically relevant dose of ethanol (1.5 g/kg body weight) in rats resulted in inhibition of NMDA-evoked electrophysiological activity in the MS [164]. This inhibition of NMDA-evoked electrophysiological activity, however, was observed only in a subset of neurons. Administration of an intoxicating dose of ethanol (2.5 g/kg body weight) by the systemic route profoundly suppressed behavioral activity of rats but inhibited only 60% of NMDA-evoked neuronal activity. In contrast, a dose of NMDA antagonist MK-801 (0.6 mg/kg body weight) that augmented behavioral activity, totally inhibited NMDA-evoked neuronal activity [164]. These results indicated that (a) inhibition of NMDA-evoked activity alone can not account for all of the behavioral effects of ethanol, (b) inhibition of NMDA-mediated synaptic activity contributes to the effects of ethanol on the CNS, and (c) ethanol has a direct action on NMDA receptor function [164]. In an extension of their study, Simson and colleagues [165] demonstrated that ethanol applied locally via electro-osmosis also inhibited NMDA-evoked electrophysiological activity in the inferior colliculus and hippocampus of adult rats but not in the lateral septum. Thus, inhibition of NMDA-evoked neuronal activity by ethanol varies regionally in the brain [165]. Yang et al. [166] also observed similar brain region specificity for ethanol's effect in adult rats. They reported that in unanesthetized and urethane-anesthetized rats, not all neurons in the medial septum and cortex responed to ethanol [166]. It is interesting to note that Lovinger et al. [153] also observed a variable response of cultured hippocampal neurons to acute ethanol treatment. In yet another study, ethanol produced a discriminative stimulus effect similar to that produced by NMDA antagonists [167].

Taken together, these *in vivo* observations suggest that the response to acute ethanol exposure is restricted to specific brain regions rather than being a global effect in the CNS. This regional specificity of ethanol's effect on the brain may stem from differences in the composition of NMDA receptors in various neurons (see section 2). Direct evidence for such a concept came from a study where investigators compared the ability of ethanol to inhibit NMDA responses in the presence or absence of ifenprodil using the same neurons. Results of this study showed that ethanol preferentially acts on an ifenprodil-sensitive NMDA receptor [166]. Previous studies have documented that sensitivity to ifenprodil is restricted to NMDA receptors containing NR2B subunit [168, 169]. This perhaps explains why ethanol antagonizes NMDA responses only in some neurons. Those neurons that showed response to ethanol, may have NMDA receptors with the NR2B subunit subtype.

The role of various binding sites on the NMDA receptor in transducing the effects of acute ethanol treatment *in vivo* has also been addressed. The glycine and polyamine modulatory binding sites on the NMDA receptors do not play a role in the mediation of ethanol's effects. However, it appears that *in vivo*, the ethanol-like discriminative stimulus effects of PCP, pentazocine and (+)-N-allyl-normetazocine (NANM) which are also sigma receptor ligands, were likely to be attributed to their activity at NMDA receptors. It is suggested that some of the acute effects of ethanol are mediated via NMDA receptor anatgonism at the PCP binding site [170]. At the molecular level, acute ethanol treatment *in vivo* interferes with the transcription of cellular oncogenes such as *c-fos*. Generally, levels of *c-fos* are low in neurons. But a number of substances including NMDA are able to induce the expression of *c-fos*. For instance, treatment of rats with NMDA produced a dose- and time-dependent increase in the synthesis of *c-fos* mRNA in brain. Both MK-801 and acute ethanol treatment inhibited the NMDA-induced increase in *c-fos* mRNA in brain [171].

Acute ethanol treatment affects processes underlying learning and memory. For instance, electrophysiological recordings made using adult rat hippocampal slices in the presence of ethanol (5 mM, 15 min) demonstrated a significant reduction in LTP. It was shown that the potency of ethanol in depressing LTP correlates well with its potency in inhibiting the response to NMDA which is implicated in LTP induction [172].

3.2 *In vitro* effects

A number of electrophysiological and biochemical studies have shown that acute ethanol treatment alters neuronal function in the CNS. For example, ethanol (both acute and chronic) inhibits depolarization-dependent calcium flux and neurotransmitter release from striatal synaptosomes [173–175]. The link between NMDA receptors and the release of neurotransmitters came from the studies of Goethert and Fink [8]. They observed an inhibition of NMDA- or L-glutamate-induced [^{3}H]-noradrenaline release by ethanol in rat cortical slices that were superfused with physiologically composed salt solution lacking Mg^{2+}. In contrast, [^{3}H]-noradrenaline release occurring in response to electrical stimulation, reintroduction of Ca^{2+} ions or veratridine was not affected by ethanol up to a concentration of 320 mM/l when the above experiments were performed in the presence of a physiological concentration of Mg^{2+}. These results suggested that the NMDA receptor-ion channel complex is one of the sites of action underlying the ethanol-induced inhibition of neurotransmitter release [8]. Inhibition of neurotransmitter release in response to acute ethanol is not a global effect but varies in different brain regions. For instance, no inhibition of dopamine release was seen in cortical slices when incubated with 25 mM ethanol for 6 min. However, under similar conditions, ethanol inhibited NMDA-stimulated dopamine release from striatal slices suggesting a region-specific distribution of NMDA receptor subtypes exhibiting variable ethanol sensitivity [176].

Acute ethanol treatment alters NMDA receptor function in synaptosomes as well as intact neurons. Exposure to ethanol for 10 min increased the intracellular calcium concentration ($[Ca^{2+}]_i$) in synaptosomes isolated from the anterior part of the adult rat cerebrum but decreased the Ca^{2+} uptake by synaptosomes under polarized and depolarized conditions [177]. It was speculated that ethanol perhaps prevents the binding of Ca^{2+} to cytoplasmic buffers, and at the same time, inhibits the uptake of Ca^{2+} by mitochondria as suggested in *Aplysia* neurons [177, 178]. NMDA treatment (25 μM) stimulated an increase in $[Ca^{2+}]_i$ in brain cells freshly isolated from whole brain of newborn rat pups [10] as well as in cultured cerebellar granule cells isolated from 8-day-old rat pups [9]. Exposure to ethanol for 50 s was sufficient to inhibit NMDA-induced increase in $[Ca^{2+}]_i$ in freshly isolated neurons [10] and in cultured cortical neurons [179]. Similarly, exposure to ethanol to as low as 10 mM for 60 s significantly inhibited NMDA-stimulated Ca^{2+} uptake by the cultured cerebellar granule cells [9]. Thus, inhibition of NMDA-stimulated calcium uptake by acute ethanol is a phenomenon seen in intact neurons as well as synaptosomes. It appears from these studies that acute ethanol exposure affects the NMDA receptor itself.

Further support to the notion that ethanol inhibits NMDA receptor function came from studies performed by Lovinger et al. [7]. Using a whole-cell patch-clamp approach, they documented the effect of ethanol on NMDA receptors. Their electrophysiological results indicated that acute ethanol treatment (50 mM, 3 min) is a potent inhibitor of NMDA-gated ion currents in cultured hippocampal neurons isolated from mouse fetuses, adult hippocampus, spinal cord, neocortex and dorsal root ganglia. It is important to note that the inhibition of NMDA-activated current by ethanol in neurons was not a consequence of activation of $GABA_A$ receptors [7, 180]. Ethanol (25 and 50 mM) also inhibited excitatory synaptic transmission mediated by NMDA receptors in hippocampal slices of adult rodents [153]. Thus, ethanol acts as an inhibitor of NMDA receptor function in cultured neurons as well as freshly isolated neuronal preparations from fetal and adult brains [181].

Lovinger and co-workers [7] also documented the selectivity of ethanol's action on NMDA receptors. They found that ethanol (50 mM) was less effective in inhibiting kainate and AMPA receptors-mediated responses in neurons isolated from both fetal and adult hippocampus [7]. However, with the recent development and use of a highly selective AMPA receptor antagonist, it has become apparent that ethanol inhibits kainate-mediated glutamatergic synaptic transmission in rat hippocampal CA_3 pyramidal neurons at relatively low doses (20 mM) [182].

Does ethanol produce its inhibitory action on NMDA receptors via a direct interaction with NMDA receptors? Interaction between ethanol and the modulatory sites on the NMDA receptor has been repeatedly examined. Ethanol does not appear to interact with the glutamate binding site or the phencyclidine site on the NMDA receptor [163]. With respect to interactions at the glycine binding site of the NMDA receptor, conflicting results had been reported. Two independent studies performed using cultured cerebeller granule cells [183] and freshly isolated brain cells [184] suggested that the inhibitory effect of ethanol on NMDA-stimulated response decreased with increasing concentrations of glycine. Comparable results were observed with recombinant NMDA receptors expressed in *Xenopus* oocytes [185]. Using similar combinations of recombinant receptors in *Xenopus* oocytes, however, it was observed that ethanol did not compete for the glycine site on the NMDA receptor [186, 187]. In addition, inhibition of NMDA-activated ion current by ethanol (50 mM) in cultured rat hippocampal neurons was shown not to involve a competitive interaction with glycine [188]. Furthermore, using a different approach, Bhave and colleagues reported that glycine did not reverse ethanol-mediated inhibition of NMDA-induced increase in intracellular calcium in cultured cortical neurons [179]. These observations suggest that ethanol acts at a site on the NMDA receptor-ion channel complex distinct from the glycine modulatory site [179, 188]. Ethanol treatment (60 mM) significantly inhibited the NMDA-stimulated release of neurotransmitter from slices of hippocampus, cerebral cortex and striatum, and glycine reversed this effect of ethanol only in the striatum. Based on these results, Gonzales and Brown [189] suggested that interaction between glycine and ethanol may be a region-specific effect. Chu and colleagues [158] showed that the presence of zinc, magnesium, and redox modulatory agents did not alter the ethanol sensitivity of heteromeric NMDA receptors (NR1b/NR2A; NR1b/NR2B; NR1b/NR2C). Taken together these studies suggest that ethanol acts at a site distinct from any of the known modulators of the NMDA receptor.

Acute ethanol treatment also interferes with NMDA receptor mediated intracellular events in neurons. In cultured cerebellar granule cells, the production of cyclic GMP (cGMP) is a calcium-dependent process and involves activation of soluble guanylate cyclase. NMDA treatment increased the production of cGMP while ethanol treatment (10–50 mM, 60 s) inhibited NMDA-stimulated cGMP production in a dose-dependent manner. Acute ethanol (up to 100 mM concentration) treatment did not inhibit kainate-stimulated cGMP production in cerebellar granule cells grown under identical conditions. These observations suggest that physiologically relevant concentrations of ethanol specifically altered the NMDA receptor mediated cellular processes in these neurons [9]. Activation of protein kinase C (PKC) may underlie ethanol-mediated inhibition of NMDA receptor function in cerebellar granule cells. Treatment of cerebellar granule cells with an activator of PKC, phorbol-12-myristate 13-acetate (PMA) inhibited NMDA receptor function in a similar manner as acute ethanol treatment. This inhibition could be reversed by high concentrations of glycine and PKC inhibitors (staurosporine and calphostin C) [32]. This apparent role of PKC in ethanol inhibition of NMDA responses is highly brain-region specific. For example, in cultured cortical neurons, PMA did not inhibit the response to NMDA or decrease glycine potency, but instead produced a small increase in the NMDA receptor response at low glycine concentrations [179]. In mouse striatal neurons, PMA increased NMDA-induced responses only in the presence of submaximal concentrations of NMDA and/or the glycine site agonist, D-serine [190]. PMA treatment thus can affect co-agonist activation of NMDA receptor in ways that depend upon the origin of the cultured neurons, e.g. cerebellum, hippocampus. This regional specificity reflects upon the subunit composition of the NMDA receptors in the cell types employed in these studies. Other factors that could also contribute to the observed differences are a variation in the age of fetuses employed for cell isolation, cell culture conditions, number of days in culture, and the development and differentiation of cells *in vitro* as evidenced by the pattern of expression of various NMDA receptor subunits [141, 191, 192].

The identification of various NMDA receptor subunits and their heterogenic nature as well as differential ethanol sensitivity is based on initial experiments utilizing the *Xenopus* oocyte expression system [63, 99, 106, 193, 194]. The NR1 subunit when expressed in *Xenopus* oocytes formed homomeric functional NMDA receptors [99, 193]. These homomeric assemblies of the NR1 subunit exhibited ethanol sensitivity similar to that observed in intact neurons [7, 180]. However, the sensitivity to ethanol depended upon the NR1 splice variant (Fig. 1) forming the functional homomeric receptors. The reduction of total current produced by physiologically relevant concentration of ethanol was found to be greatest for NR1-1b and the order of sensitivity to ethanol was NR1-1b > NR1-2b > NR1-1a > NR1-2a [160]. Recent studies however suggested that the ethanol sensitivity of the NR1 splice variant was a characteristic of the *Xenopus* oocyte expression system only. Striatal neurons naturally express functional NMDA receptors that are comprised of NR1-1a or NR1-1b and NR2B subunits. The response of NMDA receptors to ethanol remained the same whether striatal neurons had NR1-1a or NR1-1b splice variant. Similar results were obtained with transfected HEK cells expressing NR1-1a/NR2B or NR1-1b/NR2B receptor subunits. These observations demonstrated that ethanol sensitivity of NR1 subunit does not depend upon the presence or absence of the N-terminal cassette (or exon 5) [161]. Results obtained in another independent study using mesencephalon neurons are in agreement with the above observations that alternatively spliced exons of the NR1 subunit do not contribute sensitivity towards ethanol [72] as had been shown previously using the *Xenopus* oocyte expression system [160]. Most of the neurons in the mesencephalon express NR1 splice variants lacking exons 5, 21 and 22 (NR1-4a) and only 25% of the mesencephalic neurons express NR1 with exon 21 only (NR1-3a) [72]. Ethanol (50 and 100 mM) inhibited NMDA-stimulated increase in intracellular calcium in all the mesencephalic neurons tested in this study [72].

The magnitude of the NMDA-activated current was greatly enhanced when NR1 and members of NR2 subunits were co-expressed in *Xenopus* oocytes. The heteromeric channels thus formed exhibit different agonist, antagonist and ethanol sensitivity [195–197]. Studies performed on recombinant heteromeric NMDA receptors expressed in *Xenopus* oocytes suggested that ethanol preferentially affected heteromers containing the NR2A or NR2B subunit, while the least effect was observed on NR1/NR2C combinations

[157, 159, 186, 187]. The NR1/NR2A and NR1/NR2B receptors expressed in *Xenopus* oocytes did not significantly differ from each other in their response to acute ethanol treatment. It is thus not surprising that trimeric receptors (NR1/NR2A/NR2B) show similar response as any of the parent receptors, i.e. NR1/NR2A or NR1/NR2B. Furthermore, NR1/NR2A/NR2C combinations show the same response to ethanol as NR1/NR2C in combination [187]. However, it is yet to be established whether expression of three different mRNAs in *Xenopus* oocytes generated trimeric receptors as shown for the native NMDA receptors [114, 119, 127]. It is interesting that ethanol's inhibitory effect on recombinant NR1/NR2A receptors was decreased when wild type NR1 was replaced with mutant NR1 subunit (N616R and N616Q) [187]. This decrease was attributed to the ability of mutant NR1 subunit to cause a reduced or complete lack of divalent cation permeability and sensitivity to Mg^{2+} block [198, 199]. More recent studies suggested that the ethanol sensitivity of NR1/NR2A receptors was modulated by a calcium-dependent signal pathway and required the presence of C0 domain of the NR1 subunit [200]. It is likely that sensitivity to acute ethanol depends upon activation of specific signal pathways involving intracellular calcium.

4   Chronic effects of ethanol on NMDA receptors

4.1   *In vivo* effects

The development of ethanol dependence and the associated withdrawal syndrome in humans requires continuous consumption of large quantities of ethanol for a long period of time. When ethanol intake is abruptly decreased or stopped, a withdrawal syndrome occurs, and the symptoms of CNS excitation manifest themselves. In the early stages of ethanol withdrawal, up to 72 h, signs of CNS hyperexcitability, such as tremor, increased autonomic activity, and convulsions are observed [201].

Similar physical dependence and ethanol withdrawal symptoms were also seen in laboratory bred rodents. For instance, cessation of ethanol intake in mice resulted in ethanol withdrawal-associated (handling-induced) seizures [202]. The severity of the handling-induced seizures increased as a function of time following removal of ethanol. The most severe seizure activity was observed at 6–10 h after ethanol withdrawal, when blood levels of ethanol became undetectable. All signs of ethanol withdrawal-associated seizures disappeared 48 h after the last ethanol intake [203–205]. Administration of the NMDA receptor antagonist, MK-801, decreased the occurrence and severity of the ethanol withdrawal seizures in a dose-dependent manner without producing sedation [206, 207]. These observations suggested that the ethanol withdrawal syndrome is a result of an adaptive response of the CNS to the intoxicating effects of ethanol. This "(mal)adaptation" is evidenced as CNS hyperexcitability once ethanol is removed from the system [205, 208].

Prolonged exposure to ethanol results in neuropathological changes in brain [209–212]. A significant loss of pyramidal cells in hippocampus and granule cells in dentate gyrus was observed in hematoxylin and eosin stained brain sections of rats exposed to ethanol for 5 months and 2 months of ethanol withdrawal period [212–214]. The density of synapses on dendritic spines in the striatum oriens of the CA_1 hippocampal region of normal mice and mice genetically selected for sensitivity to ethanol, also decreased following exposure to ethanol for several months [215, 216]. In addition to changes in hippocampus, loss of neurons was also detected in cerebellum following chronic ethanol treatment in animals [217, 218]. In the aging brain, the gradual loss of neurons is compensated by an increase in synaptic efficacy. Whether the neuronal loss observed following chronic ethanol exposure is accompanied by a similar alteration in synaptic efficacy was therefore addressed [219, 220]. Results of an *in vivo* study indicated that synaptic efficacy did indeed increase in rodents which were exposed to chronic ethanol treatment. Since these animals were anesthetized during the course of the experiments [220], it was possible that anesthetics could have confounded the results. However, *in vitro* studies utilizing hippocampal slices [221] provided similar results as observed *in vivo* [220]. More recently, neurodegeneration in the entorhinal cortex, dentate gyrus and olfactory bulbs accompanied by cerebrocortical edema and electrolyte accumulation was observed following 5–10 days of ethanol treatment of adult rats [222]. Co-administration of MK-801, non-NMDA receptor and Ca^{2+} channel antagonists could not prevent ethanol-induced brain damage [222]. However, cotreatment with the electrolyte transport inhibitor/diuretic furosemide reduced ethanol-dependent cerebrocortical damage by 75–85% but not in olfactory bulbs [222].

One of the first clues that the glutaminergic system may be involved in the neuropathological and neurochemical alterations observed following exposure to chronic ethanol came from studies performed by Michaelis and his group [223]. They demonstrated an increase in the total number of L-glutamate binding sites in whole brain homogenates of rats exposed to chronic ethanol (14–21 days) pointing to an alteration in the glutaminergic function in the brain of treated rats [223, 224]. Although these preliminary biochemical studies did not indicate whether the increase in L-glutamate binding sites was accompanied by an overall increase of receptors in the CNS or was restricted to specific brain regions, their observations initiated a series of studies leading to identification of the role of the glutaminergic system in the alcohol field. Subsequently, the design and use of novel natural and synthetic agonists and antagonists both *in vivo* and *in vitro* has provided evidence for the existence of different types of ionotropic glutamate receptors and their involvement in ethanol-mediated alterations in brain structure and function. Thus there was a need to identify and characterize which glutamate receptors are affected by chronic ethanol exposure.

Further evidence that the glutaminergic system mediates some of the chronic effects of ethanol came from several studies. When adult rodents were chronically treated with ethanol, an increase in MK-801 binding sites in hippocampus occurred [225–227]. Similar observations were made by Gulya et al. [204]. They demonstrated that chronic ethanol administration for 7 consecutive days to adult mice significantly increased MK-801 binding in the membrane fraction of hippocampus, cerebral cortex, striatum, and thalamus. Twenty-four hours after ethanol withdrawal, MK-801 binding was comparable to untreated control animals [204]. It should be noted that during the ethanol treatment period, mice received vitamin supplements to prevent complications due to malnutrition [203]. In another study, Snell and colleagues found an increase in hippocampal [^{3}H]-MK-801 and NMDA specific [^{3}H]-glutamate binding sites in ethanol-dependent mice. Since this increase in [^{3}H]-MK-801 and [^{3}H]-glutamate binding sites occurred without affecting strychnine-insensitive glycine or a competitive NMDA antagonist, CGS 19755 binding sites, it was suggested that not all binding sites on the NMDA receptor complex respond to chronic ethanol treatment [228]. Furthermore, they also demonstrated that [^{3}H]-kainate binding sites in the cortex and hippocampus were not increased following chronic ethanol exposure of mice [228]. This suggested that the increased hyperexcitability observed following ethanol withdrawal is a specific effect on NMDA receptors and not due to a general increase in excitatory neurotransmission.

Interestingly, no increase in MK-801 binding was observed in cerebral cortex of mice exposed to chronic ethanol treatment [228]. Similarly, no increase in MK-801 binding occurred following 7 days of ethanol treatment of withdrawal seizure-prone mice and withdrawal seizure-resistant mice [229]. In rats, no change in MK-801 binding was reported in all the brain regions tested following 48 h of ethanol withdrawal after 28 weeks of chronic ethanol treatment. It is possible that 48 h after ethanol withdrawal, NMDA receptor number returned to control levels. A time-course of MK-801 binding during 48 h of ethanol withdrawal should help resolve this issue. Nevertheless, it is apparent that there is some controversy regarding alterations of NMDA receptor binding sites following chronic ethanol exposure. Whether the observed controversy in NMDA receptor binding was due to different ethanol treatment paradigms was examined by Rudolph and colleagues [230]. They reported a significant increase in NMDA receptor binding in CA_1 and dentate gyrus region of the hippocampus after 30 days of ethanol treatment. A small increase in MK-801 and CGP binding was also observed in select frontal brain regions after 3 weeks of ethanol liquid diet [230]. It was thus concluded that perhaps differences in receptor binding assays contributed to the observed discrepancy in binding results. It is possible that the NMDA receptor supersensitivity observed during ethanol tolerance and dependence may not only be due to changes in the density of NMDA receptors, but may rather involve several different mechanisms. As pointed out by Crews and colleagues [30], the differences observed in binding could also result from changes in receptor subunit composition rather than actual increases in the number of binding sites.

Identification of NMDA receptor subunits by molecular cloning helped, at least in part, to address this controversy. Highly specific polyclonal antibodies raised against NMDA receptor subunits and radiolabeled cRNA probes were used to determine the distribution, alteration in expression, and composition of NMDA receptors by co-immunoprecipitation/co-localization in the brain [106, 119, 124, 125, 127]. One of the first reports that showed an increase in NR1 subunit following chronic ethanol treatment (12 weeks) of adult rats came from Trevisan and colleagues [231]. Using Western blot analysis, they observed a 65% increase in NR1 receptor subunit polypeptide levels in hippocampus without any dramatic change in cerebral cortex, nucleus accumbens and striatum. They also documented that the upregulation of NR1 subunit was an ethanol-specific response seen in rat hippocampus [231]. A minimum of 6 days of chronic ethanol treatment in adult rats appeared to be sufficient to observe an upregulation of NR1, NR2A and NR2B polypeptide levels in hippocampus and cerebral cortex [232]. Similar changes in polypeptide levels of NR1 and NR2A subunits were observed in mice following chronic ethanol treatment [233]. However at the molecular level, chronic ethanol treatment (6 days) in rats had no effect on the NR1 mRNA levels in any of the brain regions examined [234]. Hardy and colleagues reported an alteration in the expression of NR1 splice variants in cortex without any apparent change in the total amount of NR1 mRNA levels. The NR1 variant containing the 5' insert (exon 5) was more predominant and this alteration was persistent even after 48 h of ethanol withdrawal [235]. In contrast NR2A, and NR2B mRNA levels in the cerebral cortex and hippocampus were elevated by ~ 40% and 30%, respectively. The NR2A and NR2B mRNA levels returned to control levels within 48 h of ethanol withdrawal. No change in NR1, NR2A and NR2C mRNA levels was reported in cerebellum [234].

It is thus apparent that polypeptide and mRNA levels of NMDA receptor subunits are differentially upregulated in response to chronic ethanol treatment. Also, this upregulation of protein and mRNA levels occurs in a region-specific manner in the brain. It is yet to be established *in vivo* whether this increase is due to an increase in transcription and/or translation rate of the respective receptor subunits. It may be difficult to obtain an answer to some of these questions, as certain techniques require manipulations that are not possible *in vivo*. Recently, however, attempts in this direction have been made using cultured neurons (see section 4.2).

4.2 *In vitro* effects

In the early 1980's, primary cultures of neurons isolated from various regions of fetal, neonatal or adult brain, were employed to determine the effects of acute ethanol treatment on electrophysiological response of cells and these results were correlated with ethanol-mediated changes in brain morphology and function of intact animals. Over the years, culture conditions for neurons have been refined and their use has been extended to delineate the effects of chronic ethanol treatment. Fetal neurons when cultured under optimal conditions, show signs of development and differention as evidenced by the expression of genes whose transcription and translation products are seen only at specific stages of development [141, 191, 192]. Most importantly, the effects of chronic ethanol treatment on cultured neurons are comparable to the results obtained *in vivo* [204, 234, 237]. An added advantage is that it is easy to manipulate cultured cells and experiments that cannot be performed in intact animals, but can be performed using *in vitro* systems. Primary cultures of various regions of fetal brain have been especially beneficial in the advancement of our knowledge in the alcohol field. Specifically, two important interrelated aspects of ethanol-mediated effects are being examined in detail using primary cultures of neurons: (1) molecular mechanisms underlying ethanol-mediated upregulation of NMDA receptor function, and (2) ethanol-mediated excitotoxicity.

Chronic ethanol treatment of neonatal cerebellar granule cells, fetal hippocampal and fetal cortical neurons upregulated the NMDA receptor function as measured by an increase in Ca^{2+} influx [236–238]. This increased function of neurons in response to chronic ethanol treatment was due to an actual increase in the number of NMDA receptors as shown by [^{3}H]MK-801 binding rather than a change in NMDA receptor properties [236, 237, 239]. The enhanced NMDA response and MK-801 binding was reversed following 48 h of ethanol withdrawal [43, 237]. Supporting evidence for the increased number of NMDA receptors came from Western blot analyses. Chronic ethanol treatment (75 mM, 5 days) increased NR1 and NR2B polypeptide levels in cultured fetal cortical neurons [43]. Exposure to 100 mM ethanol for 4 days increased the expression of NR1, NR2A and NR2B subunits of the NMDA receptor in neonatal cortical neurons grown in the presence of low glutamine. A similar increase in NMDA receptor subunits was not seen when neurons were grown in the presence of high glutamine [240]. The significance of glutamine concentration on the expression of NMDA receptors is not known at present [237, 240].

At the molecular level, chronic ethanol treatment of fetal cortical neurons augmented NR2B mRNA levels (~ 40%) without any alterations in the NR1 and NR2A mRNA levels. The NR2B mRNA levels returned to control levels with in 72 h of ethanol withdrawal [241]. Nuclear run-on analysis demonstrated that upregulation of NR2B mRNA levels was due to an increase in the rate of *nmdar2b* gene transcription in fetal cortical neurons following chronic ethanol treatment. At the same time, chronic ethanol treatment increased the half-life of the NR1 mRNA in these neurons [48]. At the present time very little is known as to how ethanol affects gene expression of different NMDA receptor subunits. To this end, progress has been made with regard to delineation of the structural organization of various NMDA receptor subunit genes [104, 108–110, 146, 242]. Interestingly, alternate splicing of exons was observed for NR1, NR2B, NR2C receptor subunits. Alternate splicing of exons for the NR1 subunit (Fig. 1) results in mRNA's with different coding regions [103, 104]. Whereas alternative splicing of NR2B and NR2C subunit mRNAs (Figs. 3 and 4) generates mRNA's with different 5' untranslated regions (5'

175

UTRs) [108, 110, 243]. In the case of the NR2B subunit, a differential expression of NR2B splice variants was seen in the cortex, hippocampus, thalamus and striatum [110]. The significance of 5' UTRs lies in the fact that they control the translational efficiency of the respective mRNA [244, 245]. A differential expression of the NR2B splice variants is suggestive of such a post-transcriptional control mechanism as has been shown for the NR2A subunit mRNA. The 5' UTR of the NR2A subunit severely restricted its protein translation in both *Xenopus* oocytes and in an *in vitro* translation system [246].

More recently, attempts have been made to understand the complex mechanisms that direct tissue- and region-specific expression of *nmdar1*, *nmdar2b* and *nmdar2c* [110, 242, 243, 247–250]. The interplay between ubiquitous transcription factors such as Sp1, and tissue-specific transcription factors such as fushi tarazu factor 1, steroidogenic factor, cyclic AMP response element, myocyte enhancer factor 2C appear to regulate expression of NMDA receptor subunit genes. Further complexity is added by factors such as NGF and neuregulin that modulate gene expression in a tissue specific manner [247, 248]. At present, we know that chronic ethanol treatment upregulated *nmdar2b* gene expression in cultured cortical neurons [48]. The exact mechanisms as to how ethanol brings about such transcriptional changes need to be further explored.

Excessive stimulation of NMDA receptors can trigger a series of events that results in delayed neuronal cell death and this process is termed excitotoxicity. Neuronal excitotoxicity is implicated in several neuropathological conditions such as stroke and several chronic neurodegenerative conditions such as Huntington's disease. As mentioned in section 4.1, chronic ethanol treatment *in vivo* also results in a loss of neurons and dendritic processes in various parts of brain [212–218, 222]. A number of investigators have made attempts to identify mechanisms involved in ethanol-induced excitotoxicity using cultured neurons.

Excitotoxic effects observed *in vivo* in intact animals (section 4.1) had been duplicated *in vitro* in cultured neurons (see below). For instance, exposure to the NMDA receptor agonist, glutamate, for 30 min caused a dose-dependent death of cerebellar granule cells pre-exposed to 100 mM ethanol for 3 days [251]. Similarly, NMDA-mediated neuronal cell death was reported in cultured hippocampal neurons after a minimum of 2 days of ethanol treatment. Extension of exposure to ethanol treatment for 7 days enhanced the magnitude of NMDA-mediated cell death. Neuronal cell death was seen to be specifically mediated by NMDA receptors as AMPA receptors, kainic acid or nifedipine failed to induce cell death [238]. Additional evidence for the involvement of NMDA receptors in excitotoxicity came from antagonist treatment studies. Excitotoxicity caused by glutamate in cerebellar granule cells was blocked by simultaneous addition of glutamate and antagonists, acting at different sites on the NMDA receptor, to the culture medium. The blockade of excitotoxicity by antagonists was observed both in control and ethanol-treated cells, supporting the hypothesis that the enhanced susceptibility to glutamate-induced excitotoxicity after chronic ethanol treatment was a consequence of enhanced activity of NMDA receptors [239]. Recently it was shown that glutamate-induced increase in intracellular Mg^{2+} in fetal neurons could also result in neuronal cell death. Exposure to glutamate increased both intracellular Ca^{2+} and Mg^{2+} in cortical neurons isolated from 16-day-old rat fetuses and cultured for 2 weeks. When these neurons were grown in the absence of Ca^{2+} but in the presence of 9 mM Mg^{2+}, exposure to glutamate (100 µM) or NMDA (200 µM) for 20 min produced delayed neuronal death. NMDA or glutamate mediated excitotoxic effects on fetal cortical neurons were blocked when NMDA receptor antagonists and agonists were added together to the culture medium. It was also observed that rat cortical neurons grown under different serum conditions developed an altered sensitivity to Mg^{2+}-dependent NMDA receptor-mediated excitotoxicity [252]. However, it is not yet known whether ethanol plays a role in Mg^{2+}-dependent NMDA receptor-mediated excitotoxicity.

It is thus clear that ethanol mediates some of its deleterious effects on neurons via NMDA receptors. But how these deleterious effects are transduced eventually leading to cell death, is not yet known. Changes in intracellular calcium can disrupt normal cellular function and can contribute to cell death. Both ethanol and nerve growth factor (NGF) independently and collectively affected the regulation of calcium homeostasis in embryonic hippocampal neurons [253]. It was suggested that alteration of calcium homeostasis may be an underlying mechanism involved in ethanol excitotoxicity [253]. In an earlier study, blockage of glutamate-induced increase in intracellular calcium was correlated with prevention of the excitotoxic effects [239]. Thus, calcium appears to be a good candidate as a signaling molecule. In addition, increase in intracellular calcium seems to be the key event in the induction of signal pathways in neurons [254]. To this end, a recent report showed that ethanol-induced upregulation of NMDA receptors was associated with the influx of calcium through NMDA receptors [255].

Glutamate induced a delayed increase in Ca^{2+} influx resulting in sustained activation of protein kinase C (PKC) [256] while downregulation of PKC attenuated glutamate-induced cytotoxicity in cerebellar granule cells [41]. Activation of PKC in turn could potentiate NMDA-induced current by about 2.5 fold in *Xenopus* oocytes. Kainate or quisqualate-mediated currents were not potentiated in oocytes [257, 258]. It was hypothesized that PKC potentiated NMDA response by increasing the probability of channel openings and by reducing the voltage-dependent magnesium block of NMDA receptor channels [39]. Whether chronic ethanol treatment of cultured neurons will activate PKC is not known as yet. However, it may be noted here that acute ethanol treatment did reduce the frequency and duration of ion channel opening in electrophysiological experiments using the membrane fraction of rat cortex and hippocampus [259].

A number of studies have shown that NMDA receptor subunits are phosphorylated at their C-terminal ends by a variety of kinases such as protein kinase A, protein kinase C, protein tyrosine kinases, and cam kinase II in neurons and in transfected cells [32, 38, 40, 256, 260–265]. Phosphorylation of NMDA receptor subunits result in initiation of certain cellular events. For instance, phosphorylation of serine 890 of the NR1 subunit by PKC resulted in dispersion of surface-associated clusters of the NR1 subunit expressed in quail fibroblasts [38]. Similar trafficking of distinct NMDA receptor subunits was also observed in cultured hippocampal neurons following phosphorylation of NMDA receptor subunits (NR1 and NR2B) [266]. More recently, Lieberman and Mody [265] demonstrated that the NMDA receptor complex is a target of cam kinase II (CKII) in hippocampal neurons of adult rats [265]. Interestingly, like PKC, CKII also controls NMDA channel gating through phosphorylation. Inhibition of dephosphorylation by calcineurin enhances the NMDA channel activity [40, 265]. Given the potentially important role of phosphorylation on regulation of NMDA receptors, it is of particular interest to examine possible signal pathways that may be activated in response to ethanol.

A recent study indicated that acute tolerance to ethanol involving NMDA receptors might involve phosphorylation of tyrosine on the NMDA receptor by Fyn kinase, a member of Src family of tyrosine kinases [33]. Csk, a novel cytoplasmic protein-tyrosine kinase, phosphorylates tyrosine residues at the carboxy terminal of Fyn kinase rendering Fyn kinase inactive [267] indicating an inverse relation between Src and Fyn kinases. Miyakawa et al. [33] showed that acute ethanol treatment (5 min) *in vivo* increased phosphorylation of the NR2B subunit in hippocampus of heterozygous (+/fyn^z) but not in Fyn-deficient (fyn^z/fyn^z) mice. Similar increase in phosphorylation of the NR2B subunit in hippocampus of adult mice following acute ethanol treatment was also observed by Kalluri and Ticku [36]. Ethanol-mediated increase in phosphorylation of the NR2B subunit by Fyn kinase is highly brain region specific as ethanol treatment of adult mice had no effect on phosphorylation of the NR2B subunit in cerebral cortex. Both acute and chronic ethanol treatment of cultured cortical neurons also did not affect total or tyrosine phosphorylation of the NR2B subunit [35]. This is an interesting observation since high levels of Fyn kinase polypeptide were detected in adult mouse cortex and in cultured fetal cortical. High levels of CSK polypeptide were detected only in fetal cortical neurons and not in adult cortex [36]. However at this time it is not known whether these two enzymes (Fyn and Csk kinases) are active in these tissues.

Nevertheless, these studies suggest that tyrosine phosphorylation of the NR2B subunit plays a role in the development of ethanol tolerance and that Fyn-kinase-mediated phosphorylation of the NR2B subunit is not a universal phenomenon involved in the regulation of the NR2B subunit. Interestingly, Fyn-deficient mice exhibited an increased hypnotic effect to ethanol, but did not exhibit acute tolerance to ethanol. Miyakawa et al. [33] correlated the changes in Fyn kinase mediated phosphorylation of the NR2B subunit in hippocampus to the hypnotic effect of ethanol in mice. In an independent *in vitro* study, it was observed that tyrosine phosphorylation of NMDA receptors by c-Src did not modulate the inhibitory effects of ethanol on NMDA activated currents in HEK 293 cells expressing both NMDA receptor subunits and c-Src [34]. Additional studies are required to establish the significance of Fyn kinase dependent phosphorylation of the NR2B subunit in ethanol treated animals and whether phosphorylation by Fyn kinase indeed plays a role in excitotoxicity.

More recently, the importance of phosphatidylinositol 3′-OH kinase (PI 3-kinase) signal pathway in cerebellar granule cell death was documented. It was observed that NMDA treatment of cultured cerebellar granule cells induced expression of brain-derived neurotrophic factor (BDNF). BDNF in turn increased phosphorylation of protein kinase B (or Akt) which is a target of PI 3-kinase. Acute ethanol treatment (100 mM, 24 h) inhibited the NMDA-induced increase in BDNF levels in cultured cerebellar granule cells, but did not block the neuroprotective effect of BDNF on these cells. Investigators suggested that deleterious effects of ethanol on cerebellar granule cells were mediated by PI 3-kinase signal transduction pathway via BDNF [268]. Additional investigations are required to determine if different signal pathways are utilized by neurons in different regions of the brain.

Recently, another potential signaling molecule in the CNS has gained importance as a mediator of ethanol's neuropathological effects. Nitric oxide (NO) is a short-lived gas and has been recognized as a novel neurotransmitter. The enzyme, nitric oxide synthase (NOS) is responsible for NO synthesis in various tissues including the CNS. NOS activity is calcium dependent [269] and is coupled to activation of glutamate receptors [270]. It is speculated that NO plays a role in alcohol dependence, withdrawal, and alcohol-associated brain damage. Biochemical studies demonstrated that acute ethanol treatment (25–200 mM) inactivated NOS activity in a dose-dependent manner and this was achieved by modulating the conformation of NOS [271, 272]. It is therefore not surprising to observe a reduction in NMDA-stimulated NO formation in cultured cortical neurons following acute ethanol treatment (100 mM, 10 min) [270]. In contrast, chronic ethanol treatment (100 mM, 4 days) of cultured cortical neurons enhanced NMDA-mediated NOS activity while AMPA, kainate or the calcium ionophore ionomycin had no effect on NOS activity [273]. It is possible that the increased NOS activity may also contribute to the development of ethanol dependence, withdrawal and the associated excitotoxicity. That increased NO production following chronic ethanol exposure perhaps contributes to ethanol's excitotoxic effects was suggested by Adam et al. [274]. Specifically, they observed that inhibitors of NOS were able to suppress convulsions and tremors associated with ethanol withdrawal in rats while NO donors seemed to worsen symptoms of ethanol withdrawal. It should be noted, however, that NO's potential excitotoxic effects *in vivo* are not without controversy. Studies by Zou et al. [275] showed that in intact animals, inhibition of NOS enhanced the neurodegeneration observed following ethanol withdrawal.

5   Conclusions

From the foregoing review it is clear that over the years numerous studies have implicated the NMDA receptor system in ethanol's effect on brain function. Inhibition of NMDA receptor function by acute ethanol exposure probably underlies some of the symptoms of ethanol intoxication. Chronic ethanol exposure on the other hand, results in upregulation of NMDA receptor number and function, and contributes to the development of ethanol tolerance, dependence, ethanol withdrawal syndrome and excitotoxicity. Thus much has been learned, but many questions remain and the precise molecular mechanisms that bring about ethanol's effect on the CNS remain to be elucidated. The heterogeneity of NMDA receptors and their regional-specificity are all factors that lead to their differential sensitivity to ethanol and add further complexity to ethanol's effect on neurotransmission in the brain. The involvement of second messenger pathways and the role of phosphorylation in mediating ethanol's effects are at present not completely understood and need further exploration. Perhaps with recent advances in techniques in molecular biology, signal transduction and development of more selective ligands, we may be able to solve some of the mysteries that lie before us.

Acknowledgement

We thank Sadie Phillips for excellent secretarial assistance, and Elena Wright and Kamran Shaik for their help. We offer special thanks to Ruby Kainth for preparing figures and Dr. Antje Anji for helpful comments.

References

1   F. Fadda and Z.L. Rossetti: Prog. Neurobiol. *56*, 385 (1998).
2   P.J. Langalis and R.G. Mair: J. Neurosci. *10*, 1664 (1990).
3   R.F. Butterworth, J.J. Kril and C.G. Harper: Alcohol Clin. Exp. Res. *17*, 1084 (1993).
4   A.M. Allan and R.A. Harris: Life Sci. *39*, 2005 (1986).
5   M.K. Ticku, P. Lowrimore and P. Lehoullier: Brain Res. Bull. *17*, 123 (1986).
5   D.D. Suzdak, R.D. Schwartz, P. Skolmick and S.M. Paul: Proc. Natl. Acad. Sci. *83*, 4071 (1986).
7   D.M. Lovinger, G. White and F.F. Weight: Science *243*, 1721 (1989).
8   M. Goethert and K. Fink: Naunyn-Schmiedeberg's Arch. Pharmacol. *340*, 516 (1989).
9   P.L. Hoffman, C.S. Rabe, F. Moses and B. Tabakoff: J. Neurochem. *52*, 1937 (1989).
10   J.E. Dildy and S.W. Leslie: Brain Res. *499*, 383 (1989).
11   J. Anwar and M.S. Dar: Alcohol Clin. Exp. Res. *19*, 777 (1995).
12   S.G. Madamba, M. Hsu, P. Schweitzer and G.R. Siggins: Brain Res. *685*, 21 (1995).
13   L.G. Aguayo, J.C. Tapia and F.C. Pancetti: J. Pharmacol. Exp. Ther. *279*, 1116 (1996).
14   I.R. Coe, L.N. Yao, I. Diamond and A.S. Gordon: J. Biol. Chem. *271*, 29468 (1996).
15   A. Concas, M.P. Masci.a, T. Cucheddu, S. Floris, M.C. Mostallino, C. Perra, S. Satta and G. Bibbio: Pharmacol. Biochem. Behav. *53*, 249 (1996).
16   T.V. Dunwiddie, in: R.A. Dietrich and V.G. Erwin (eds): Pharmacological effects of ethanol on the nervous system, CRC Press, Florida 1996, pp. 147–161.

17   M.P. Mascia, S.J. Mihic, C.F. Valenzuela, P.R. Schofield and R.A. Harris: Mol. Pharmacol. *50*, 402 (1996).

18   K. Nagata, G.L. Aistrup, C.S. Huang, W. Marszalec, H.J. Song, J.Z. Yeh and T. Narahashi: Neurosci. Lett. *217*, 189 (1996).

19   A.H.L. Lau and G.D. Frye: Brain Res. *731*, 12 (1996).

20   C. Wang, W.-F. Pralong, M.-F. Schulz, G. Rougon, J.-M. Aubry, S. Pagliusi, A. Robert and J. Z. Kiss: J. Cell Biol. 135, 1565 (1996).

21   D. Mullikin-Kilpatrick and S.N. Treistman, in: R.A. Dietrich and V.G. Erwin (eds): Pharmacological effects of ethanol on the nervous system, CRC Press, Florida 1996, pp. 29–49.

22   K.T. Eggeman and M.D. Browning, in: R.A. Deitrich and V.G. Erwin (eds.): Pharmacological effects of ethanol on the nervous system, CRC Press, Florida 1996, pp. 117–133.

23   S.J. Mihic and R.A. Harris, in: R.A. Dietrich and V.G. Erwin (eds): Pharmacological effects of ethanol on the nervous system, CRC Press, Florida 1996, pp. 1–72.

24   G.F. Koob, in: R.A. Dietrich and V.G. Erwin (eds.): Pharmacological effects of ethanol on the nervous system, CRC Press, Florida 1996, pp. 1–12.

25   I. Diamond and A.S. Gordon: Physiol. Rev. *77*, 1 (1997).

26   H.H. Kerschbaum and A. Hermann: Brain Res. *765*, 30 (1997).

27   M. Solem, T. McMahon and R.O. Messing: J. Pharmac. Exp. Ther. *282*, 1487 (1997).

28   L.J. Chandler, R.A. Harris and F.T Crews: Trends Pharmacol. *19*, 491 (1998a).

29   C.L. Faingold, P. N'Gouemo and A. Riaz: Prog. Neurobiol. *55*, 509 (1998).

30   F.T. Crews, A.L. Morrow, H. Criswell and G. Breese: Int. Rev. Neurobiol. *39*, 283 (1996).

31   R.O. Messing, P.J. Petersen and C.J. Henrich: J. Biol. Chem. *26*, 23428 (1991).

32   L.D. Snell, B. Tabakoff and P.L. Hoffman: Alcohol Clin. Exp. Res. *18*, 81 (1994).

33   T. Miyakawa, T. Yagi, H. Kitazawa, M. Yasuda, N. Kawai, K. Tsuboi and H. Niki: Science *278*, 698 (1997).

34   D.L. Anders, T. Blevins, G. Sutton, L.J. Chandler and J.J. Woodward: Alcohol Clin. Exp. Res. *23*, 357 (1999).

35   H.S.G. Kalluri and M.K. Ticku: Mol. Brain Res. *65*, 206 (1999a).

36   H.S.G. Kalluri and M.K. Ticku: Mol. Brain Res. *68*, 159 (1999b).

37   D.M. Lovinger: Naunyn-Schmiedberg's Arch. Pharmacol. *356*, 267 (1997).

38   W.G. Tingley, M.D. Ehlers, K. Kameyama, C. Doherty, J.B. Ptak, C.T. Riley and R.L. Huganir: J. Biol. Chem. *272*, 5157 (1997).

39   L. Chen and L.-Y.M. Huang: Nature *356*, 521 (1992).

40   Z.-G. Xiong, R. Raouf, W.-Y. Lu, L.-Y. Wang, B.A. Orser, E.M. Dudek, M.D. Browning and J.F., McDonald: Mol. Pharmacol. *54*, 1055 (1998).

41   M. Favaron, H. Manev, R. Siman, M. Bertolino, A.M. Szekely, G. DeErausquin, A. Guidotti and E. Costa: Proc. Natl. Acad. Sci. *87*, 1983 (1990).

42   P. Candeo, M. Favron, I. Lengyel, R.M. Manev, J.M. Rimland and H. Manev: J. Neurochem. *59*, 1558 (1992).

43   P. Follesa and M.K. Ticku: J. Biol. Chem. *271*, 13297 (1996).

5   D.M. Lovinger: Naunyn-Schmiedeberg's Arch. Pharmacol. *356*, 267 (1997).

45   M.F. Miles, J.E. Diaz and V.X. Deguzman: J. Biol. Chem. *266*, 2409 (1991).

46   M.F. Miles, N. Wilke, M. Elliot, W. Taanner and S. Shah: Mol. Pharmacol. *46*, 873 (1994).

47   J.R. Dave, B. Tabakoff and P.L. Hoffman: Mol. Pharmacol. *37*, 367 (1990).

48   M. Kumari and M.K. Ticku: J. Neurochem. *70*, 1467 (1998).

49   D.R. Beier, A. Sledziewski and E.T. Young: Mol. Cell Biol. *5*, 1743 (1985).

50   T. Liesen, C.P. Hollenberg and J.J. Heinisch: Mol. Microbiol. *21*, 621 (1996).

51   N. Wilke, M. Sganga, S. Barhite and M.F Miles, in: B. Jansson, H. Jörnvall, U. Rydberg, L. Terenius and B.L. Vallee (eds.): Toward a molecular basis of alcohol use and abuse, Birkhäuser Verlag, Basel 1994, pp. 49–59.

52   J. Ekblom, Q.-S. Zhu, K. Chen, and J.C. Shih: J. Neural Transm. *103*, 681 (1996).

53   K.-P Hsieh, N. Wilke, A. Harris and M.F. Miles: J. Biol. Chem. *271*, 2709 (1996).

54   S. Rahman, B. Doung and M.F. Miles: Alcohol Clin. Exp. Res. *23*, 534 (1999).

55   E.H.F. Wong and J.A. Kemp: Annu. Rev. Pharmacol. Toxicol. *31*, 407 (1991).

56   C.J. McBain and M.L. Mayer: Physiol. Rev. *74*, 723 (1994).

57   R. Robichon and M.K. Ticku: Indian J. Exp. Biol. *36*, 947 (1998).

58   M.L. Mayer and G.L. Westbrook: Prog. Neurobiol. *8*, 197 (1987).

59   J.C. Watkins: J. Med. Pharm. Chem. *5*, 1187 (1962).

60   J. Davies, A.A. Francis, A.W. Jones and J.C. Watkins: Neurosci. Lett. *12*, 77 (1981).

61   H. Betz: Neuron *5*, 383 (1990).

62   Tanabe, M. Masu, T. Ishii, R. Shigemota and S. Nakanishi: Neuron *8*, 169 (1992).

63   M. Hollmann and S. Heinemann: Annu. Rev. Neurosci. *17*, 31 (1994).

64   M. Recasens, J. Guiramand, N. Nourigat, I. Sassetti and G. Deviliers: Neurochem. Int. *13*, 463 (1988).

65   H. Sugiyama, I. Ito and M. Watanabe: Neuron *3*, 129 (1989).

66   J.-P. Pin and R. Duvoisin: Neuropharmacology *34*, 1 (1995).

67   L. Nowak, P. Bregestovski, P. Ascher, A. Herbert and A. Prochiantz: Nature *307*, 462 (1984).

68   A.B. MacDermott, M.L. Mayer, G.L. Westbrook, S.J. Smith and J.L. Barker: Nature *321*, 519 (1986).

69   S.G. Cull-Candy and M.M. Usowicz: Nature *325*, 525 (1987).

70   C.E. Jahr and C.F. Stevens: Nature *325*, 522 (1987).

71   X.-M. Yu and M.W. Salter: Nature *396*, 469 (1998).

72   C. Allgaier, P. Scheibler, D. Mueller, T.J. Feuerstein and P. Illes: Br. J. Pharmacol. *126*, 121 (1999).

73   J.C. Watkins, P. Krogsgaard-Larsen and T. Honore: Trends Pharmacol. Sci. *11*, 25 (1990).

74   R. Schoepfer, H. Monyer, B. Sommer, W. Wisden, R. Sprengel, T. Kuner, H. Lomeli, A. Herb, M. Koehler, N. Burnashev et al.: Prog. Neurosci. *42*, 353 (1994).

75   M. Benveniste and M.L. Mayer: Biophys. J. *59*, 560 (1991).

76   J.D. Clements and G.L. Westbrook: Neuron *7*, 605 (1991).

77   J. Johnson and P. Ascher: J. Physiol. *455*, 339 (1992).

78   M.L. Mayer, G.L. Westbrook and P.B. Guthrie: Nature *325*, 261 (1984).

79   P. Ascher and L. Nowak: J. Physiol. *377*, 35 (1986).

80   B. Gustafsson, H. Wigstrom, W.C. Abraham and Y.-Y. Huang: J. Neurosci. *7*, 774 (1987).

81   G.L. Collingridge and W. Singer: Trends Pharmacol Sci. *11*, 42 (1990).

82   T.V.P. Bliss and G.L. Collingridge: Nature *361*, 31 (1993).

83   H. Komuro and P. Rakic: Science *260*, 95 (1993).

84   Y. Wang, C.H. Jeng, J.C. Lin and J.Y. Wang: Alcohol Clin. Exp. Res. *20*, 1229 (1996).

85   K. Gottmann, A. Mehrle, G. Gisselmann and H. Hatt: J. Neurosci. *17*, 2766 (1997).

86   B. Meldrum and J. Garthwaite: Trends Pharmacol Sci. *11*, 379 (1990).

87   E.K. Michaelis, in: S. Grisolia and V. Felipo (eds): Cirrhosis, hyperammonemia, and hepatic encephalopathy, Plenum Press, New York 1994, pp. 119–128.

88   D.T. Monaghan, D. Yao, H.J. Oliverman, J.C. Watkins and C.W. Cotman: Neurosci. Lett. *52*, 253 (1984).

89   D.T. Monaghan, H.J. Oliverman, L. Nguyen, J.C. Watkins and C.W. Cotman: Proc. Natl. Acad. Sci. *85*, 9836 (1988).

90   M.F. Jarvis, D.E. Murphy and M. Williams: Eur. J. Pharmacol. *141*, 149 (1987).

91   D.T. Monaghan and J.A. Beaton: Eur. J. Pharmacol. *194*, 123 (1991).

92   B. Ebert, E.H.F. Wong and P. Krogsgaard-Larsen: Eur. J. Pharmacol. *208*, 49 (1991).

93   L.J. Reynolds and A.M. Palmer: J. Neurochem. *56*, 1731 (1991).

94   Y. Yoneda and K. Ogita: J. Pharmacol. Exp. Ther. *259*, 86 (1991).

95   J.A. Beaton, K. Stemsrud and D.T. Monaghan: J. Neurochem. *14*, 5202 (1992).

96   S.Y. Sakurai, J.B. Penney and A.B. Young: J. Neurochem. *60*, 1344 (1993).

97   T. Matsunaga, A.G. Mukhin and E.D. London: NeuroReport *7*, 833 (1996).

98   F.T. Mugnaini, M. van Amsterdam, E. Ratti, D.G. Trist and N.G. Bowery: Br. J. Pharmacol. *119*, 819 (1996).

99   K. Moriyoshi, M Masu, T. Ishii, R. Shigemoto, N. Mizuno and S. Nakanishi: Nature *354*, 31 (1991).

100   H. Meguro, H. Mori, K. Araki, E. Kushiya, T. Kutsuwada, M. Yamazaki, T. Kumanishi, M. Arakawa, K. Sakimura and M. Mishina: Nature *357*, 70 (1992).

101   H. Monyer, R. Sprengel, R. Schoepfer, A. Herb, M. Higuchi, H. Lomeli, N. Burnashev, B. Sakman and P. Seeburg: Science *256*, 1217 (1992).

102   T. Ishii, K. Moriyoshi, H. Sugihara, K. Sakurada, H. Kadotani, M. Yokoi, C. Akazawa, R. Shigemoto, N. Mizuno, M. Masu and S. Nakanishi: J. Biol. Chem. *268*, 2836 (1993).

103   H. Sugihara, K. Moriyoshi, T. Ishii, M. Masu and N. Nakanishi: Biochem. Biophys. Res. Comm. *185*, 826 (1992).

104   M. Hollman, J. Boulter, C. Maron, L. Beasley, J. Sullivan, G. Pecht and S. Heinemann: Neuron *10*, 943 (1993).

105   T. Kutsuwada, N. Kashiwabuchi, H. Mori, K. Sakimura, E. Kushiya, K. Araki, H. Meguro, H. Masaki, T. Kumanishi, M. Arakawa and M. Mishina: Nature *358*, 36 (1992).

106   H. Mori and M. Mishina: Neuropharmacology *34*, 1219 (1995).

107   S.D. Hess, L.P. Daggett, J. Crona, C. Deal, C.-C. Lu, A. Urrutia, L. Chavez-Noriega, S.B. Ellis, E.C. Johnson and G. Velicelebi: J. Pharmacol. Exp. Ther. *278*, 808 (1996).

108   B. Suchanek, P.H. Seeburg and R. Sprengel: J. Biol. Chem. *270*, 41 (1995).

109   M. Nagasawa, K. Sakimura, K.J. Mori, M.A. Bedell, N.G. Copeland, N.A. Jenkins and M. Mishina: Mol. Brain Res. *36*, 1 (1996)

110   M. Klein, I. Pieri, F. Uhlmann, K. Pfizenmaier and U. Eisel: Gene *208*, 259 (1998).

111   H. Monyer, N. Burnashev, D.J. Laurie, B. Sakmann and P.H. Seeburg: Neuron *12*, 529 (1994).

112   N. Nakanishi, R. Axel, and N.A. Shneider: Proc. Natl. Acad. Sci. USA *89*, 8552 (1992).

113   M. Mishina, H. Mori, K. Araki, E. Kushiya, H. Meguro, T. Kutsuwada, N. Kashiwabuchi, K. Ikeda, M. Nagasawa, M. Yamazaki et al.: Ann. N.Y. Acad. Sci. *707*, 136 (1993).

114   P.L. Chazot, S.K. Coleman, M. Cik and F.A. Stephenson: J. Biol. Chem. *269*, 24403 (1994).

115   J.C. Brimecombe, F.A. Boeckman and E. Aizenman: Proc. Natl. Acad. Sci. *94*, 11019 (1997).

116   S. Vicini, J.F. Wang, J.H. Li, W.J. Zhu, Y.H. Wang, J.H. Luo, B.B. Wolfe and D.R. Grayson: J. Neurophysiol. *79*, 555 (1998).

117   G. Kohr, S. Eckardt, H. Luddens, H. Monyer and P.H. Seeburg: Neuron *12*, 1031 (1994).

118   J.M. Sullivan, S.F. Traynelis, H.-S.V. Chen, W. Escoboar, S.F. Heinemann and S. Lipton: Neuron *13*, 929 (1994).

119   N. Brose, G.P. Gasic, D.E. Vetter, J.M. Sullivan and S.F. Heinemann: J. Biol. Chem. *268*, 22663 (1993).

120 K.A. Wafford, C.J. Bain, B. LeBourdelles, P.J. Whiting and J.A. Kemp: NeuroReport 4, 1347 (1993).

121 A.L. Buller, H.C. Larson, B.E. Schneider, J.A. Beaton, R.A. Morrisett and D.T. Monaghan: J. Neurosci. 14, 5471 (1994).

122 J. Luo, Y. Wang, R.P. Yasuda, A.W. Dunah and B.B. Wolfe: Mol. Pharmacol. 51, 79 (1997).

123 A.W. Dunah, J. Luo, Y-H. Wang, R.P. Yasuda and B.B. Wolfe: Mol. Pharmacol. 53, 429 (1998).

124 R.S. Petralia, N. Yokotani and R.J. Wenthold: J. Neurosci. 14, 667 (1994a).

125 R.S. Petralia, Y.-X. Wang and R.J. Wenthold: J. Neurosci. 14, 6102 (1994b).

126 L.S. Premkumar and A. Auerbach: J. Gen. Physiol. 110, 485 (1997).

127 M. Sheng, J. Cummings, L.A. Roldan, Y.N. Jan and L.Y. Jan: Nature 368, 144 (1994).

128 J.W. Kusiak and D.D. Norton: Brain Res. Mol. Brain Res. 20, 64 (1993).

129 K. Wedzony and A. Czyrak: Brain Res. 768, 333 (1997).

130 D.G. Standaert, C.M. Testa, J.B. Penney Jr. and A.B. Young: Neurosci. Lett 152, 161 (1993).

131 T.R. Tolle, A. Berthele, D.J. Laurie, P.H. Seeburg and W. Zieglgansberger: Eur J. Neurosci. 7, 1235 (1995).

132 M. Rigby, B. Le Bourdelles, R.P. Heavens, S. Kelly, D. Smith, A. Butler, R. Hammans, R. Hills, J.H. Xuereb, R.G. Hill, P.J. Whiting and D.J.S. Sirinathsinghji: Neurosci. 73, 429 (1996).

133 G.D. Rudolph, C.A. Cronin, G.B. Landwehrmeyer, D.G. Standaert, J.B. Penney, Jr. and A.B. Young: Neurosci. 73, 417 (1996).

134 D.J. Goebel and M.S. Poosch: Mol. Brain Res. 69, 164 (1999).

135 M. Watanabe, Y. Inoue, K. Sakimura and M. Mishina: NeuroReport 3, 1138 (1992).

136 J.D. Mikkelsen, P.J. Larsen and F.J.P. Ebling: Brain Res. 632, 329 (1993).

137 J. Zhong, D.P. Carrozza, K. Williams, D.B. Pritchett and P.B. Molinoff: J. Neurochem. 64, 531 (1995).

138 M.-C. Paupard, L.K. Friedman and R.S. Zukin: Neurosci. 79, 399 (1997).

139 M. Didier, M. Xu, S.A. Berman and S. Bursztajn: NeuroReport 6, 2255 (1995).

140 T. Takahashi, D. Feldmeyer, N. Suzuki, K. Onodera, S.G. Cull-Candy, K. Sakimura and M. Mishina: J. Neurosci. 16, 4376 (1996).

141 M.L. Vallano, B. Lambolez, E. Audinat and J. Rossier: J. Neurosci. 16, 631 (1996).

142 R. Sprengel and F.N. Single: Ann. N Y Acad Sci. 868, 494 (1999).

143 Ito, K. Futai, H. Katagiri, M. Watanabe, K. Sakimura, M. Mishina and H. Sugiyama: J. Physiol. (Lond.) 500, 401 (1997).

144 A.K. Ebralidze, D.J. Rossi, S. Tonegawa and N.T. Slater: J. Neurosci. 16, 5014 (1996).

145 H. Kadotani, T.Hirano, M. Masugi, K. Nakamura, K. Nakao, M. Katsuki and S. Nakanishi: J. Neurosci. 16, 7859 (1996).

146 Y. Li, R.S. Erzurumlu, C. Chen, S. Jhaveri and S. Tonegawa: Cell 76, 427 (1994).

147 D. Forrest, M. Yuzaki, H.D. Soares, L. Ng, D.C. Luk, M. Sheng, C.L. Stewart, J.I. Morgan, J.A. Connor and T. Curran: Neuron 13, 325 (1994).

148 T. Kutsuwada, K. Sakimura, T. Manabe, C. Takayama, N. Katakura, E. Kushiya, R. Natsume, M. Watanabe, Y. Inoue, T. Yagi et al.: Neuron 16, 333 (1996).

149 J.Z. Tsien, P.T. Huerta and S. Tonegawa: Cell 87, 1327 (1996).

150 T.J. Mchugh, K.I. Blum, J.Z. Tsien, S. Tonegawa and M.A. Wilson: Cell 87, 1339 (1996).

151 M.T.R. Lima-Landman and E.X. Albuquerque: FEBS Lett. 247, 61 (1989).

152 S.K. Kulkarni, A.K. Mehta and M.K. Ticku: Life Sci. 46, 481 (1990).

153 D.M. Lovinger, G. White and F.F. Weight: Ann. Med. 22, 247 (1990).

154 D.M. Lovinger: J. Pharmacol. Exp. Ther. 274, 164 (1995).

155   A.C. Engblom, M.J. Courtney, J.P. Kukkonen and K.E.O. Akerman: J. Neurochem. *69*, 2162 (1997).

156   S.V. Bhave, L.D. Snell, B. Tabakoff and P.L. Hoffman: Eur. J. Pharmacol. *369*, 247 (1999).

157   T. Kuner, R. Schoepfer and E.R. Korpi: NeuroReport *5*, 297 (1993).

158   B. Chu, V. Anantharam and S.N. Treistman: J. Neurochem. *65*, 140 (1995).

159   N.J. Sucher, M. Awobuluyi, Y.-B. Choi and S.A. Lipton: Trends Pharmacol. Sci. *17*, 348 (1996).

160   V. Koltchine, V. Anantharam, A. Wilson, H. Bayley and S.N. Treistman: Neurosci. Lett. *152*, 13 (1993).

161   R.L. Popp, R. Lickteig, M.D. Browning and D.M. Lovinger: Neuropharmacology *37*, 45 (1998).

162   M. Sheng and D.T. Pak: Ann. N.Y. Acad. Sci. *868*, 483 (1999).

163   D.M. Lovinger, in: M. Soyka (ed.): Acamprosate in relapse: prevention of alcoholism, Springer Verlag, New York 1996, pp. 1–26.

164   P.E. Simson, H.E. Criswell, K.B. Johnson, R.E. Hicks and G.R. Breese: J. Pharmacol. Exp. Ther. *257*, 225(1991).

165   P.E. Simson, H.E. Criswell and G.R. Breese: Brain Res. *607*, 9 (1993).

166   X. Yang, H.E. Criswell, P. Simson, S. Moy and G.R. Breese: J. Pharmacol. Exp. Ther. *278*, 114 (1996).

167   K.A. Grant and G. Colombo: J. Pharmacol. Exp. Ther. *264*, 1241 (1993).

168   K. Williams, S.L. Russell, Y.M. Shen and P.B. Molinoff: Neuron *10*, 267 (1993).

169   C. Nicolas and C. Carter: J. Neurochem. *63*, 2248 (1994).

170   W. Hundt, W. Danysz, S.M. Hoelter and R. Spanagel: Psychopharmacology *135*, 44 (1998).

171   F. Le, P.A. Wilce, D.A. Hume and B.C. Shanley: J. Neurochem. *59*, 1309 (1992).

172   R.D. Blitzer, O. Gil and E.M. Landau: Brain Res. *537*, 203 (1990).

173   R.A. Harris and W.F. Hood: J. Pharmacol. Exp. Ther. *213*, 562 (1980).

174   S.W. Leslie, J.J. Woodward, R.E. Wilcox and R.P. Farrar: Brain Res. *386*, 174 (1986).

175   J.J. Woodward and R.A. Gonzales: J. Neurochem. *54*, 712 (1990).

176   R.A. Gonzales and J.J. Woodward: J. Pharmacol. Exp. Ther. *253*, 1138 (1990).

177   M. Davidson, P. Wilce and B. Shanley: Neurosci. Lett. *89*, 165 (1988).

178   M.H. Schwatz: Brain Res. *22*, 99 (1982).

179   S.V. Bhave, L.D. Snell, B. Tabakoff and P.L. Hoffman: Alcohol Clin. Exp. Res. *20*, 934 (1996).

180   G. White, D.M. Lovinger and F.F. Weight: Brain Res. *507*, 332 (1990).

181   P.L. Hoffman, in: H. Kranzler (ed): Handbook of experimental pharmacology, Vol 114, The pharmacology of alcohol abuse, Springer Verlag, Heidelberg 1995, pp. 75–102.

182   J.L. Weiner, T.V. Dunwiddie and C.F. Valenzuela: Mol. Pharmacol. *56*, 85 (1999).

183   C.S. Rabe and B. Tabakoff: Mol. Pharmacol. *38*, 753 (1990).

184   J.E. Dildy-Mayfield and S.W. Leslie: J. Neurochem. *56*, 1536 (1991).

185   A.L. Buller, H.C. Larson, R.A. Morisett, and D.T. Monaghan: Mol. Pharmcol. *48*, 717 (1995).

186   K. Masood, C. Wu, U. Brauneis and F.F. Weight: Mol. Pharmacol. *45*, 324 (1994).

187   T. Mirashahi and J.J. Woodward: Neuropharmacology *34*, 347 (1995).

188   R.W. Peoples and F.F. Weight: Brain Res. *571*, 342 (1992).

189   R.A. Gonzales and L.M. Brown: Life Sci. *56*, 571 (1995).

190   N.P. Murphy, J. Cordier, J. Glowinski, and J. Premont: Eur. J. Neurosci. *6*, 854 (1994).

191 J. Zhong, S.L. Russell, D.R. Pritchett, P.B. Molinoff and K. Williams: Mol. Pharmacol. *45*, 846 (1994).
192 R.L. Popp, R.L. Lickteig and D.M. Lovinger: J. Pharmacol. Exp. Ther. *289*, 1564 (1999).
193 V. Anantharam, R. Panchal, A. Wilson, V.V. Koltchine, S.N. Treistman and H. Bayley: FEBS Lett. *305*, 27 (1992).
194 M. Yamazaki, H. Mori, K. Araki, J. Mori and M. Mishina: FEBS Lett. *300*, 39 (1992).
195 T. Yamakura, H. Mori, H. Masaki, K. Shimoji and M. Mishina: NeuroReport *4*, 687 (1993).
196 D.J. Laurie and P.H. Seeburg: J. Neurosci. *14*, 3180 (1994).
197 D.R. Lynch, N.J. Anegawa, T. Verdoorn and D.B. Pritchett: Mol. Pharmacol. *45*, 540 (1994)
198 S. Kawajiri and R. Dingledine: Neuropharmacology *32*, 1203 (1993).
199 K. Sakurada, M. Masu and S. Nakanishi: J. Biol. Chem. *268*, 410 (19930.
200 T. Mirshahi, D.L. Anders, K.M. Ronald and J.J. Woodward: J. Neurochem. *71*, 1095 (1998).
201 G.F. Koob and F.E. Bloom: Science *242*, 715 (1988).
202 B. Tabakoff and P.L. Hoffman: Behav. Genet. *23*, 231 (1993).
203 R.F. Ritzmann and B. Tabakoff: J. Pharmacol. Exp. Ther. *199*, 158 (1976).
204 K. Gulya, K.A. Grant, P. Valverius, P.L. Hoffman and B. Tabakoff: Brain Res. *547*, 129 (1991).
205 T. Ibbotson, M.J. Field and P.R. Boden: Br. J. Pharmacol. *122*, 956 (1997).
206 S. Liljequist: Eur. J. Pharmacol. *192*, 197 (1991).
207 K.A. Grant, L.D. Snell, M.A. Rogawski, A. Thurkauf and B. Tabakoff: J. Pharmacol. Exp. Ther. *260*, 1017 (1992).
208 J.C. Walker and S.F. Zornetzer: Clin. Neurophysiol. *36*, 233 (1974).
209 A. Cadete-Leite, M.A. Tavares, M.M. Volk and M.M. Paula-Barbosa: Alcohol *6*, 303 (1989).
210 D. Durand, J.A. Saint-Cyr, N. Guervich and P.L. Carlen: Brain Res. *477*, 373 (1989).
211 M.E. Charness, R.P. Simon and D.A. Greenberg: New Engl. J. Med. *321*, 442 (1989).
212 D.W. Walker, M.A. King and B.E. Hunter, in: W.A. Hunt and S.J. Nixon (eds): Alcohol-induced brain damage, NIAAA Research Monograph, U.S. Government Printing Office, Washington D.C. 1993, pp. 231–248.
213 D.W. Walker, D.E. Barnes, S.F. Zornetzer, B.E. Hunter and P. Kubanis: Science *209*, 711 (1980)
214 L. Lescaudron and A. Verna: Exp. Brain Res. *58*, 362 (1985).
215 J.N. Riley and D.W. Walker: Science *201*, 646 (1978).
216 A.J. Scheetz, J.A. Markham and E. Fifkova: Brain Res. *409*, 329 (1987).
217 D.W. Walker, W.H. Hunter, C. Wickliffe and B.A. Abraham: Alcohol Clin. Exp. Res. *5*, 267 (1981).
218 M.A. Tavares, M.M. Paula-Barbarosa and A. Cadete-Leite: Alcohol Clin. Exp. Res. *11*, 315 (1987).
219 W.C. Abraham, B.E. Hunter, S.F. Zornester and D.W. Walker: Brain Res. *221*, 271 (1981).
220 C.J. Rogers, W.C. Abraham, B.E. Hunter and D.W. Walker: Soc Neurosci. Abstr. *8*, 741 (1982).
221 D. Durand and P.L. Carlen: Brain Res. *308*, 325 (1984).
222 M.A. Collins, J.Y. Zou and E.J. Neafsey: FASEB J. *12*, 221 (1998).
223 E.K. Michaelis, M.J. Mulvaney and W.J. Freed: Biochem. Pharmacol. *27*, 1685 (1978).
224 W.J. Freed and E.K. Michaelis: Pharmacol. Biochem. Behav. *8*, 509 (1978).
225 K.A. Grant, P. Valverius, M. Hudspith and B. Tabakoff: Eur. J. Pharmacol. *176*, 289 (1990).

226 E. Sanna, M. Serra, A. Cossu, G. Colombo, P. Follesa and G. Biggio, in: G. Biggio, A. Concas and E. Costa (eds): GABAergic synaptic transmission, Raven Press, New York 1992, pp. 317–324.
227 E. Sanna, M. Serra, A. Cossu, G. Colombo, P. Follesa, T. Cuccheddu, A. Concas and G. Biggio: Alcohol Clin. Exp. Res. *17*, 115 (1993).
228 L.D. Snell, B. Tabakoff and P.L. Hoffman: Brain Res. *602*, 91 (1993).
229 P. Valverius, J.C. Crabbe, P.L. Hoffman and B. Tabakoff: Eur. J. Pharmacol. *184*, 185 (1990).
230 J.G. Rudolph, D.W. Walker, Y. Iimuro, R.G. Thurman and F.T. Crews: Alcohol Clin. Exp. Res. *21*, 1508 (1997).
231 L. Trevisan, L.W. Fitzgerald, N. Brose, G.P. Gasic, S.F. Heinemann, R.S. Duman and E.J. Nestler: J. Neurochem. *62*, 1635 (1994).
232 H.S.G. Kalluri, A.K. Mehta and M.K. Ticku: Mol. Brain Res. *58*, 221 (1998).
233 L.D. Snell, K.R. Nunley, R.L. Lickteig, M.D. Browning, B. Tabakoff and P.L. Hoffman: Mol. Brain Res. *40*, 71 (1996).
234 P. Follesa and M.K. Ticku: Mol. Brain Res. *29*, 99 (1995).
235 P.A. Hardy, W. Chen and P.A. Wilce: Brain Res. *819*, 33 (1999).
236 K.R. Iorio, L. Reinlib, B. Tabakoff and P.L. Hoffman: Mol. Pharmacol. *41*, 1142 (1992).
237 X.-J. Hu and M.K. Ticku: Mol. Brain Res. *30*, 347 (1995).
238 C.T. Smothers, J.J. Mrotek and D.M. Lovinger: J. Pharmacol. Exp. Ther. *283*, 1214 (1997).
239 P.L. Hoffman, K.R. Iorio, L.D. Snell and B. Tabakoff: Alcohol Clin. Exp. Res. *19*, 721 (1995).
240 L.J. Chandler, D. Norwood and G. Sutton: Alcohol Clin. Exp. Res. *23*, 363 (1999).
241 X.-J. Hu, P. Follesa and M.K. Ticku: Mol. Brain Res. *36*, 211 (1996).
242 M. Sasner and A. Bounannno: J. Biol. Chem. *271*, 21316 (1996).
243 Pieri, M. Klein, C. Bayertz, J. Gerspach, A. van der Ploeg, K. Pfizenmaier and U. Klein: Eur J. Neurosci. *11*, 2083 (1999).
244 M. Kozak: J. Biol. Chem. *266*, 19867 (1991).
245 D. Curtis, R. Lehmann and P.D. Zamore: Cell *81*, 171 (1995).
246 M.W. Wood, H.M.A. VanDongen, and A.M.J. VanDongen: J. Biol. Chem. *270*, 8115 (1996).
247 G. Bai and J.W. Kusiak: J. Biol. Chem. *272*, 5936 (1997).
248 M. Ozaki, M. Sasner, R. Yano, H.S. Lu and A. Buonanno: Nature *390*, 691 (1997).
249 G. Bai, D.D. Norton, M.S. Prenger and J.W. Kusiak: J. Biol. Chem. *273*, 1086 (1998).
250 D. Krainc, G. Bai, S. Okamoto, M. Carles, J.W. Kusiak, R.N. Brent and L.A. Lipton: J. Biol. Chem. *273*, 26218 (1998).
251 K.R. Iorio, B. Tabakoff and P.L. Hoffman: Eur. J. Pharmacol. *248*, 209 (1993).
252 K.A. Hartnett, A.K. Stout, S. Rajdev, P.A. Rosenberg, I.J. Reynolds and E. Aizenman: J. Neurochem. *68*, 1836 (1997).
253 B. Webb, M.B. Heaton and D.W. Walker: Alcohol Clin. Exp. Res. *21*, 1643 (1997).
254 H. Bito: Cell Calcium *23*, 143 (1998).
255 S. Chen, D. Moore-Nichols, H. Nguyen and E.K. Michaelis: J. Neurochem. *72*, 1969 (1999).
256 H. Manev, A. Favaron, A. Guidotti and E. Costa: Mol. Pharamcol. *36*, 106 (1989).
257 H. Urushihara, M. Tohda and Y. Nomura: J. Biol. Chem. *267*, 11697 (1992).
258 S.-J. Chen and J.P. Leonard: J. Neurochem. *67*, 194 (1996).
259 K. Spuhler-Phillips, J. Gonzalez, P.K. Randall and S.W. Leslie: Alcohol Clin. Exp. Res. *19*, 305 (1995).

260   T.J. O'Dell, E.R. Kandel and S.G.N. Grant: Nature *353*, 558 (1991).
261   W.G. Tingley, K.W. Roche, A.K. Thompson and R.L. Huganir: Nature *364*, 70 (1993).
262   I.S. Moon, M.L. Apperson and M.B. Kennedy: Proc. Natl. Acad. Sci. *91*, 3954 (1994).
263   L.F. Lau and R.L. Huganir: J. Biol. Chem. *270*, 20036 (1995).
264   X.-M. Yu, R. Askalan, G.J. Keil I and M.W. Salter: Science *275*, 674 (1997).
265   D.N. Lieberman and I. Mody: Nature Neurosci. 2, *125* (1999).
266   R.A. Hall and T.R. Soederling: J. Biol. Chem. *14*, 4135 (1997).
267   M. Inomata, Y. Takayama, H. Kiyama, S. Nada, M. Okada and H. Nakagawa: J. Biol. Chem. *116*, 386 (1994).
268   S.V. Bhave, L. Ghoda and P.L. Hoffman: J. Neurosci. *19*, 3277 (1999).
269   D.S. Bredt and S.H. Snyder: Neuron *8*, 3 (1992).
270   L.J. Chandler, N.J. Guzman, C. Sumners and F.T. Crews: J. Pharmacol. Exp. Ther. *271*, 67 (1994).
271   L. Volicer and B.A. Klosowicz: Biochem. Pharmacol. *28*, 2677 (1979).
272   A.P. Ferko, E. Bobyock and W.S. Chernick: Toxicol. Applied Pharmacol. *64*, 447 (1982).
273   L.J. Chandler, G. Sutton, D. Norwood, C. Sumners and F.T. Crews: Mol. Pharmacol. *51*, 733 (1997).
274   M.L. Adam, B.N. Sewing, J. Chen, E.R. Meyer and T.J. Cicero: Alcohol Clin. Exp. Res. *19*, 195 (1995).
275   J.Y. Zou, D.B. Martinez, E.J. Neafsey and M.A. Collins: Alcohol Clin. Exp. Res. *20*, 1406 (1996).

Progress in Drug Research, Vol. 54 (E. Jucker, Ed.)
© 2000 Birkhäuser Verlag, Basel (Switzerland)

Troglitazone and emerging glitazones: New avenues for potential therapeutic benefits beyond glycemic control

By Hiroyoshi Horikoshi[1],
Toshihiko Hashimoto[2] and
Toshihiko Fujiwara[3]

[1]Sankyo Pharma Research Institute,
La Jolla, CA 92037, USA;
[2]Sankyo Co., Ltd., R & D Planning
and Management Dept.
[3]Molecular Biology and Pharmacology Research Laboratories, Tokyo
140-8761, Japan

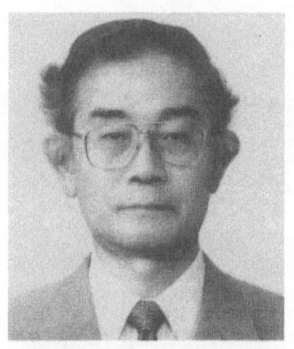

Hiroyoshi Horikoshi

was born in 1941 and obtained a D.V.M. in 1966 and a Ph.D. in 1973 from the University of Tokyo. He was a visiting scientist at the Washington University School of Medicine, St. Louis from 1968–1971, and at the University of Colorado Health Sciences Center, Denver from 1981– 1983. He joined Sankyo Co., Ltd., Tokyo, in 1973 and has worked as a pharmacologist in charge of research on diabetes and endocrine diseases. He is President of Sankyo Pharma Research Institute, La Jolla, California, and Senior Research Director of the Research Institute at Sankyo Co., Ltd., Tokyo, Japan.

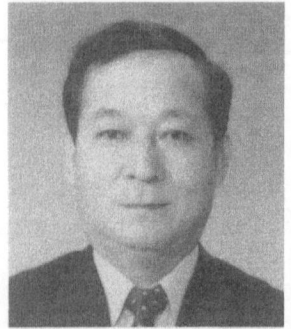

Toshihiko Hashimoto

was born in 1946 and obtained a Ph.D. in 1978 from the University of Tokyo. He was a visiting scientist at the University of Southern California, Hydrocarbon Research Institute, Los Angeles from 1984–1986. He joined Sankyo Co., Ltd., Tokyo, in 1972 and has worked as medicinal chemist and coordinator on diabetes research. He is Deputy Director of Sankyo's Licensing Department.

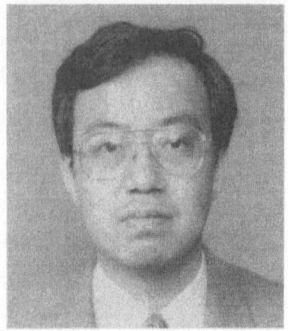

Toshihiko Fujiwara

was born in 1954 and obtained his Ph.D. in 1990 from the University of Tokyo. He was a visiting scientist at the Vanderbilt University School of Medicine, Nashville from 1990–1992. He joined Sankyo Co., Ltd., Tokyo, in 1979, and has worked as pharmacologist in charge of diabetes research. He is Group Leader of the Pharmacology and Molecular Biology Research Laboratories.

Summary

Insulin resistance is characterized as one of the major pathogeneses of type 2 diabetes and has been associated with these same cardiovascular risk factors. Troglitazone, rosiglitazone, and pioglitazone are a new class of oral antidiabetic agents which can ameliorate peripheral insulin resistance in type 2 diabetes. There is considerable evidence that trogliterazone may have beneficial effects on cardiovascular and metabolic abnormalities associated with insulin resistance. There is supportive evidence for positive effects of the other glitazones, but they have been less well studied. These potential benefits span effects ranging from molecular events in the arterial wall to amelioration and/or improvement in lipid parameters known to be associated with atherosclerosis.

Contents

Keywords

Insulin sensitizer, troglitazone, pioglitazone, rosiglitazone, type 2 diabetes mellitus, insulin resistance, dyslipidemia, atherosclerosis, thrombosis, cardiovascular disease

Glossary of abbreviations

FAA, free fatty acid; HDL, high density lipoprotein; IMT, intimal medical thickness; LDL, low density lipoprotein; MMP, matrix metalloproteinases; NE, norepinephrine; PAI-1, plasminogen activator inhibitor-1; PDGF, platelet-derived growth factor; PPARγ, peroxisome proliferator-activated receptor γ; SMC, smooth muscle cells; TG, triglyceride; TNFα, tumor necrosis factor α

1 Introduction

Type 2 diabetes mellitus is an incurable, chronic, life-threatening disease. The majority of diabetic patients have heart disease with death rates approximately two to four times higher than adults without diabetes [1]. Coronary artery disease is the most common life-threatening disease associated with diabetes, accounting for approximately 75% of diabetes-related deaths. Diabetic retinopathy causes blindness, and diabetic neuropathy can lead to lower extremity amputation. The risk of stroke is two to four times higher in people with diabetes than in the general population. Diabetic nephropathy causes end-stage renal failure.

One of the major underlying causes of type 2 diabetes is insulin resistance, which is associated with several metabolic abnormalities known as the insulin-resistance syndrome. Insulin resistance is characterized by impaired responsiveness to endogenous or exogenous insulin, resulting in hyperinsulinemia in conjunction with normoglycemia or hyperglycemia. The insulin resistance syndrome has been associated not only with type 2 diabetes, but also with impaired glucose tolerance, hyperinsulinemia, thrombosis, dyslipidemia, atherosclerosis, and hypertension, all of which have been identified with cardiovascular risk factors [2]. Insulin resistance and/or hyperinsulinemia are also risk factors for coronary heart disease [3].

Two long-term major studies, the Diabetic Control and Complication Trial (DCCT) in type 1 diabetes and the United Kingdom Prospective Diabetes Study (UKPDS) in type 2 diabetes, demonstrated that intensive glycemic control can delay the development of macrovascular events, microvascular complications, retinopathy, nephropathy, and neuropathy [4, 5]. However, in many patients with type 2 diabetes, it is difficult to attain adequate glycemic control. Their therapeutic treatments often begin with diet and exercise alone and progress to oral hypoglycemic agents and then to insulin. Oral antidiabetic agents showed failure of their effectiveness year by year, causing many patients to lose appropriate glycemic control. Even when using these therapies in various combinations, there has often been a requirement for increasing amounts of insulin. The UKPDS study epidemiologically confirmed that in spite of intensive or conventional use of sulfonylurea agents, metformin, acarbose and/or insulin, glycemic control gradually deteriorated in many patients over time.

Troglitazone and structurally related emerging thiazolidinediones, such as rosiglitazone and pioglitazone, are novel antidiabetic drugs for treating insulin resistance. They are not related chemically or functionally to the sulfonylurea agents or to metformin.

Glitazones are insulin sensitizers. However, they do not stimulate insulin release and ameliorate the insulin-resistant state by their abilities to enhance impaired insulin-mediated glucose utilization and reduce abnormal hepatic glucose production in type 2 diabetic patients. These glitazones offer several benefits over conventional oral hypoglycemic agents. The major advantage of therapy with insulin-sensitizers includes significant improvements in hyperglycemia concomitant with reduction in hyperinsulinemia.

Troglitazone, the first of the thiazolidinedione class of oral antidiabetic drugs [6], was available for the treatment of Type 2 diabetes in 1997. Subsequent glitazones, such as rosiglitazone and pioglitazone, became available in 1999. These insulin sensitizers have the potential to treat the insulin-resistant disease states in type 2 diabetes.

The potential benefits of insulin sensitizer have been to decrease major risk factors for coronary artery disease by improving insulin resistance and to reduce mortality from cardiovascular disease among type 2 diabetes. Since troglitazone was the first in the glitazone class to be on the market, its effects have been studied most relative to several of these disease states. Rosiglitazone and pioglitazone are being increasingly studied and they are emerging as potential therapeutic agents that may also have value as insulin sensitizers.

This article reviews the potential benefits of troglitazone, pioglitazone and rosiglitazone as insulin sensitizers on cardiovascular diseases and considers other non-hypoglycemic effects of these agents.

2 Effects of insulin sensitizers on risk factors for cardiovascular disease

2.1 Effects on dyslipidemia

2.1.1 Triglycerides (TG)

Hypertriglyceridemia has been strongly identified as one of the major cardiovascular risk factors, and this risk is amplified by diabetes.

In human studies, troglitazone at doses between 400 and 800 mg/day reduced TG levels in more than a thousand patients in at least 16 large and small studies in Japan, the USA, and Europe. The first randomized, double-blind, placebo-controlled trials were conducted in Japan. Troglitazone monotherapy in 284 diet-failure type 2 patients, and troglitazone in combination therapy with sulfonylurea in 291 sulfonylurea-failure type 2 diabetic patients significantly decreased plasma TG levels [7, 8].

Results have been confirmed by clinical trials in the USA and Europe. Troglitazone used as a treatment for 6 months in 93 type 2 diabetic patients who were previously uncontrolled by diet or antidiabetic therapy, significantly decreased fasting and postprandial triglyceride levels [9]. Troglitazone at 400–600 mg/day given over 6 months in 402 type 2 diabetes patients significantly decreased TG [10]. In 330 type 2 diabetes patients previously treated with diet or oral antidiabetic agents, troglitazone given at dosages of 200– 800 mg/day decreased TG levels when doses reached 600 and 800 mg/day [11]. Decreased triglyceride levels effected by troglitazone were also observed in several other controlled, double-blind, placebo-controlled trials of patients with Type 2 diabetes [10–17], impaired glucose tolerance [18], and poorly controlled type 2 diabetes on insulin [19]. Decreases in fasting TG levels ranged from 1.1 to 2.14 mmol/L (13–26%) (package insert for Rezulin). Decreased triglyceride levels were attributed to improvement of insulin resistance.

In double-blind, placebo-controlled trials of 253 Japanese type 2 diabetes patients, pioglitazone used as monotherapy in diet-failure patients and combination therapy with sulfonylurea failure patients decreased TG levels by 1.2 to 1.5 mmol/L [20, 21]. However, in one study of 134 type 2 diabetes diet-failure patients treated for 12 weeks by pioglitazone (30 mg/day), TG levels were not significantly decreased when compared with patients on placebo [20].

Fasting lipid profiles were evaluated in 197 type 2 diabetic patients with 30 mg/day pioglitazone monotherapy for 16 weeks. Plasma TG levels were significantly decreased as compared to patients on placebo [22]. Similar results were obtained from combination therapy of pioglitazone with metformin in 328 type 2 diabetes patients [23]. In contrast, rosiglitazone monotherapy had no significant effect on plasma TG levels in type 2 diabetes patients (package inserts for Avandia).

In animal studies, troglitazone significantly decreased TG levels in ZDF rats [24], in diabetic KK mice, ob/ob mice, and Zucker fatty rats [25–27], and in fructose-fed rats [28–30], in db/db mice [31], and in aP2/DTA, fatless mice [32].

Pioglitazone decreased plasma TG levels by 50% in KKAy mice [33], but had no effect on liver or muscle TG contents [33,34]. Pioglitazone also decreased TG levels in obese aged beagle dogs [35], in obese Wistar rats [36–41], in Wistar fatty rats [42, 43], in GK rats fed high-sucrose solution [44], in Dahl salt-sensitive rats fed high-sucrose diet [45] and in spontaneously obese, insulin resistant rhesus monkeys [46].

Rosiglitazone caused a decrease in serum TG levels, but had no effect on TG production in normal rats [47]. In insulin-resistant rats fed high-fat diets, rosiglitazone decreased liver TG, but not muscle TG [48]. In comparative studies, rosiglitazone and troglitazone each decreased TG levels in obese hyperglycemic db/db mice treated for 4 weeks; rosiglitazone was much more effective than troglitazone [49].

In *in vitro* studies, troglitazone or pioglitazone administered to hepatocytes isolated from rats starved for 24 h led to inhibition of TG synthesis [50].

Troglitazone and pioglitazone appear to have similar effects in lowering TG, while rosiglitazone does not. The lack of an effect by rosiglitazone in human beings is not consistent with animal data. In human beings, the TG lowering effect of troglitazone and pioglitazone may play an important role in reducing the burden of cardiovascular disease in type 2 diabetes patients.

2.1.2 LDL concentration and size

Elevated LDL has been considered a significant risk factor for cardiovascular disease and is generally exacerbated by the presence of diabetes.

Plasma LDL concentrations were measured in four large and one small clinical trials. In 402 type 2 diabetes patients treated with troglitazone for 6 months at 100–600 mg/day, LDL increased above baseline levels by 6.5 to 10.0 mg/dl [10]. In 552 sulfonylurea-failure type 2 diabetic patients, troglitazone treatment with or without glyburide for 52 weeks caused slightly increased LDL levels. Similar results were obtained in 350 type 2 diabetes patients poorly controlled on insulin therapy [19] and in 330 type 2 patients previously treated with diet or oral antidiabetic agents [11]. LDL levels increased from 3.21 to 3.52 mmol/L with troglitazone treatment for 4 weeks in 33 type 2 diabetic patients in Japan [51].

In two studies on rosiglitazone in combination therapy with sulfonylurea or metformin, LDL levels were increased in 183 [52] and 348 type 2 diabetic patients [53]. Increased LDL levels were also seen in pioglitazone combination therapy with metformin in 328 type 2 patients [23]. LDL levels did not change in pioglitazone monotherapy in 197 type 2 patients [22].

LDL size was measured in 15 obese subjects who received 400 mg/day troglitazone for 8 weeks. Increased LDL levels were attributed to an increase in large buoyant LDL1 which were elevated from 0.45 to 0.60 mmol/L concomitant with a decrease in small density LDL3 [54]. These data support an action of troglitazone to raise LDL levels by 3–10 mg/dL through decreased small density LDL and increased large buoyant LDL. The changes in these LDL sizes may result in a pattern that is less atherogenic since it is now hypothesized that large buoyant LDL particles are not as prone to oxidative modification as small dense particles.

Simple measurements of total LDL concentrations may be misleading. The effects of these glitazones to increase LDL levels may be differential by affecting LDL size primarily. This trend may, in fact, be positive in terms of decreasing the risk of cardiovascular disease.

2.1.3 LDL oxidation

Oxidative modification of lipoproteins, including LDL and HDL, has been hypothesized to increase their atherogenic properties. In type 2 diabetes patients, increased levels of glycated LDL have been considered to be more susceptible to oxidation.

Troglitazone contains an α-tocopherol moiety and therefore may express antioxidant effects similar to vitamin E.

Troglitazone increased LDL resistance to oxidation in several human studies. In 29 type 2 diabetes patients treated with troglitazone for 8 weeks, LDL resistance to oxidation was measured by the lag phase of fluorescence development during copper treatment. Troglitazone decreased LDL oxidation in TBARS (thiobarbituric acid-reactive substances) from 5.32 nmol/L in the placebo to 3.63 nmol/L, decreased LDL hydroperoxide concentrations from 1.48 at baseline to 1.19 ng/mg, and decreased plasma E-selectin (endotherial cell-derived selectin) levels from 56.5 at baseline to 43.7 µg/L [55]. Those results were confirmed with 15 obese subjects treated with 400 mg/day troglitazone or placebo for 8 weeks [54], and in 10 healthy male subjects for 2 weeks [56].

Troglitazone-related decreases in LDL oxidation may slow down the development of atherosclerosis in patients with type 2 diabetes.

In vitro human studies with troglitazone showed the protection of LDL from oxidation. Troglitazone inhibited the formation of lipid hydroperoxides and the peroxyl radical-induced oxidation of LDL isolated from human plasma of healthy volunteers. Ascorbic acid added to the system reduced oxidized alpha-tocopherol and troglitazone moieties, verifying their antioxidant effects [57]. Troglitazone protected LDL from oxidation induced by Cu^{2+} or by 2′2′-azobis-2amidinopropanehydrochloride, and inhibited oxidation and subsequent uptake and degradation of LDL by macrophages [58]. Troglitazone inhibited lipid peroxidation of human plasma LDL more potently than α-tocopherol [59]. Troglitazone lowered copper and endothelial cell-induced oxidation of LDL and HDL isolated from human plasma, and also lowered vitamin E decay during LDL oxidative studies. Under the same oxidative stress, troglitazone was a much more potent radical scavenger than vitamin E when compared to control conditions. There were significant increases in the LDL lag phase at a troglitazone concentration of 0.50 mg/ml plasma [60].

In a comparative *in vitro* study, troglitazone and the antioxidant vitamin E, but not pioglitazone, showed scavenging effects on reactive oxygen species produced by xanthine oxidase; troglitazone showed similar effects on reactive species generated by isolated healthy human neutrophils [61].

Troglitazone may have, in addition to its insulin sensitizing effect, the ability to inhibit oxidative processes. This ability could play a crucial role in preventing the development of atherosclerotic disease.

2.1.4 Free fatty acids (FFA)

Studies of the effects of glitazones on FFA levels in human beings have been performed with troglitazone, rosiglitazone and pioglitazone.

Troglitazone reduced FFA levels by about 0.10 to 0.40 mmol/L in elderly, sulfonylurea-failure type 2 diabetic patients previously uncontrolled by diet or antidiabetic therapy type 2 diabetic patients in at least five large studies [9–11, 15, 62] and two smaller studies [12, 63]. Most studies attributed the lowering of FFA levels to a reduction in insulin resistance. Pioglitazone reduced serum FFA levels in type 2 diabetes patients [64], both in monotherapy [22] and in combination therapy with metformin [23]. Rosiglitazone also decreased serum FFA levels in type 2 diabetes patients in combination therapy with insulin [65], sulfonylurea [52], and metformin [53].

In vivo animal studies with all three glitazones showed reductions in FFA levels. Troglitazone was used in diabetic KK mice, ob/ob mice and Zucker fatty rats [24, 25, 31] and in aP2/DTA fatless mice [32]. Elevated FFA levels were decreased in all animal models. Pioglitazone normalized elevated FFA levels in Wistar fatty rats fed a high-fructose diet [36]. Rosiglitazone used as treatment in insulin-resistant rats fed high-fat diets caused normalization of FFA levels [48, 66] and reduced plasma FFA in ob/ob mice [67].

The ability to reduce FFA levels appears to be a class effect of glitazones.

2.1.5 Total cholesterol

Increased levels of various types of cholesterol, including LDL cholesterol and total cholesterol, are important risk factors for cardiovascular disease.

The available data on the effects of troglitazone on total cholesterol have given mixed results. Two studies on uncontrolled type 2 diabetic patients on sulfonylurea therapy in combination with troglitazone for 12 weeks, and in troglitazone monotherapy for 3 months showed no effect on cholesterol [8, 68]. One study in poorly controlled type 2 diabetic patients on insulin therapy for 26 weeks with troglitazone showed an increase [19] and another study on troglitazone monotherapy for 8 weeks showed a decrease in total cholesterol [12].

Pioglitazone monotherapy and combination therapy with sulfonylurea showed no significant changes on total cholesterol levels for 12 weeks [20, 21].

In animal studies, decreases of total cholesterol levels were seen with troglitazone [27, 32], while results with pioglitazone in animals were mixed. In KKAy mice, there was no effect on total cholesterol [34], but pioglitazone decreased total cholesterol levels in GK rats fed high sucrose solution [44]. In one study in normal rats given rosiglitazone, there were no effects on total cholesterol [47].

The effects that the glitazones have on total cholesterol levels are not clear at this time. However, since total cholesterol levels result from a mix of many kinds of individual cholesterol types, including HDL and LDL, differentiation of the forms of cholesterol may help simplify an understanding of specific cholesterol effects.

Glitazone therapies have been shown to decrease cholesterol levels in patients with type 2 diabetes, but the mechanism by which this is achieved is uncertain.

There is one *in vitro* comparative study in which Chinese hamster ovary cells were treated with troglitazone, rosiglitazone, pioglitazone, ciglitazone, englitazone, or PGJ2. Troglitazone, ciglitazone, and englitazone inhibited cholesterol biosynthesis in Chinese hamster ovary cells, HepG2, L6 and 3T3-L1 cells, but rosiglitazone, pioglitazone and PGJ2 showed only weak or no inhibition [69].

Peroxisome proliferation-activated receptor (PPARγ)-binding ability did not predict the potency to inhibit cholesterol biosynthesis; troglitazone's ability to inhibit cholesterol biosynthesis is likely mediated by another pathway than PPARγ. This effect may at least partially explain troglitazone's cholesterol lowering ability *in vivo* and may indicate a greater cholesterol-lowering efficacy of troglitazone over pioglitazone and rosiglitazone.

2.1.6 HDL cholesterol

HDL levels are inversely related to cardiovascular disease risk, i.e. lower levels of HDL are thought to be a risk factor for the development of cardiovascular disease.

In several human studies, troglitazone treatment in 154 type 2 patients with 800 mg/day for 48 weeks [13], in 552 sulfonylurea-failure type 2 diabetes patients with 200–600 mg/day with or without sulfonylurea for 52 weeks [15], in 330 type 2 diabetes patients previously treated with diet or oral antidiabetic agents with 100–600 mg/day for 12 weeks [11], in 402 type 2 diabetes patients previously treated with diet/exercise or sulfonylurea for 6 months [10], in 350 poorly controlled type 2 diabetes patients on insulin therapy for 26 weeks [19], and in 282 type 2 diabetes patients with or without sulfonylurea for 24 weeks [17], troglitazone significantly increased HDL levels at the 600 and 800 mg/day dosages. However, one study with troglitazone using 400 mg/day in 291 type 2 diabetes sulfonylurea-failure patients showed no effect on HDL levels [8].

The effects of pioglitazone on HDL levels were also determined by monotherapy in 20 type 2 diabetes patients [64], in 264 diet/exercise failure patients for 12 weeks with 15–45 mg/day [20], and by combination therapy in 273 sulfonylurea-failure patients for 12 weeks with 15–45 mg/day [21]. In these human studies in Japan, pioglitazone significantly increased HDL levels. Similar results were also observed in pioglitazone monotherapy in 197 type 2 patients [22].

Slight increases of HDL levels were shown in rosiglitazone combination therapy with sulfonylurea in 574 type 2 patients followed for 6 months [52].

Troglitazone, pioglitazone, and possibly rosiglitazone, appear to have the ability to increase HDL levels in patients with type 2 diabetes. The increased HDL levels may have an effect on ameliorating the risk of cardiovascular disease.

3 Effects on coagulation disorders

3.1 Plasminogen activator inhibitor-1 (PAI-1)

In patients with type 2 diabetes, basal fibrinolytic activity is impaired and plasminogen activator inhibitor-1 (PAI-1) content is increased in atherosclerotic lesions. This may accelerate not only the development of cardiovascular disease, but also the occurrence of myocardial infarction.

Two clinical studies have looked at the effect of troglitazone on PAI-1 levels. In a randomized placebo controlled trial, 18 patients with type 2 diabetes were treated with troglitazone and placebo for 26 weeks. Plasma PAI-1 concentrations decreased significantly from 68.8 ng/ml to 40.4 ng/ml in the troglitazone treated patients. Elevated plasma PAI-1 concentrations were normalized in eight of 18 patients treated with troglitazone [70]. Both plasma PAI-1 and fibrinogen levels were decreased significantly in a clinical study on 12 patients with type 2 diabetes treated with troglitazone as monotherapy and in combination with gliclazide for 12 weeks [71]. Significant decreases of plasma PAI-1 levels were also observed in women with polycystic ovary syndrome and impaired glucose tolerance who were treated with troglitazone for 12 weeks [72].

These clinical results indicate that troglitazone may be able to lower PAI-1 concentrations in patients with type 2 diabetes. Results will have to be verified in larger-scale, controlled clinical trials.

Troglitazone (3 µg/ml) inhibited PAI-1 expression by 23%, and TGFβ induced PAI-1 expression by 34% in human aortic smooth muscle cells, and by 32% in human umbilical vein endothelial cells (HUVEC) [73]. Human vascular smooth muscle cells were treated with TNFα and pioglitazone (10–1000 µM) for 24 h. Pioglitazone suppressed TNFα induced increases in PAI-1 secretion and also suppressed PAI-1 secretion by 55% and mRNA levels by 37% when compared to controls [74].

In cultured HUVEC, troglitazone and pioglitazone decreased basal and TNFα stimulated PAI-1 secretion and mRNA expression in HUVEC in a dose-dependent fashion [75]. These *in vitro* data indicate that troglitazone and pioglitazone directly inhibit PAI-1 expression in vessel walls.

Based on these *in vivo* and *in vitro* data, glitazones may have beneficial effects on fibrinolysis in preventing and treating accelerated cardiovascular disease and vascular complications in diabetic patients.

3.2 Platelet aggregation

Platelet aggregation is elevated in patients with type 2 diabetes and may thus play a role in their increased risk of cardiovascular disease.

In the only *in vitro* study on human platelet aggregation [76], platelets were treated with troglitazone, pioglitazone and vitamin E for 60 min. Troglitazone and vitamin E decreased platelet aggregation induced by ADP, collagen, and thrombin, but pioglitazone did not cause a decrease.

These results indicate that the α-tocopherol moiety may play an important role in troglitazone's ability to inhibit platelet aggregation in human platelets. However, inhibition of platelet aggregation may not be an effect of the glitazones in general.

4 Direct vascular effects

4.1 Intimal medial thickness (IMT)

Intimal medial thickness in the carotid arterial wall is generally recognized as a measurement of atherosclerotic progression in patients with and/or without type 2 diabetes, though it is still not clear whether the cause is a direct action of insulin or a result of insulin resistance.

The only human clinical trials conducted with troglitazone have been in Japan. In 57 type 2 diabetic patients treating with 400 mg/day of troglitazone for 3–6 months, IMT was decreased from 0.087 to 0.027 mm [16]. These effects were observable in 3 months. Troglitazone given for 6 months also significantly reduced neointimal hyperplasia by about 50% in 12 type 2 diabetic patients with coronary stent implants as compared with diet-only treatment [77]. These studies strongly indicate that troglitazone could reduce intimal hyperplasia in type 2 diabetes patients whether or not they have had coronary stent implants.

In animal *in vivo* studies, Zucker fatty rats were treated for 14 days with troglitazone after being subjected to balloon injury of the aorta. The neointimal area and the ratio of neointimal to medial area decreased by 53–62%. These effects were attributed to the inhibition of DNA synthesis in vascular smooth muscle cells synthesis [78, 79]. The intima density was reduced in Wistar fatty and lean rats treated for 7 days with pioglitazone after carotid arterial intimal thickening lesions induced by balloon catheter. The enhanced effects of SMC growth and proliferation in diabetic state were inhibited [80].

In these animal studies, both troglitazone and pioglitazone showed an ability *in vivo* to inhibit intimal hyperplasia.

It appears that troglitazone, and perhaps pioglitazone, is able to potently inhibit intimal hyperplasia and may thus prevent the development of atherosclerosis in type 2 diabetes patients. These effects are most often attributed to the inhibition of smooth muscle cell proliferation and migration.

4.2   Smooth muscle cells (SMC)

Vascular smooth muscle cell proliferation and migration play an important role in the pathogenesis of atherosclerosis as general cellular responses to arterial injury.

Both troglitazone and pioglitazone have been evaluated in human *in vitro* studies. Troglitazone inhibited platelet-derived growth factor (PDGF)-induced SMC proliferation by 78–91% and migration in cultured vascular cells [81, 82]. It also inhibited mitogen-activated protein kinase (MAPkinase) activity and suppressed insulin-induced increases in human aortic SMC DNA synthesis in a dose-dependent fashion [83]. The number of cultured human umbilical vein endothelial cells was reduced 36% by pioglitazone when compared to untreated control cells [84]. Those observations indicate that both glitazones were able to inhibit SMC proliferation and/or migration.

Matrix metalloproteinases (MMP) play a role in vascular SMC migration, which in turn is a critical aspect of atherosclerosis.

In a human *in vitro* study, troglitazone inhibited matrix metalloproteinase-9 secretion in human monocyte-derived macrophages and MMP-9 mRNA and protein levels in human vascular smooth muscle cells *via* PPARγ activation [82, 85].

Troglitazone inhibited MMP-9 secretion and activity in macrophages and SMC, and thus may be able to play a role in regulating atherosclerosic plaque rupture and inhibiting the progression of atherosclerosis.

Similar effects were seen in animal *in vitro* studies. High-glucose induced SMC migration and proliferation were suppressed by cultured rabbit coronary cells [86]. In cultured rat cells, DNA synthesis and SMC migration induced-angiotensin II, basic fibroblast growth factor (bFGF) and PDGF were inhibited by troglitazone or pioglitazone [79, 87–89]. These antiproliferative effects of troglitazone may be partially due to enhancement of SMC differentiation [75].

The only *in vivo* data on the effects of pioglitazone are from animals. Pioglitazone treated Wistar fatty rats at day 10 had their SMC outgrowth rate decreased by 42% compared to untreated fatty rats [80]. Pioglitazone reduced DNA synthesis in the neointima of Wistar rats subjected to injury of the common carotid artery [43].

Troglitazone and pioglitazone have shown potent effects in inhibiting SMC proliferation and/or migration. Since increased SMC proliferation and migration lead directly to increased intimal medial thickness, the effects of these glitazones on vascular tissue may prove very important in preventing the progression of atherosclerosis in patients with type 2 diabetes.

4.3 Endothelial dysfunction

Endothelial function is generally measured by vascular reactivity and peripheral resistance, and is often impaired in patients with type 2 diabetes.

Only human studies have been performed with troglitazone. Patients with peripheral vascular disease and occult diabetes treated with troglitazone for 4 months had brachial artery vasoactivity normalized after 5 min of brachial artery occlusion [90]. In nine type 2 diabetic patients treated with 400 mg/day troglitazone for 4 months, troglitazone significantly improved their responses to endothelium-dependent acetylcholine in the left coronary artery. These improvements were measured by reactive changes in coronary artery diameter (0.6 ± 3.6 % to 7.0 ± 5.7% for the troglitazone-treated group vs 1.3 ± 2.3% to 1.4 ± 2.4% for diet or sulfonyl urea-treated groups), and by coronary blood flow (48 ± 20% to 108 ± 53% for troglitazone-treated group vs 45 ± 205 to 39 ± 23% for the control group) [91].

Nondiabetic, insulin resistant male subjects treated with troglitazone for 4 weeks had improved endothelium-dependent flow-mediated dilatation in the brachial artery. Increased forearm blood flow and decreased forearm vascular resistance were observed 2 h after a single 200 mg dose of troglitazone administered to 11 lean healthy males. Forearm blood flow increased significantly from 3.66 to 4.81 ml/dl/min and forearm vascular resistance significantly decreased from 24.7 to 20.2 units [92]. Increased stroke volume index and cardiac index, significant decreases in diastolic pressure, and decreased estimated peripheral resistance were observed in a long-term clinical trial in which 154 type 2 diabetic patients were treated with troglitazone for 48 weeks [13].

However, in 15 obese subjects with insulin resistance treated with troglitazone for 8 weeks, endothelial vascular function remained normal despite impaired vasodilator responses to insulin. It was concluded that troglitazone improved insulin sensitivity, but it had no effects on endothelium-dependent and endothelium–independent vascular responses [93]. In patients with type 2 diabetes, troglitazone generally improved vascular reactivity, increased blood flow, and decreased peripheral resistance, with one exception in obese subjects.

In comparative studies, small arteries with intact endothelium from human subcutaneous fat were treated with rosiglitazone, troglitazone or α-tocopherol. Troglitazone, but not rosiglitazone or α-tocopherol, relaxed norepinephrine-constricted arteries by 69.4% [94]. In arteries from Wistar fatty rats, a similar vasorelaxant effect for troglitazone was shown and the effect was also independent of nitric oxide. Indomethacin replaced troglitazone's vasorelaxant effect with a vasoconstrictive effect and enhanced rosiglitazone's vasoconstrictive effect 58.5% over norepinephrine-constricted baseline. This NO-independent, indomethacin-sensitive vasorelaxant effect of insulin sensitizer could possibly lead to fluid retention, edema, and hemodilution [95].

Similar improvements in vascular reactivity were seen in both troglitazone (*in vivo* and *in vitro*) and pioglitazone (*in vitro*) studies. Troglitazone treatment for 7 days in streptozotocin-induced diabetic rats decreased perfusion pressure by 13% in rat hindlimb and significantly increased skin blood flow at the base of the tail. These vasodilatory effects were indomethacin sensitive, but not nitric oxide sensitive. Similar effects were attributed to increases in PGI2 and PGE2 production in aorta wall rings in rats [96].

Troglitazone, but not rosiglitazone, caused an acute increase in skin blood flow in normal Wistar-Imamichi rats; vitamin E and pioglitazone affected skin blood flow to a lesser extent in rats [96].

In other *in vitro* animal studies, troglitazone increased the EC_{50} values for phenylephrine- and KCl (depolarizing agent)-induced contractions and abolished BAY K 8644 (Calbiochem, voltage-gated Ca channel agonist)-induced contractions in rat thoracic aortic rings with no endothelium. These effects were synergistic with insulin and were attributed to inhibition of Ca^{2+} influx [97]. Troglitazone prevented or attenuated high-glucose-induced relaxation defects in normal adult rat ventricular myocytes. Results were attributed to troglitazone's ability to prevent high-glucose-induced impairment of Ca^{2+} transient decay [98]. In addition, troglitazone attenuated contractile response to norepinephrine and potassium chloride, and increased relaxant responses to sodium nitroprusside and acetylcholine in endothelium-intact rat tail artery rings. These effects were dependent on the presence of Ca^{2+}, but independent of insulin and NO [99, 100].

Pioglitazone blunted contractile responses to norepinephrine (NE) and potassium by 42% in rat aortic tail rings, but only in the presence of calcium [101, 102]. Pioglitazone blunted contractile responses to NE, but not to angiotensin II in rat thoracic aorta strips. Pioglitazone had no effect on vasoconstriction in response to NE in fructose-fed rats. Pioglitazone alone or with insulin augmented acetylcholine-induced, but not nitroprusside-induced, vasodilation in rat thoracic aorta strips [103, 104]. In spontaneous hypertensive rats, pioglitazone inhibited vasopressin-induced and NE-induced vasoconstriction in aortae and superior mesenteric arteries [105].

Troglitazone was able to improve endothelial function in patients with type 2 diabetes and in animal models of type 2 diabetes. These results were most often attributed to troglitazone's effect on calcium channels. Pioglitazone likely shares this ability. These effects may prove important in the preservation of cardiovascular health in patients with type 2 diabetes.

4.4 Cardiac output

In human clinical trials, troglitazone increased the stroke volume index from 32.43 at baseline to 34.89 after 48 weeks of treatment. The cardiac index changes ranged from 6.6–13.2% in 154 type 2 diabetic patients treated with

800 mg/day for 48 weeks as compared to glyburide; the left ventricular mass index was not affected [13]. These results appear to be maintained through 96 weeks of study [106].

In an animal study on hearts isolated from streptozotocin-induced diabetic rats treated for 6 weeks with troglitazone, there was partially normalized basal heart rate, cardiac work, and ultrastructural damage, and improved postischemic functional problems including heart rate, left ventricular developed pressure, and cardiac works [107]. Troglitazone has direct positive inotropic, positive lusitropic, negative chronotropic, and coronary artery dilating effects in isolated perfused rat hearts [108].

Troglitazone increased stroke volume and cardiac indices in humans, and had beneficial effects on basal heart rate, cardiac work, and other measures in animals.

Troglitazone may have the ability to directly improve cardiac function in patients with type 2 diabetes. This ability may or may not be shared with other members of the class.

5 Summary and conclusions

Type 2 diabetes patients are more likely than nondiabetic subjects to have or develop cardiovascular risk factors such as hypertension, dyslipidemia, atherogenic lipid abnormalities, and coagulation disorders. Insulin resistance is characterized as one of the major pathogeneses of type 2 diabetes and it has been associated with these same cardiovascular risk factors.

Troglitazone, rosiglitazone, and pioglitazone are a new class of oral antidiabetic agents which can ameliorate peripheral insulin resistance in type 2 diabetes.

There is considerable evidences that troglitazone may have benefical effects on cardiovascular and metabolic abnormalities associated with insulin resistance. There is supportive evidence for positive effects of the other glitazones, but they have been less well studied. These potential benefits span effects ranging from molecular events in the arterial wall to amelioration and/or improvement in lipid parameters known to be associated with atherosclerosis.

Such benefits need to be considered as part of antidiabetic therapies, particularly given the very high vascular and metabolic risk factors that diabetic patients face as a part of the natural history of their disease.

References

1   National Institute of Health, National Institute of Diabetes and Digestive Diseases: Diabetes Statistics, Pub. No. 96–3926 (1995).
2   Hunter S.J. and Garvey W.T.: Am. J. Med. *105*, 331–345 (1998).
3   Reaven G.M.: Physiol. Rev. *75*, 473–486 (1995).
4   DCCT Research Group: N. Engl. J. Med. *329*, 977–986 (1993).
5   UK Prospective Diabetes Study (UKPDS) Group: Lancet *352*, 837–865 (1998).
6   Iwamoto Y., Kuzuya T., Matsuda A., Awata T., Kumakura S., Inooka G. and Shiraishi I.: Diabetes Care *14*, 1083–1086 (1991).
7   Iwamoto Y., Kosaka K., Kuzuya T., Akanuma Y., Shigeta Y. and Kaneko T.: Diabetes Care *19*, 151–156 (1996).
8   Iwamoto Y., Kosaka K., Kuzuya T., Akanuma Y., Shigeta Y. and Kaneko T.: Diabet. Med. *13*, 365–370 (1996).
9   Maggs D.G., Buchanan T.A., Burant C.F., Cline G., Gumbiner B., Hsueh W.A., Inzucchi S., Kelley D., Nolan J. and Olefsky J.M.: Ann. Intern. Med. *128*, 176–185 (1998).
10 Fonseca V.A., Valiquett T.R., Huang S.M., Ghazzi M.N. and Whitcomb R.W.: J. Clin. Endocrinol. Metab. *83*, 3169–3176 (1998).
11 Kumar S., Boulton A.J., Beck-Nielsen H., Berthezene F., Muggeo M., Persson B., Spinas G.Z., Donoghue S., Lettis S. and Stewart-Long P.: Diabetologia *39*, 701–709 (1996).
12 Mimura K., Umeda F., Hiramatsu S., Taniguchi S., Ono Y., Nakashima N., Kobayashi K., Masakado M., Sako Y. and Nawata H.: Diabet Med. *11*, 685–691 (1994).
13 Ghazzi M.N., Perez J.E., Antonucci T.K., Driscoll J.H., Huang S.M., Faja B.W. and Whitcomb R.W.: Diabetes *46*, 433–439 (1997).
14 Shimizu H., Tsuchiya T., Sato N., Shimomura Y., Kobayashi I. and Mori M.: Diabetes Care *21*, 1470–1474 (1998).
15 Horton E.S., Whitehouse F., Ghazzi M.N., Venable T.C. and Whitcomb R.W.: Diabetes Care *21*, 1462–1469 (1998).
16 Minamikawa J., Tanaka S., Yamauchi M., Inoue D. and Koshiyama H.: J. Clin. Endocrinol. Metab. *83*, 1818–1820 (1998).
17 Nozue T., Minagawa F., Michishita I. and Genda A.: Diabetes Care *22*, 355–356 (1999) (Commentary).
18 Antonucci T., Whitcomb R., McLain R., Lockwood D. and Norris R.M.: Diabetes Care *20*, 188–193 (1997).
19 Schwartz S., Raskin P., Fonseca V. and Graveline J.F.: N. Engl. J. Med. *338*, 861–866 (1998).
20 Kaneko T., Baba S. Toyota T., Akanuma Y., Sakamoto N., Shigeta Y., Shichiri M. and Nakano S.: Jap. J. Clin. Exper. Med. *74*, 1491–1514 (1997).
21 Kaneko T., Baba S. Toyota T., Akanuma Y., Sakamoto N., Shigeta Y., Shichiri M. and Nakano S.: Jap. J. Clin. Exper. Med. *74*, 1515–1539 (1997).
22 Mathisen A., Geerlof J. and Houser V.: Diabetes *48* (Suppl. 1), A102–103 (1999).
23 Egan J., Rubin C. and Mathisen A.: Diabetes *48* (Suppl. 1), A106 (1999).
24 Sreenan S., Sturis J., Pugh W., Burant C.F. and Polonsky K.S.: Am. J. Pathol. *271*, E742–E747 (1996).
25 Fujiwara T., Yoshioka S., Yoshioka T., Ushiyama I., Horikoshi H.: Diabetes *37*, 1549–1558 (1988).
26 Okuno A., Tamemoto H., Tobe K., Ueki K., Mori Y., Iwamoto K., Umesono K., Akanuma Y., Fujiwara T., Horikoshi H. et al.: J. Clin. Invest. *101*, 1354–1361 (1998).

27   Yoshioka S., Nishino H., Shiraki T., Ikeda K., Koike H., Okuno A., Wada M., Fujiwara T. and Horikoshi H.: Metabolism *42*, 75–80 (1993).
28   Lee M.K., Miles P.D., Khoursheed M., Gao K.M., Mossa A.R. and Olefsky J.M.: Diabetes *43*, 1435–1439 (1994).
29   Chen S., Noguchi Y., Izumida T., Tatebe J. and Katayama S.: J. Hypertens. *14*, 1325–1330 (1996).
30   Inoue I., Katayama S., Takahashi K., Negishi K., Miyazaki T., Sonoda M. and Komoda T.: Biochem. Biophys. Res. Commun. *235*, 113–116 (1997).
31   Fujiwara T., Wada M., Fukuda K., Fukami M., Yoshioka S., Yoshioka T. and Horikoshi H.: Metabolism *40*, 1213–1218 (1991).
32   Burant C.F., Sreenan S., Hirano K., Tai T.A. , Lohmiller J., Lukens J., Davidson N.O. , Ross S. and Graves R.A.: J. Clin. Invest. *100*, 2900–2908 (1997).
33   Saha A.K., Kurowski T.G., Colca J.R. and Ruderman N.B.: Am. J. Physiol. *267*, E95–E101 (1994).
34   Castle C.K., Colca J.R. and Melchior G.W.: Arterioscler. Thromb. *13*, 302–309 (1993).
35   Ikeda H., Taketomi S., Sugiyama Y., Shimura Y., Shoda T., Meguro K. and Fujita T.: Arzneimittelforschung *40*, 156–62 (1990).
36   Ikeda T. and Fujiyama K.: Metabolism *47*, 1152–1155 (1998).
37   Kazumi T., Hirano T., Odaka H., Ebara T., Amano N., Hozumi T., Ishida Y. and Yoshino G.: Diabetes *45*, 806–11 (1996).
38   Sugiyama Y., Taketomi S., Shimura Y., Ikeda H. and Fujita T.: Arzneimittelforschung *40*, 263–267 (1990).
39   Sugiyama Y., Shimura Y. and Ideda H.: Arzneimittelforschung *40*, 436–440 (1990).
40   Suzuki M., Nomura C., Odaka H. and Ikeda H.: Jpn. J. Pharmacol. *74*, 297–302 (1997).
41   Murase K., Odaka H., Suzuki M., Tayuki N. and Ikeda H.: Diabetologia *41*, 257–64 (1998).
42   Odaka H., Sano Y., Amano N. and Ikeda H.: Jap. Pharmacol. Ther. *25*, 355–361 (1997).
43   Yoshimoto T., Naruse M., Seki T., Nishikawa M., Naruse K., Tanabe A., Seki T., Aikawa E. and Demura H.: Hypertension *29*, 909 (1997) (Abstract).
44   Odaka H., Kataoka O., Suwa Y., Tayuki N., Amano N. and Ikeda H.: Jap. Pharmacol. Ther. *25*, 345–353 (1997).
45   Kurowski T.G., Saha A.K., Cunningham B.A., Holbert R.I., Colca J.R., Corkey B.E. and Ruderman N.B.: Metabolism *45*, 519–525 (1996).
46   Kemnitz J.W., Elson D.F., Roecker E.B., Baum S.T., Bergman R.N. and Meglasson M.D.: Diabetes *43*, 204–11 (1994).
47   Lefebvre A.M., Peinado-Onsurbe J., Leitersdorf I., Briggs M.R., Paterniti J.R., Fruchart J.C., Fievet C., Auwerx J. and Staels B.: Arterioscler. Thromb. Vasc. Biol. *17*, 1756–64 (1997).
48   Oakes N.D., Camilleri S., Furler S.M., Chisholm D.J. and Kraegen E.W.: Metabolism *46*, 935–942 (1997).
49   Berger J., Bailey P., Biswas C., Cullinan C.A., Doebber T.W., Hayes N.S., Saperstein R., Smith R.G. and Leibowitz M.D.: Endocrinology *137*, 4189–4195 (1996).
50   Fulgencio J.P., Kohl C., Girard J. and Pegorier J.P.: Diabetes *45*, 1556–62 (1996).
51   Matsumoto K., Miyake S., Yano M., Ueki Y. and Tominaga Y.: Metabolism *48*, 1–2 (1999).
52   Gomis R., Jones N.P., Vallance S.C. and Patwardhan R.: Diabetes *48* (Suppl. 1), A63 (1999).
53   Forseca V., Biswas N. and Salzman A.: Diabetes *48* (Suppl. 1), A100 (1999).
54   Tack C.J., Smits P., Demacker P.N. and Stalenhoef A.F.: Diabetes Care *21*, 796–799 (1998).
55   Cominacini L., Garbin U., Fratta-Pasini A., Campagnola M., Davoli A., Foot E., Sighieri G., Sironi A.M., Lo-Cascio V. and Ferrannini E.: Diabetes *47*, 130–133 (1998).

56   Cominacini L., Young M.M. , Capriati A., Garbin U., Fratta-Pasini A., Campagnola M., Cavoli A., Gigoni A., Contessi G.B. and Lo-Cascio V.: Diabetologia 40, 1211–1218 (1997).

57   Noguchi N., Sakai H., Kato Y., Tsuchiya J., Yamamoto Y., Niki E., Horikoshi H. and Kodama T.: Atherosclerosis 123, 227–234 (1996).

58   Crawford R.S., Mudaliar S.R., Henry R.R. and Chait A.: Diabetes 48, 783–790 (1999).

59   Nagasaka Y., Daku K., Nakamura K. and Kaneko T.: Biochem. Pharmacol. 50, 1109–1111 (1995).

60   Cominacini L., Garbin U., Pastorina A.M. , Campagnola M., Fratta-Pasini A., Davoli A., Rigoni A. and Lo-Cascio V.: Diabetologia 40, 165–172 (1997).

61   Kumar S., Prange A., Schulze J., Lettis S. and Barnett A.H.: Diabet. Med. 15, 772–779 (1998).

62   Suter S.L., Nolan J.J., Wallace P., Gumbiner B. and Olefsky J.M.: Diabetes Care 15, 193–203 (1992).

63   Yamasaki Y., Kawamori R., Wasada T., Sato A., Omori Y., Eguchi H., Tominaga M., Sasaki H., Ikeda M., Kubota M. et al.: Tohoku J. Exp. Med. 183, 173–183 (1997).

64   Raskin P., Dole J.F. and Rappaport E.B.: Diabetes 48 (Suppl. 1), A94 (1999).

65   Oakes N.D., Kennedy C.J., Jenkins A.B., Laybutt D.R., Chisholm D.J. and Kraegen E.W.: Diabetes 43: 1203–1210 (1994).

66   Young P.W., Cawthorne M.A., Coyle P. J., Holder J.C., Holman G.D., Kozka I.J., Kirkham D.M., Lister C.A. and Sith S.A.: Diabetes 44, 1087–1092 (1995).

67   Sironi A.M., Vichi S., Gastaldelli A., Pecori N., Anichini R., Foot E., Seghieri G. and Ferrannini E.: Clin. Pharmacol. Ther. 62, 194–202 (1997).

68   Wang M., Wise S.C., Leff T., Su T.-Z.: Diabetes 48, 254–260 (1999).

69   Inoue I., Takahashi K., Katayama S., Harada Y., Negishi K., Itabashi A. and Ishii J.: Metabolism 44, 1626–1630 (1995).

70   Fonseca V.A., Reynolds T., Hemphill D., Randolph C., Wall J., Valiquet T.R., Graveline J. and Fink L.M.: J. Diabetes Complications 12, 181–186 (1998).

71   Kubo K.: Curr. Ther. Res. 59, 537–544 (1998).

72   Ehrmann D.A., Schneider D.J., Sobel B.E., Cavaghan M.K., Imperial J., Rosenfield R.L. and Polonsky K.S.: J. Clin. Endocrinol. Metab. 82, 2108–2116 (1997).

73   Nordt T.K., Gelmann C., Peter K., Bode C. and Sobel B.E.: J. Am. Coll. Cardiol. 33 (Suppl. A): 301A (1999) (Abstract).

74   Yamakawa K., Hosoi M., Fukumoto S., Koyama H., Inaba M., Okuno Y., Nishizawa Y. and Morii H.: Diabetes 47 (Suppl. 1): A366 (1998) (Abstract).

75   Kato K., Sato H., Endo Y., Yamada D., Midorikawa S. Sato W., Mizuno K., Fujita T., Tsukamoto K., Watanabe T.: Biochem. Biophys. Res. Commun. 258, 431–435 (1999).

76   Ishizuka T., Itaya S., Wada H., Ishizawa M., Kimura M., Kajita K., Kanoh Y., Miura A., Muto N. and Yasuda K.: Diabetes 47, 1494–1500 (1998).

77   Takagi T., Yoshida K., Akasaka T., Hozumi T., Yamamuro A. and Morioka S.: JACC 33 (Suppl A): 100A (1999) (Abstract).

78   Shinohara E., Kihara S., Ouchi N., Funahashi T., Nakamura T., Yamashita S., Kameda-Takemura K. and Matsuzawa Y.: Atherosclerosis 136, 275–279 (1998).

79   Law R.E., Meehan W.P., Xi X.P., Graf K., Wuthrich D.A., Coats W., Faxon D. and Hsueh W.A.: J. Clin. Invest. 98, 1897–1905 (1996).

80   Igarashi M., Takeda Y., Ishibashi N., Takahashi D., Mori S., Tominaga M. and Saito Y.: Horm. Metab. Res. 29, 444–449 (1997).

81   Morikang E., Benson S.C., Kurtz T.W. and Pershadsingh H.A.: Am. J. Hypertens. 10, 440–446 (1997).

82   Marx N., Schonbeck U., Lazar M.A., Libby P. and Plutzky J.: Circ Res. *83*, 1097–1103 (1998).

83   Kihara S., Ouchi N., Funahashi T., Shinohara E., Tamura R., Yamashita S. and Matsuzawa Y.: Atherosclerosis *136*, 163–168 (1998).

84   Marx N., Sukhova G., Murphy C., Libby P. and Plutzky J.: Am. J. Pathol. *153*, 17–23 (1998).

85   Notoya Y., Fukuda G., Shirabe S., Tanaka A., Inamura T., Kanazawa M. and Hayashi T.: Diabetes 47 (Suppl. 1), A365 (1998).

86   Yasunari K., Kohno M., Kano H., Yokokawa K., Minami M. and Yoshikawa J.: Circ. Res. *81*, 953–962 (1997).

87   Graf K., XI X.P., Hsueh W.A. and Law R.E.: FEBS Lett. *400*, 119–121 (1997).

88   Katoh Y., Itho S., Kimura T., Konishi H. and Yamaguchi H.: Circulation 98 (Suppl.), I–798 (1998) (Abstract).

89   Dubey R.K., Zhang H.Y., Reddy S.R., Boegehold M.A. and Dotchen T.A.: Am. J. Physiol. *265*, R726–32 (1993).

90   Avena R., Mitchell M.E., Nylen E.S., Curry K.M. and Sidawy A.N.: J. Vasc. Surg. *28*, 1024–1031 (1998).

91   Fujishima S., Ohya Y., Nakamura Y., Onaku U., Abe I. and Fujishima M.: Am. J. Hypertens. *11*, 1134–1137 (1998).

92   Tack C.J., Ong M.K., Lutterman J.A. and Smits P.: Diabetologia *41*, 569–576 (1998).

93   Walker A.B., Naderali E.K., Chattington P.D., Buckingham R.E. and Williams G.: Diabetes *47*, 810–814 (1998).

94   Fujiwara T., Ohsawa T., Takahashi S., Ikeda K., Okuno A., Ushiyama S., Matsuda K. and Horikoshi H.: Life Sci. *63*, 2039–2047 (1998).

95   Fujiwara T., Ohsawa T., Miyamoto M., Ushiyama S., Matsuda K. and Horikoshi H.: Diabetes *44* (Suppl. 1), 72A (1995).

96   Goud C., Pitt B., Webb R.C. and Richey J.M.: Am. J. Physiol. *275*, E882–E887 (1998).

97   Ren J., Dominguez L.J., Sowers J.R. and Davidoff A.J.: Diabetes *45*, 1822–1825 (1996).

98   Ali S.S., Igwe R.C., Walsh J.F. and Sowers J.R.: Metabolism *48*, 125–130 (1999).

99   Song J., Walsh M.F., Igwe R., Ram J.L., Barazi M., Dominguez L.J. and Sowers J.R.: Diabetes *46*, 659–664 (1997).

100   Buchanan T.A., Meehan W.P., Jeng Y.Y., Yang D., Chan T.M., Nadler J.L., Scott S., Rude R.K. and Hsueh W.A.: J. Clin. Invest. *96*, 354–60 (1995).

101   Peuler J.D., Miller J.A., Bourghli M., Zammam H.Y., Soltis E.E. and Sowers J.R.: Metabolism *46*, 1199–1205 (1997).

102   Kotchen T.A., Zhang H.Y., Reddy S. and Hoffmann R.G.: Am. J. Physiol. *270*, R660–666 (1996).

103   Kotchen T.A., Reddy S. and Zhang H.Y.: Am. J. Hypertens. *10*, 1020–1026 (1997).

104   Verma S., Bhanot S., Arikawa E., Yao L. and McNeill J.H.: Pharmacology *56*, 7–16 (1998).

105   Driscoll J., Ghazzi M., Perez J., Huang S. and Whitcomb R.: Diabetes *46* (Suppl 1.), A149 (1997) (Abstract).

106   Shimabukuro M., Higa S., Shinzato T., Nagamine F., Komiya I. and Takasu N.: Metabolism *45*, 1168–1173 (1996).

107   Shimoyama M., Ogino K., Tanaka Y., Ikeda T. and Hisatome I.: Diabetes *48*, 609–615 (1999).

108   Murakami T., Mizuno S., Kaku B. and Ohnaka M.: J. Am. Coll. Cardiol. *33* (Suppl. A), 301A (1999) (Abstract).

Progress in Drug Research, Vol. 54 (E. Jucker, Ed.)
©2000 Birkhäuser Verlag, Basel (Switzerland)

Applications of developmental biology to medicine and animal agriculture

By Rosamund C. Smith[1,2] and
Simon J. Rhodes[1]

[1]Department of Biology, Indiana
University-Purdue University
Indianapolis (IUPUI),
723 W. Michigan Street,
Indianapolis IN 46202-5132, USA;
[2]Lilly Research Laboratories,
Eli Lilly and Company,
Lilly Corporate Center,
Indianapolis, IN 46285, USA

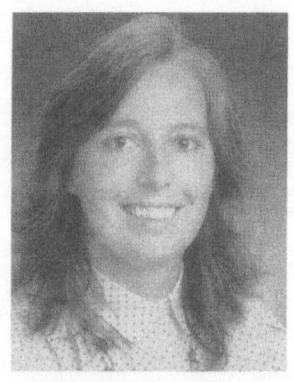

Rosamund C. Smith

studied at Cambridge University and earned her doctoral degree in biochemistry at the University of Oxford for her work on the molecular biology of amphibian development. After post-doctoral fellowships at Indiana University in Bloomington, Indiana and at Columbia University in New York, she joined Boehringer-Ingelheim in Vienna, Austria. She currently is a Research Scientist at Lilly Research Laboratories, holds an adjunct assistant professorship in the Department of Biology at Indiana University-Purdue University Indianapolis (IUPUI) and is a Visiting Scientist in the Indiana Molecular Biology Institute, Bloomington, Indiana.

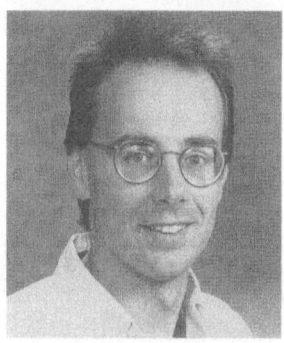

Simon J. Rhodes

received a B.Sc. Hons. degree from the University of Sheffield. He earned his doctoral degree in Biochemistry from Purdue University, Indiana, USA, for studies of transcriptional regulation during skeletal muscle development. He was a post-doctoral fellow at the University of California, San Diego, where he investigated the molecular pathways that control pituitary organogenesis in mammals. He currently is an assistant professor at Indiana University-Purdue University Indianapolis and a member of the Cancer Center at the Indiana University School of Medicine.

Summary

With the complete sequence of the human genome expected by winter 2001, genomic-based drug discovery efforts of the pharmaceutical industry are focusing on finding the relatively few therapeutically useful genes from among the total gene set. Methods to rapidly elucidate gene function will have increasing value in these investigations. The use of model organisms in functional genomics has begun to be recognized and exploited and is one example of the emerging use of the tools of developmental biology in recent drug discovery efforts. The use of protein products expressed during embryogenesis and the use of certain pluripotent cell populations (stem cells) as candidate therapeutics are other applications of developmental biology to the treatment of human diseases. These agents may be used to repair damaged or diseased tissues by inducing or directing developmental programs that recapitulate embryonic processes to replace specialized cells. The activation or silencing of embryonic genes in the disease state, particularly those encoding transcription factors, is another avenue of exploitation. Finally, the direct drug-induced manipulation of embryonic development is a unique application of developmental biology in animal agriculture.

Contents

Keywords

Functional genomics, model organisms, developmental biology, stem cells, embryonic proteins, drug discovery

Glossary of abbreviations

AI, aromatase inhibitor; ALS, amyotrophic lateral sclerosis; AP, anterior pituitary gland; APL, acute promyelocytic leukaemia; BDNF, brain-derived neutrophic factor; BHLH, basic helix-loop-helix; BMP, bone morphogenetic protein; CBP, CREB-binding protein; CGAP, cancer genome anatomy project; EKLF, erythroid Krüppell-like factor; FGF, fibroblast growth factor; GDF, growth and differentiation factor; GDNF, glial derived neurotrophic factor; GH, growth hormone; GPCR, G protein coupled receptor; HAT, histone acetyltransferase; HDAC, histone deacetylase; HSC, haematopoietic stem cell; IGF, insulin-like growth factor; IP, intermediate pituitary gland; KGF, keratinocyte growth factor; Mb, megabase; MSC, marrow stromal cell; NR, nuclear receptor; PERV, porcine endogenous retrovirus; PP, posterior pituitary gland; pST, porcine somatotropin; PRL, prolactin; RAR, retinoic acid receptor; SAGE, serial analysis of gene expression; TF, transcription factor; TGFβ, transforming growth factor beta; TSH, thyroid stimulating hormone; VEGF, vascular endothelial-derived growth factor; YS-HSC, yolk sac haematopoietic stem cell.

1   Introduction

This review examines the use of developmental biology approaches in drug discovery efforts by the pharmaceutical industry for both human and animal applications. These approaches will be divided into five main sections for ease of discussion:

(1) The use of model organisms in functional genomic studies
(2) The therapeutic use of embryonic proteins
(3) The reactivation or silencing of developmental genes
(4) Embryonic cells as therapeutic agents
(5) Embryos as direct targets for drug delivery in animal agriculture

2   Post-genomic drug discovery

The Human Genome Project plans to have sequenced approximately 90% of the human genome (3500 Megabases (Mb)) by spring 2000 and to have completed sequencing of the entire genome by winter 2001. Using a shotgun sequencing strategy, Celera Genomics, a subsidiary of Perkin Elmer, plans to independently achieve this goal within a similar timeframe. The total number of human genes is still unknown, but estimates are within the range of 80 000–140 000. The majority of these genes will likely not have any therapeutic or disease connection. It has been estimated that 3000–10 000 of these genes may be useful therapeutically or be causal in disease onset or progression [1]. This represents an order of magnitude over the approximately 500 genes or targets that drug companies are currently focusing their drug discovery efforts upon. How will these rare gene targets be identified from amidst the vast number of gene sequences coming from the human genome sequencing efforts? Many approaches have focused on identifying genes whose expression pattern correlates with a particular disease state. Differential display, DNA microarray (DNA chip) analysis and serial analysis of gene expression (SAGE) are methods that allow comparison of gene expression profiles within large populations of genes, and in some cases such as yeast, within the entire genome [2–6]. Some of these analyses have been published and are also available on the internet, e.g. CGAP, the Cancer Genome Anatomy Project web site is a database of the known active and silent genes in normal, precancerous and tumour cells (www.ncbi.nlm.nih.gov/ncicgap) [7]. Proteomics, the study of all the protein products from the genome, allows for large-scale comparison, most often based on two-dimensional (2D) gel electrophoretic methods, of the expression of proteins in normal and diseased tissues [8]. Mass spectrometry allows for identification of candidate proteins. Although these methods are valuable and can give a short-list of candidate disease-associated genes, they do not distinguish between genes that are causal in disease onset and progression and those that are a consequence of disease. Obviously it is those genes that play a causal role in disease that are the most interesting therapeutically. In order to distinguish between these two categories of disease-associated genes, it is necessary to understand more about the function of candidate genes [9–11]. Bioinformatic searches *in silico* for sequence homologies between candidate genes and genes of known function are a way to suggest possible function. The presence of certain motifs or blocks in the sequence of the gene of interest can predict many features including intra- or extracellular location, transcriptional activity or protein-protein interactions [12]. This information can be used to help design ways to test predicted functions experimentally *in vitro* in cell-based assays, or *in vivo* in a variety of model organisms.

2.1 Use of model organisms in functional genomics

Developmental biologists study a variety of non-human species in order to understand the processes of differentiation, tissue specification, pattern formation and gene regulation during embryogenesis. These studies are based on the premise that due to high conservation of gene structure and function between vertebrate and invertebrate species, research on these mechanisms in lower organisms will provide information that is directly applicable to our understanding of human development, gene regulation and disease. With the need to rapidly determine gene function in the postgenomic era, the utility of model organisms to aid in this endeavor has become apparent [13]. The fruitfly, *Drosophila melanogaster*, and the nematode worm, *Caenarhabitis elegans*, are the two invertebrate multicellular organisms most studied in developmental biology. Their fast generation times, practicality of production of mutants and ability to incorporate foreign DNA into their genomes make both organisms ideal for genetic screening and analysis of genetic pathways and gene interactions. The lineage of each of the 959 cells in the adult *C. elegans* is known and facilitates analyses of mutant phenotypes. Studies in the worm are also aided in that the full sequence of the 97 Mb of the *C. elegans* genome was made publicly available at the end of 1998 [14]. This was the first full sequence of a multicellular organism to be reported. The worm genome contains 19 099 predicted protein-coding genes, which is about three times that found in yeast and about one-fifth to one-third the number predicted for humans. 42% of the predicted protein products find significant matches in other organisms [14]. There are, somewhat surprisingly, a number of vertebrate gene families that do not have orthologs in *C. elegans*. For example, there appear to be no nerve growth factor or PDGF receptor genes. In addition, the "hedgehog" protein signaling molecule is missing. This is surprising since hedgehog-encoding genes are present in *Drosophila* as well as many vertebrate species. Further, there appear to be no Janus kinase enzyme sequences in the *C. elegans* genome, although this signal pathway component is present in many vertebrate species in addition to the fly [15]. However, these differences appear to be the exception rather than the rule, and the high conservation of genes between *C. elegans* and higher species confirms the utility of *C. elegans* in functional genomic studies of human gene function. The *Drosophila* genome (150 Mb) is currently being sequenced by a federally funded effort, the Berkeley *Drosophila* Genome project, in collaboration with Celera Genomics. At this time, approximately 20% of the *Drosophila* genome is sequenced with plans to have the full genomic sequence available by the end of 1999.

Given the conservation in gene sequence from worms and flies to mouse and man, especially as it relates to drug discovery, it is important to know whether the genes known to cause disease in man are conserved in these invertebrate species. In one study, it was found that the majority of known human disease genes do have counterparts in *C. elegans* or *Drosophila* [16]. Because this study was performed prior to completion of the sequencing of the worm genome, however, it is possible that the conservation of human disease genes in model organisms may be higher than reported. A number of tools are available for searching for homologous genes in model organisms [17].

Developmental biologists also study several vertebrate species that are proving useful for studies of gene function. The mouse (*Mus musculus*) is the standard mammalian model organism. The ability to make transgenics, and to knock-out and knock-in specific genes through homologous recombination and to regulate the spatial and temporal expression of transgenes using such systems as cre-lox makes the mouse a powerful system for gene function studies. However, the generation time of the mouse is relatively long;

early development is not easily accessible; and such studies are relatively expensive to perform. The chick, the frog *Xenopus laevis* and the zebrafish *Brachydanio rerio* all will be useful in functional genomic studies. The zebrafish is a new and emerging model organism that is likely to become more prominent in the future. It is one of the few vertebrate species that is amenable to genetic analysis as well as standard embryological manipulation. The results of a saturation mutagenesis study in zebrafish and a description of some of the mutants isolated by the laboratories of C. Nusslein-Volhard and W. Driever in 1996 clearly showed the potential of this model organism [18]. Unfortunately, to date there is no genetic map and little genomic sequence available for the zebrafish. Further, the cloning of genes identified in mutant screens is not routine. Both the chick and the frog also have their place as model organisms. Although neither species is currently routinely amenable to genetic analysis, and there is only sparse genome sequence available, their strength lies in the ability to manipulate the developing embryo without the confines of *in utero* development. More recently, there is an effort to use the frog species *Xenopus tropicalis* (instead of *Xenopus laevis*) because of its shorter generation time and diploid genome (*laevis* is effectively tetraploid) that makes transgenesis more feasible [19].

The genomic sequence of the budding yeast *Saccharomyces cerevisiae* has been known for a number of years. A high-throughput strategy to systematically knockout each known open reading frame (ORF) is underway and the results of the production of yeast strains representing 2026 individual knockouts (representing more than one-third of the total genes in the yeast genome) have recently been reported [20]. Obviously, yeast is amenable to powerful genetic analyses. Such analyses, however, are usually limited to analyses of intracellular pathways rather than to the exploration of gene function involved in intercellular communication and/or tissue differentiation.

2.2 Functional studies in model organisms

No one single model organism is ideal in contributing information about the function of unknown genes. Rather, each has strengths and weaknesses, and a number of model organisms should be used when gathering information about gene function. The power of *C. elegans* and *Drosophila* lies in the ability to perform genetic analyses. It is possible to identify the functional *Drosophila* counterpart of a human gene of interest by the ability of the human gene to rescue the fly mutant. It is then possible to identify upstream and downstream members of the genetic pathway in which this gene lies by screening for suppressors or enhancers of this particular mutation. Not only does this provide useful information about the signaling system or functional complex in which a gene works, but it can be useful for identifying possible new targets for drug discovery. When a gene known to be causal in the generation of a particular human disease is identified it can often be that, apart from gene therapy approaches, the gene defect cannot be overcome by direct drug modulation. Rather, it is necessary to modulate downstream members of the mutated gene or activate a parallel signaling pathway. Such members can perhaps be identified through the use of fly and worm genetics.

Expression patterns of orthologous target genes during embryonic development of model organisms, such as the frog and chick, can often give clues to their function. An increasing number of genes that are known to be normally expressed only during development are re-expressed under disease conditions. Elucidation of the normal function of a protein during development may shed light on its role in disease. Proteome Inc. has a number of protein databases from model organisms, including yeast and *C. elegans*, that facilitate gene function analyses (www.proteome.com).

The effects of overexpression of human genes, or their lower species orthologs, in developing embryos of the zebrafish, frog, chick or mouse can often be illuminating in terms of function. Mouse overexpression is usually achieved through transgenic analysis, whereas overexpression in fish and frogs is routinely performed by microinjection of RNA or DNA into fertilized eggs or early embryos. Retroviral expression is commonly used to overexpress genes of interest in regions of the developing chick embryo. Downregulation of gene activity is often achieved through the use of reverse genetic methods such as the use of antisense RNA or DNA oligonucleotides in frogs, fish and the chick. The recent advent of "RNAi" technology, first described in the worm, which allows for the specific ablation of mRNAs of interest by the delivery of double stranded RNA homologous to the gene of interest, has increased the tools available for underexpression studies (reviewed in [21] and at www.macalester.edu/~montgomery/RNAi). There is much excitement about the applicability of RNAi to vertebrate species, but as yet no positive results have been reported.

A number of biotechnology companies founded around the use of model organisms for gene function analysis have formed over the last few years. Axys Pharmaceuticals (www.axyspharm.com) and DevGen (www.devgen.

com), based in Belgium, are using *C. elegans* in developmental biology-based efforts for target identification in drug discovery. Exelixis Pharmaceuticals Inc. (www.exelixis.com) focuses on the use of *Drosophila* and *C. elegans* and is allied with Artemis Pharmaceuticals (www.artemispharmaceuticals.com), a German company that focuses on the zebrafish and mouse as genetic models for human disease. Artemis uses the zebrafish and its utility in large-scale genetic screens to isolate mutants that could be potential models for human disease. DeveloGen (www.develogen.de), also based in Germany, is pursuing developmental biology approaches to develop a treatment for diabetes, obesity and pancreatic cancer by using the mouse, zebrafish and *Drosophila* as model organisms. In its diabetes program, the company is attempting to generate insulin-producing cells by activating transcription factor genes, specifically Pax-4 and Pax-6, normally expressed in the pancreas during embryogenesis. Ontogeny Inc. (www.ontogeny.com), in addition to developing therapeutic uses for the hedgehog proteins and genes, also has a proprietary screening system called "Ontoscreen" that uses a variety of model organism functional approaches to identify genes or proteins with therapeutic potential. Using the power of mouse transgenesis, Lexicon Genetics is generating banks of embryonic stem (ES) cells with individual genes knocked out that can be used to generate specific knock-out mice. Some companies including Exelixis and Axys, are using *C. elegans* mutants for direct screening for small molecule therapeutics. Cadus Pharmaceuticals (www.cadus.com) is using yeast to express human G protein coupled receptors (GPCRs) and then engineering the yeast cell to produce and excrete a ligand for the receptor. It is thus possible to identify a surrogate agonist for an orphan GPCR. The surrogate ligand can be used to develop an assay to identify small molecule antagonists of the same receptor.

3 Use of embryonic proteins as therapeutic drugs or as drug targets

Many of the proteins that have been characterized as important regulators of embryonic development, especially intercellular signalling molecules and growth factors, may have application as therapies to treat human diseases. Examples of the applications and current status of some of these protein factors are given in Table 1. As drugs, such proteins would stimulate specific developmental processes resulting in the replacement of differentiated cell

Table 1
Examples of embryonic proteins under development or in use as therapeutic agents or as the targets of therapies. Information was obtained from public company web sites and news releases. The testing and approval status of a particular drug changes frequently: the data given here are meant to convey the diversity of potential protein therapeutics at various stages of testing and approval.

Protein	Application
Erythropoeitin (*Epogen*)	Chronic renal failure
Granulocyte colony stimulating factor (G-CSF) (*Neupogen*)	Chemotherapy or marrow transplant-induced neutropenia
Interleukin 11 (*Neumega*)	Thrombocytopenia
Stem cell factor (*Stemgen*)	Stem cell transplantation
Basic fibroblast growth factor (bFGF) (*FIBLAST*)	Stroke Coronary heart disease Peripheral vascular disease
Osteogenic protein-1 (OP-1/BMP-7)	Repair of bone and cartilage Stroke, neurodegenerative diseases Chronic renal disease
Myeloid progenitor inhibitory factor-1 (MPIF 1)	Bone marrow cell protection during chemotherapy
Vascular endothelial growth factor (VEGF)	Coronary arterial disease
Vascular endothelial growth factor–2 gene (gtVEGF-2)	Coronary arterial disease
Brain-derived neurotrophic factor (BDNF)	Amyotrophic lateral sclerosis (ALS)
Glial cell line-derived neurotrophic factor (GDNF)	Parkinson's disease
Keratinocyte growth factor (KGF)	Wound healing and mucositis
Keratinocyte growth factor-2 (KGF-2)	Wound healing and mucositis
Bone morphogenetic protein-2 (BMP2)	Repair of bone and cartilage
Interleukin 12	Cancer, hepatitis
Sonic hedgehog (Shh)	Neurological diseases
Indian hedgehog (Ihh)	Orthopedic diseases
Desert hedgehog (Dhh)	Multiple sclerosis, neuropathy diseases
Patched (Ptc)	Basal cell nevus syndrome Basal cell carcinoma
Growth and differentiation factor 1 (GDF-1)	Neurological disorders
Growth and differentiation factor 8/ myostatin (GDF-8)	Muscle-wasting diseases
Growth and differentiation factor 9 (GDF-9)	Fertility diseases

Status	Company
On the market	Amgen
On the market	Amgen
On the market	Genetics Institute
Phase III clinical trials	Amgen
Phase II/III clinical trials	Scios/Wyeth-Ayerst
Phase II clinical trials	
Phase II clinical trials	
Phase III clinical trials complete	Creative BioMolecules/Stryker
Preclinical trials	Creative BioMolecules
Preclinical trials	Biogen/Creative BioMolecules
Phase II clinical trials	Human Genome Sciences
Phase II clinical trials	Genentech
Phase I/II clinical trials	Human Genome Sciences/Vascular Genetics
Phase I/II clinical trials	Amgen/Regeneron
Phase I/II clinical trials	Amgen
Phase I/II clinical trials	Amgen
Phase I/II clinical trials	Human Genome Sciences
Phase I clinical trials	Genetics Institute
Phase I clinical trials	Genetics Institute/Wyeth-Ayerst
Research/Preclinical trials	Ontogeny/Biogen
Research/Preclinical trials	Ontogeny/Biogen/Roche
Research/Preclinical trials	Ontogeny/Biogen
Research	Ontogeny
Research	Creative BioMolecules/Cambridge Neuroscience
Research	MetaMorphix
Research	MetaMorphix

types lost through disease or injury. This approach requires that any receptors, cofactors and signalling pathways required for the actions of the protein drug remain intact in the target tissues.

The requirement for delivery by direct injection into the bloodstream is currently a limitation on the widespread use of proteins and some peptides as drugs. Many companies are pursuing methods to make effective oral formulations of protein drugs. Successful protocols will prevent degradation by proteases in the gut and subsequently will allow the absorption of active protein drugs into the bloodstream of the patient. Methods under testing include the encapsulation of proteins to protect them from protease enzymes and the addition of protease inhibitor molecules to drug formulations. Other approaches are more direct, involving the use of protease-resistant, covalently-modified proteins. Recent approaches also have added viral transduction domains to proteins to mediate the passage of biologically active proteins into target cells and organs, including the brain [22]. These techniques will extend the types of proteins that can be used as therapies to include those with intracellular actions. The use of directly modified proteins requires that the altered proteins must retain their biological activity in addition to having increased delivery effectiveness. Other approaches that are under consideration for the delivery of protein drugs include the formulation of proteins in fine powders for inhalation delivery via the lungs, the development of depot delivery systems using skin patches, and devices that allow needleless injection through the skin.

Several proteins already are widely used drugs. For example, recombinant human erythropoietin (Epogen) from Amgen is used to treat patients with chronic kidney diseases that develop anemia due to lack of erythrocytes. Erythropoietin, a protein normally produced by the kidney, stimulates progenitor cells found in the bone marrow to form mature erythrocytes. A second Amgen product, Neupogen, is a recombinant form of granulocyte colony stimulating factor used to treat neutropenia caused by chemotherapy or marrow transplantation. An interleukin 11-based drug (Neumega) is being sold by Genetics Institute for use in the treatment of thrombocytopenia disorders.

3.1 Growth and signalling factors

The many secreted protein molecules of the fibroblast growth factor, transforming growth factor β (TGFβ), hedgehog, and other signalling protein families offer significant promise as drugs in the treatment of many diseases. These factors have been demonstrated to play specific roles in the development of many organs, tissues and specialized cell types. The components of the multiple intracellular pathways activated by these factors, including their receptors and downstream signalling partners, may also provide candidates for direct protein therapies or may provide targets for therapy.

3.1.1 Fibroblast growth factor family

The fibroblast growth factor family comprises at least 18 members with demonstrated roles in the development of cells of ectodermal, mesodermal and endodermal origin (reviewed in [23]). Basic fibroblast growth factor (bFGF or FGF-2), found in tissues such as the pituitary gland and the placenta, affects the growth and proliferation of most mesodermal cell types, as well as some ectodermal and endodermal cells. In therapeutic applications, bFGF may have neuroprotective and angiogenic (blood vessel forming) properties. For example, Scios is developing recombinant forms of bFGF for the treatment of stroke, coronary artery disease and peripheral vascular disease. Keratinocyte growth factor (KGF or FGF-7) and the related KGF-2 protein are in clinical trials by Amgen and Human Genome Sciences, respectively, as agents to promote epidermal growth and wound healing. These proteins are also being tested in the treatment of mucositis: a painful condition of the mucosal tissues of the intestine, colon, bladder and lung that can result as a side effect of some cancer treatments. There are four fibroblast growth factor receptors that mediate intracellular signalling of this class of proteins through their tyrosine kinase activity (reviewed in [23, 24]). Mutations of some of these genes are well characterized as underlying human developmental diseases, including birth defects involving skeletal and cranial abnormalities. An increased understanding of the biochemistry of the fibroblast growth factor receptors and their pathways will likely present additional protein molecules or targets for therapeutic intervention.

3.1.2 Transforming growth factor β family

Transforming growth factor β (TGFβ) and members of the large superfamily of TGFβ-related proteins are under widespread investigation by many companies as potential drugs to treat cancers and other diseases (reviewed in [25]). This structurally related group of proteins includes the bone morphogenetic proteins (BMPs) and the growth/differentiation factors (GDFs). BMPs have diverse effects during development, including regulation of cell differentiation, proliferation, apoptosis and morphogenesis (reviewed in [26, 27]). They are involved in development of the nervous system, the lungs, kidneys, gonads, skin, and somite-derived structures such as muscle and the skeleton. For example, BMPs under investigation as agents for the repair and augmentation of bone and cartilage include osteogenic protein-1 (OP-1/BMP-7) produced by Creative BioMolecules/Stryker, and BMP-2 produced by Genetics Institute. OP-1 is also being developed as a therapeutic agent for acute and chronic kidney failure by Creative BioMolecules/Biogen. The GDFs are also important regulators of tissue growth and development. For example, GDF-11 (also known as BMP-11) is required for patterning of the axial skeleton in mice [28]. GDF-8 is specifically expressed in skeletal muscle and mice with disrupted *GDF-8* genes have significantly increased muscle mass, suggesting that GDF-8 is a negative regulator of skeletal muscle growth [29]. MetaMorphix Inc. is investigating whether antagonists of GDF-8 action would be useful in the treatment of muscle wasting. GDF-9 is an oocyte-derived growth factor that is required for early ovarian folliculogenesis [30] and this protein may be a useful agent in the treatment of fertility diseases. GDF-1 is being investigated by Creative BioMolecules/Cambridge Neuroscience as a therapy for neurological diseases. The receptors and signalling pathways used by the superfamily of TGFβ-related proteins are currently being deciphered. It appears that this class of protein recognizes two classes of receptors, the type I and type II receptors. Many receptor molecules have been identified and cloned. The receptor proteins are serine/threonine kinase molecules, and both types of receptors may need to be present on a target cell for a complete response to some ligands [26]. The signalling pathways activated downstream of the TGFβ-related protein receptors are poorly understood, but clearly involve intracellular signalling molecules known as "SMAD" proteins [31, 32]. SMADs have been shown to have both stimulatory and inhibitory activities in the signalling pathways. Specific TGFβ-related protein receptors and signalling proteins, such as the SMAD molecules, may therefore be targets for future drug therapies. However, present evidence suggests that there may be some crosstalk between TGFβ-family protein signalling pathways and it will therefore be important to better understand the mechanisms that confer specificity before drugs can be used to target components of these pathways.

3.1.3 Hedgehog protein family

The *"hedgehog"* gene was discovered by the genetic screens of Nüsslein-Volhard and Wieschaus [33] as encoding an important regulator of segmentation during *Drosophila* embryonic development. Several forms of the hedgehog protein have been found in higher organisms. In humans, three forms of this inducing protein have been found: they are known as Desert hedgehog, Indian hedgehog, and Sonic hedgehog (reviewed in [34]). Studies in rodent model animals indicate that Desert hedgehog is essential for development of the male reproductive system [35]. Indian hedgehog is required for the proliferation and differentiation of chondrocytes and therefore bone formation and the skeletal system [36]. Sonic hedgehog is broadly important for development: mutants display defects of the nervous system, axial structures, and the foregut [37, 38]. Ontogeny Inc. is exploring the use of hedgehog proteins as therapies to treat neurodegenerative diseases (such as Parkinson's and Alzheimer's diseases), multiple sclerosis, and bone and cartilage disorders such as fractures, implant fixation, osteoarthritis and osteoporosis. Mutations of the patched and smoothened genes, which encode the hedgehog receptor and a target of the hedgehog signalling pathway, respectively (reviewed in [39, 40]), are associated with basal-cell carcinomas, the most common human cancer [41–43] and Ontogeny Inc. is investigating the use of the patched protein in the treatment of this and related diseases.

3.1.4 Vascular endothelial growth factors

Vascular endothelial growth factor (VEGF) is a specific mitogen for vascular endothelial cells (reviewed in [44–46]). Five distinct VEGF isoforms are generated as a result of alternative splicing from a single *VEGF* gene. The isoforms differ in their molecular mass and in biological properties. VEGF proteins recognize two tyrosine kinase receptors, VEGFR-1 (also known as flt-1) and VEGFR-2 (KDR/flk-1), which are expressed almost exclusively in endothelial cells. Like bFGF, VEGF-1 can promote angiogenesis and is in clinical trials by Genentech as an agent to promote blood vessel growth during the treatment of coronary arterial disease. Human Genome Sciences are using gene therapy approaches to target the VEGF-2 protein for the treatment of cardiac diseases and atherosclerosis. By contrast, specific inhibitors of VEGF growth factors may be useful in counteracting the neovascularization associated with diseases such as diabetic retinopathy [47]. In addition, overexpression of VEGF proteins has been associated with the development of solid tumours by promoting tumour angiogenesis, and anti-VEGF therapies may therefore have important applications in cancer treatment [46].

3.1.5 Nervous system growth factors

Nerve growth factor and ciliary neurotrophic factor have been explored as possible therapies for peripheral neuropathies (progressive nerve fiber damage in the hands and feet often suffered by diabetic patients) and for neurodegenerative disorders, but several of these studies have not produced positive results. Other proteins under testing for the treatment of neurodegenerative diseases include glial cell line-derived neurotrophic factor (GDNF) and brain-derived neurotrophic factor (BDNF) for the treatment of Parkinson's disease, Alzheimer's disease, Huntington's disease and amyotrophic lateral sclerosis (ALS, Lou Gehrig's disease).

3.2 Nuclear proteins: transcription factors and chromatin modifying enzymes

Many of the pathways that guide the development of specialized cell types, tissues or whole organ systems are controlled by the actions of transcription factors (proteins that regulate gene activity). Some transcription factors are widely expressed throughout the body and during development. By contrast, other transcription factors are cell- or tissue-specific and often are only expressed at specific developmental stages. The actions of these factors are essential for the determination and differentiation of distinct cell phenotypes. Such transcriptional regulatory proteins activate or repress specific sets of target genes to establish the proteome profiles of specialized cells during development. For example, the IPF-1 homeodomain transcription factor is required for development of the pancreas: mice with deleted *IPF-1* genes completely lack this organ [48]. Similarly, the SF-1 nuclear receptor is essential for gonadal and adrenal organogenesis [49]; the Pit-1 homeodomain protein controls the differentiation of three hormone-secreting pituitary cell types (reviewed in [50]); and the Cbfa1 transcription factor is required for bone formation [51, 52]. Some transcription factors have the remarkable capacity to alone activate entire developmental processes. For example, the four muscle regulatory factors (MyoD, myogenin, Myf-5, MRF4) can convert many varied cell types to differentiated skeletal muscle fates (reviewed in [53, 54]). Only a limited number of developmental transcription factors can alone activate specific developmental cascades: alternately, some tissues or cell types appear to use "committees" of transcription factors to regulate developmental processes rather than the sequential actions of individual factors. Such combinatorial codes of transcription factors, which may include both tissue-specific and broadly expressed members, will likely present challenging targets for drug therapy because of their complex nature. Table 2 lists examples of transcription factors that regulate developmental processes in mammals.

Therapeutic drugs that target gene transcription are already in use, for example, in the treatment of certain inflammation or endocrine disorders. In many cases, however, these drugs were not originally designed to target transcription factors: they were identified by virtue of their effects on specific biological processes and were only subsequently shown to target transcription (reviewed in [101]). Future therapies designed to specifically modulate transcriptional processes might target the transcription factors themselves by affecting their transcription and synthesis or by regulating their post-translational modification. Other protocols may target the protein interaction partners or ligands of specific transcription factors or may directly regulate their transcriptional functions by modulating their coactivator/corepressor factors or their binding to DNA recognition elements (reviewed in [102–104]). The remarkable properties of developmental transcription factors make them exciting potential targets for drug therapies designed to repair damaged organs by promoting the determination and differentiation of specialized cell types from precursor cells. For example, Ontogeny Inc. is investigating the use of IPF-1 as an agent or target in therapies to replace damaged pancreatic cells in diabetes. However, developmental transcription factors may be difficult direct targets for drug therapies because they are often transiently expressed in tissue-restricted patterns at early stages of development. In addition, these factors often do not bind natural small molecule ligands and therefore may not be readily activated or inhibited by small molecules. If suitable, however, small molecule drugs might be used to interfere with the DNA binding of specific transcription factors or to modulate their protein/protein interactions. Such molecules also would have to be amenable to delivery to the nucleus. Companies such as Oncogene Science Inc. have performed screens for low molecular weight compounds that can modulate the tran-

Table 2
Examples of transcription factors with roles in the development of specific organs or differentiated tissue types.

Tissue/Organ	Factor	Transcription factor class
Adipose	C/EBP α	Basic coiled coil (bZIP)
	PPARγ2	Nuclear receptor
Adrenals	SF-1	Nuclear receptor
Blood/immune system	c-Myb	Myb-type helix-turn-helix
	EBF/Olf-1	Zinc helix-loop-helix
	EKLF	Zinc finger
	GATA-3	GATA-type zinc finger
	Pax-5/BSAP	Paired box
	PU.1/Ets-1 family	Ets domain
Bone	Cbfa1/Osf2	Runt homology domain
Germ cells	Sperm-1	POU homeodomain
Gonads	SF-1	Nuclear receptor
Heart	dHand	Basic helix-loop-helix (bHLH)
	eHand/Hand1	bHLH
	GATA-4	GATA-type zinc finger
	Nkx-2.5/Csx	Homeodomain
	RXR α	Nuclear receptor
Kidneys	Pax-2	Paired box
	WT-1	Zinc finger
Nervous system	Brn-2	POU homeodomain
	Brn-3.0	POU homeodomain
	Brn-3.1	POU homeodomain
	Brn-3.2	POU homeodomain
	Brn-4	POU homeodomain
	Isl-1	LIM-homeodomain
	Lhx3	LIM-homeodomain
	Lhx4	LIM-homeodomain
	Lhx5	LIM-homeodomain
	Pax-6	Paired/homeodomain
	SIM1	bHLH-PAS
	Tst-1/SCIP/Oct-6	POU homeodomain
Pancreas	IPF-1/PDX-1/STF-1	Homeodomain
	Isl-1	LIM homeodomain paired/
	Pax-4	Paired/homeodomain
	Pax-6	
Pituitary gland	Lhx3	LIM-homeodomain
	Lhx4	LIM-homeodomain
	Pit-1	POU homeodomain
	Prop-1	Homeodomain
Skeletal muscle	MyoD	bHLH
	Myogenin	bHLH
	Myf-5	bHLH
	MRF4	bHLH
Skin/epidermis	Skn1a/i	POU homeodomain
Smooth muscle/vasculature	MEF2C	MADS box

Knockout/mutant phenotype	References
Lethal – adipose/metabolism defects	[55]
Colon cancer in humans	[56, 57]
Lethal – no adrenals, gonads	[49]
Lethal – defective liver hematopoiesis	[58]
Lethal – defective B cells	[59]
Lethal – β thallassemia	[60]
Lethal – defective liver hematopoiesis	[61]
Lethal – defective B cells	[62]
Lethal – defective hematopoiesis; osteopetrosis	[63, 64]
Lethal - no bone	[51, 52]
Reduced fertility	[65]
Lethal – no adrenals, gonads	[49]
Lethal – cardiac defects	[66]
Lethal – cardiac defects	[67, 68]
Lethal – cardiac defects	[69]
Lethal – cardiac defects	[70, 71]
Lethal – cardiac defects	[72]
Lethal – no kidneys	[73]
Lethal – no kidneys	[74]
Lethal – hypothalamic defects; no PP	[75]
Lethal – behavioral/coordination problems	[76]
Auditory defects	[77]
Visual defects	[77]
Inner ear defects	[78]
Lethal – motor neuron defects	[79]
Lethal – motor neuron defects	[80]
Lethal – motor neuron defects	[80, 81]
Lethal – hippocampus defects	[82]
Lethal – eye/brain defects	[83, 84]
Lethal – hypothalamic defects; no PP	[85]
Lethal – myelination defects	[86]
Lethal – no pancreas	[48]
Lethal – pancreas defects	[87]
Lethal – no glucagon/α cells	[88]
Lethal – no insulin/β cells	[89, 90]
Lethal – no AP, IP	[91]
Lethal – no AP, IP and neural defects	[91]
Dwarfed – lack GH, PRL, TSH	[92]
Dwarfed – lack GH, PRL, TSH	[93]
Viable as single knockout	[94]
Lethal – reduced muscle	[95, 96]
Lethal – normal muscle	[97]
Variable – normal muscle	[98]
Defective epidermal differentiation	[99]
Lethal – vascular defects	[100]

scription of specific target genes [105]. These researchers hope that these studies will lead to the development of new therapies for sickle cell disease and β thalassemia. Future therapies also may use genes encoding transcription factors in gene therapy strategies in order to activate specific developmental programs.

Transcription factors such as the nuclear receptors, may be more useful direct targets for drug therapies. These factors bind small ligand molecules, and then the activated receptors act as specific transcription factors in the activation and repression of target genes in the nucleus (reviewed in [106]). Many companies are exploring the use of ligands that activate or modulate the activity of transcription factors that regulate specific developmental pathways. For example, peroxisome proliferator-activated receptor-γ (PPARγ) is a nuclear receptor transcription factor that, in combination with CAAT/enhancer-binding proteins, is important for adipocyte differentiation (reviewed in [56]). PPARγ activity may play a role in lipid metabolism and insulin sensitivity and the *PPARγ* gene is therefore a candidate gene for human disorders such as obesity and type 2 diabetes mellitus [106]. PPARγ binds prostaglandin-derivative ligands and known anti-diabetic drugs may work by modulating PPARγ function [107]. Other nuclear receptors that have roles in development and might be potential targets in therapies include the retinoid/retinoid X receptors in skin and heart diseases, the thyroid hormone receptors in neural diseases, and the glucocorticoid receptor in lung diseases.

Recently, some aspects of the biochemical mechanisms by which many transcription factors activate and repress target genes have been elucidated. Elegant studies by many laboratories have established that transcription factors recruit coactivator and corepressor proteins to their transcriptional complexes (Fig. 1) (reviewed in [108–113]). Coactivator and corepressor factors can acetylate or deacetylate chromatin histone proteins, respectively, either directly or by the recruitment of additional factors with histone acetyltransferase (HAT) or histone deacetylase (HDAC) activities. HATs acetylate lysine residues within the amino termini of chromatin histone proteins [109, 110]. Modification of histones is assumed to allow greater accessibility of chromatin regions containing transcription factor binding sites, thereby promoting gene activation. Histone deactylases catalyze the removal of acetyl groups from histones, promoting tighter assembly of chromatin complexes and reduced transcriptional activity. Some coregulatory proteins, such as the nuclear receptor coactivators SRC-1 and GRIP1, appear to be ligand-dependent coactivators for specific classes of transcription factors such as the

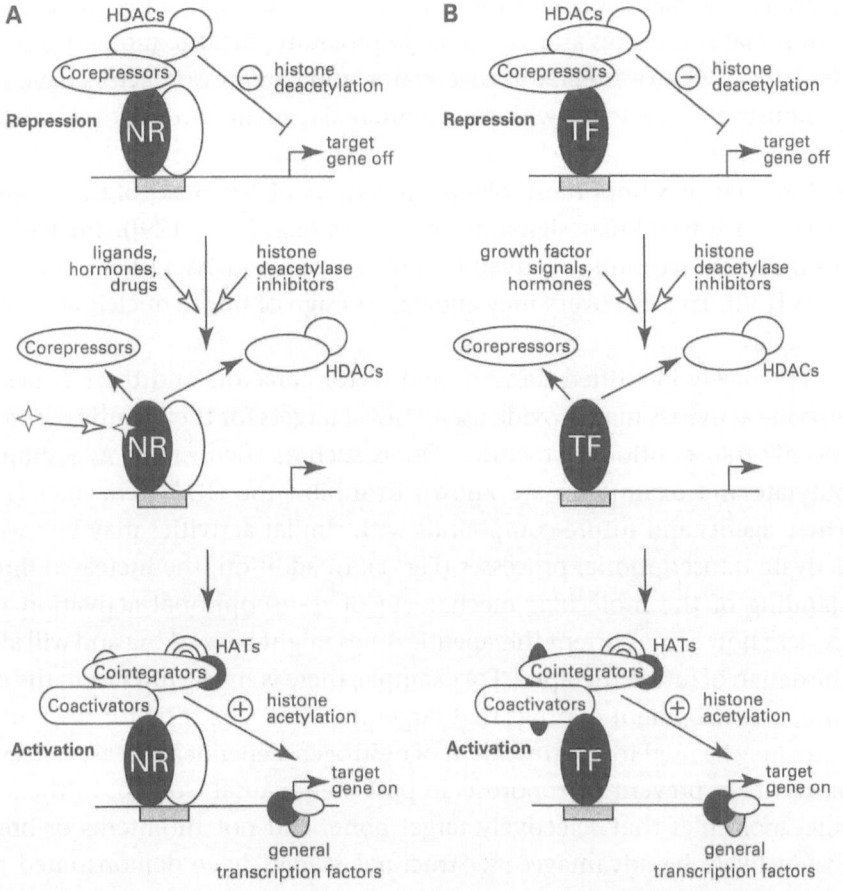

Fig. 1
Involvement of histone modifying proteins in the activation of eukaryotic genes.
Panel A. In the absence of their ligands, nuclear receptor (NR) transcription factors interact with response elements of repressed or silent target genes as complexes with corepressor and histone deacetylase (HDAC) proteins. In the presence of the ligand or drugs, the corepressor and HDAC molecules are released and replaced by coactivators, cointegrators and histone acetylases (HATs) leading to gene activation.
Panel B. A similar scheme of gene activation may occur involving some non-nuclear receptor transcription factors (TF).

nuclear receptors [114, 115]. Others, such as the CREB-binding protein (CBP) and p300 co-integrator proteins, the p/CAF and p/CIP coactivator proteins, and the N-CoR/SMRT and mSIN3 corepressor proteins, may have broader interactions with many types of transcription factors [116–121]. The co-integrator factors may serve multiple roles, acting as bridging molecules in transcriptional complexes and also directly providing histone-modifying activities [122–126]. Co-integrator, coactivator, and corepressor factors have been demonstrated to interact with developmental regulatory transcription factors such as Pit-1 [127], MyoD [128], and the oestrogen receptor [129]. Such interactions may play important roles in mediating the responses of transcription factors to intracellular signalling pathways (e.g. [127, 129]). Intriguingly, some nuclear receptor coactivators may even act as RNAs, rather than as proteins [130]. This discovery may allow the design of future nucleic acid-based therapies.

The newly identified transcription factor cofactors and their associated enzyme activities may provide useful novel targets for therapeutic control of specific transcriptional processes. Drugs such as trichostatin A, sodium n-butyrate and oxamflatin are known to inhibit the HDAC enzymes [131]. These agents and future compounds with similar activities may be used to activate transcriptional processes (Fig. 1). In addition, the increased understanding of the molecular mechanism of transcriptional activation may explain how some current therapeutic drugs might be working and will allow the design of future therapies. For example, there is strong interest in the continued development of drugs that target the oestrogen receptor. Such molecules may be used in the treatment of oestrogen-dependent breast cancers or as agents to prevent osteoporosis in post-menopausal women. In the latter role, molecules that selectively target bone, and not the uterus or breast, would likely be advantageous. Structural studies have demonstrated that coregulatory proteins interact with the carboxyl terminal ligand-binding domain of nuclear receptors such as the oestrogen receptor [132]. This domain presumably adopts distinct functional conformations depending on the presence or type of ligand. Recent experiments have shown that the cellular levels of oestrogen receptor coactivator and corepressor molecules modulate the effects of oestrogen-like ligands, such as the breast cancer drug tamoxifen, thus providing a possible mechanism to explain why such molecules can display both agonistic and antagonistic activities in different tissues [129, 133]. Consistent with these observations, studies of other nuclear receptors also have demonstrated that receptor/coregulator stoichiometry and the nature of the target gene DNA response are also critical determinants of receptor activity [134].

Interactions with chromatin-modifying transcriptional cofactors also appear to be important for other developmental diseases. In certain acute promyelocytic leukaemia (APL) patients, the aberrant actions of retinoic acid receptor (RAR) fusion proteins (caused by chromosomal translocations) lead to the promotion of proliferation instead of differentiation during haematopoiesis. Two types of fusion protein exist: one type, PML-RARα, causes a leukaemia that can often be treated with retinoic acid; the second type, PLZF-RARα, causes a leukaemia that is resistant to retinoic acid treatment. Recent studies have demonstrated that interactions of the two fusion protein types with the HDAC complexes are critical for their pathogenic activities [135, 136]. These results suggest that HDAC inhibitors might be promising agents in the treatment of both types of APL. Consistent with this hypothesis, HDAC inhibitors have been used in the treatment of PML-RARα APL patients and appear to be able to restore sensitivity to retinoic acid therapy in patients that have developed resistance [137].

The processes that lead to the modification of histones during transcription factor activities are not the only potential targets of therapeutic drugs. The methylation status of DNA is also important in gene activity, and a link between DNA methylation, histone deacetylation and gene silencing has clearly been established [138, 139]. Transcriptional complexes also contain methyltransferase enzymes that can methylate histone proteins and appear to act as secondary coactivators [140]. These enzymes also may likely provide targets for therapeutic intervention such as in the reactivation of genes in cancer therapy as described below.

4   Therapeutic reactivation and silencing of developmental genes

The molecular control of pathways of cell commitment and differentiation involves gene activation, repression and silencing. Certain tissues and organs express distinct genes encoding proteins with identical or similar functions at different times during development. These include blood, the heart and skeletal muscle. Therapeutic reactivation of foetal genes in patients carrying mutations in adult genes may be a powerful way to treat diseases of these tissues. If expression of reactivated genes in the correct tissues were achieved, this approach would have the advantage of involving isogenic (i.e. non-foreign) therapy. By contrast, in some diseases, including certain cancers, developmental genes are inappropriately activated: for these disorders, strategies designed to specifically inactivate such genes are required.

One of the best characterized systems in which discrete genes are activated during specific phases of development is the haematopoietic system. In humans, two distinct clusters of eight globin genes encode the oxygen carrying haemoglobin proteins. These genes are differentially regulated to produce distinct haemoglobin molecules for the embryo, the foetus and the adult. A major genomic DNA regulatory element, the locus control region, in collaboration with activating and silencing elements, mediates many aspects of globin gene switching. Transcription factors, such as the erythroid Krüppell-like factor (EKLF, Tab. 2), that interact with globin gene regulatory elements have been identified. The switches between the various globin genes are not absolute: traces of foetal haemoglobin can be detected in normal adults. Patients with diseases such as β thalassemia and sickle cell anemia have somewhat elevated levels of foetal haemoglobins, but still suffer debilitating symptoms. Therapeutic reactivation of embryonic or foetal globin genes in these patients may therefore improve their condition (reviewed in [141, 142]). For example, treatments with erythropoeitin (discussed above) may help in promoting higher numbers of rapidly regenerating erythrocytes that are known to produce foetal hemoglobin. Other indirect therapies that induce foetal hemoglobin include the use of cell-cycle inhibitors such as hydroxyurea that can be administered orally. Small molecules such as butyrate also have shown promise in the induction of foetal globin genes. Future therapies that directly activate globin genes may include treatments with compounds that activate genes by inducing hypomethylation of globin genomic loci or which enhance the acetylation of (or inhibit the deacetylation of) globin locus chromatin histone proteins, thereby promoting gene activation as discussed above.

Another potential target of developmental gene reactivation/silencing therapies is the diseased heart. Cardiac tissues express both foetal and adult isoforms of proteins important in the contractile process. In patients with congestive heart disease, pathological stimuli cause hypertrophy of the differentiated cardiomyocytes of the heart. The cardiac response to the increased workload of the hypertrophied heart includes a reactivation of foetal genes. Stimuli including α_1-adrenergic receptor activities promote cardiac cell hypertrophy and promote the reactivation of foetal genes such as β-myosin heavy chain and skeletal α-actin through transcriptional mechanisms (e.g. [143]). Transcription factors involved in this process include broadly expressed factors such as TEF-1 and RTEF-1, and cardiac factors such as GATA-4, dHand, eHand, Nkx-2.5 and MEF2C (Tab. 2) (reviewed in [144]). In addition, chromatin remodeling factors, such as the HAT and HDAC enzymes, are required during transcriptional reprogramming and some types of these transcriptional coregulatory proteins may be preferentially expressed in cardiac cells (reviewed in [145]). The chromatin of the cardiac β-myosin heavy chain genes, for example, has been shown to be remodeled during development [145]. Intensive studies also have been made of the role of calcium signalling in the diseased heart. Calcineurin, a calcium-regulated phosphatase enzyme is associated with cardiac hypertrophy in human patients [146] and calcineurin inhibitors such as cyclosporin and FK506 can prevent cardiac hypertrophy ([147], reviewed in [148]). Calcineurin dephosphorylates the NF-AT3 transcription factor, allowing it to translocate to the nucleus where, in synergy with GATA-4, it activates cardiac genes [149]. Other conditions and procedures also appear to lead to inappropriate activation of foetal genes in the heart. For example, foetal gene activation is associated with chronic rejection of heart transplants [150] and with the decreased workload of the unloaded heart [151]. Successful therapeutic silencing of foetal genes may therefore provide useful treatments for many forms of heart disease.

In some disease states, such as tumour formation and metastasis, embryonic and developmental genes also may be inappropriately (re)activated. These genes include the *telomerase* gene and the insulin-like growth factor II (*IGF-II*) gene. The telomerase enzyme is a ribonucleoprotein whose RNA and protein components synthesize the hexameric DNA repeats of telomeres. Telomerase is expressed in human embryonic cells but is not detected in adult somatic tissues. Telomeres are proposed to protect the ends of linear chromosomes and to promote genetic stability. In the absence of telomerase activity, progressive shortening of telomeres occurs with successive cell divisions, leading to decreased proliferation. This mechanism has been suggested to contribute to changes in cellular functions during aging. Reactivation of the *telomerase* gene has been documented in ~90% of human cancers: telomerase may help tumour cells extend their lifespan (reviewed in [152–154]). Inappropriate reactivation of the foetal promoters of the *IGF-II* gene, which encodes a potent foetal growth factor, has been associated with hepatitis C virus-related chronic hepatitis, cirrhosis and hepatocellular carcinoma in adult patients [155]. Distinct therapeutic strategies from those designed to activate developmental genes will be required to repress genes such as *telomerase* and *IGF-II* in cancer treatment protocols.

In cancerous cells, genes also are inappropriately inactivated in order to promote proliferation, rather than the differentiated state. As mentioned earlier, patched, a member of the hedgehog signalling pathway, is a developmental gene that when mutated can lead to skin cancer [41–43]. Other genes include those encoding proteins such as the tissue inhibitor of metalloproteinase 3, TIMP3 [156], DNA mismatch repair enzymes such as MLH1, [157], and the CDKN2A/CDKN2B inhibitors of the cyclin D/cyclin-dependent cell cycle kinases [158]. An increased understanding of the developmental mechanisms that control the activation of genes expressed in adult differentiated tissues may guide therapies designed to reactivate genes silenced in cancers. As described above, gene activation is a complex process involving the presence of specific transcription factors and is highly dependent upon the states of modification of chromatin components. Recent experiments have suggested that future therapies designed to activate genes that are silenced in cancer may seek to promote both the demethylation of inactive gene loci and the acetylation of chromatin-associated histones using histone deacetylase inhibitors [138, 159].

5 Embryonic cells as therapeutic agents

True primordial embryonic stem cells are undifferentiated, totipotent cells that can produce daughter cells of all cell types. The description "stem cells" also is often applied to precursor cells that have a more restricted, yet still pluripotent, capacity to form differentiated progeny (reviewed in [160]). In some systems, these cells may be called "progenitor cells". In this article, we will use the term "embryonic primordial stem cells" (or ES cells) to define the totipotent cells of the early embryo and the term "stem cells" to define other pluripotent cells. Stem cells in embryos and adult organisms serve as a source of cells for populations of differentiated cell lineages. These cells are capable of self-renewal: they can create more stem cells as well as providing differentiated progeny. Some adult tissues contain stem cells that serve as a reserve population of cells which respond, at different rates, to accidents or changing environments to provide cells that can undergo further development within the organism. Recent studies clearly demonstrate that stem cell populations are present in many more tissues of the adult mammal than was previously considered. Transplanted stem cells are potentially powerful therapeutic agents for the treatment of many human diseases. They have been proposed as regenerative therapies for wound repair, neurological diseases, cardiac disease, liver diseases, blood/immune system diseases, and other disorders (reviewed in [161]). In such applications, transplanted stem cells would replace lost or diseased cells and develop into functional tissue. In addition, the transplanted stem cells and their progeny may release important signalling molecules that facilitate the function of existing cells and tissues. The differentiated progeny of transplanted stem cells should express the correct repertoire of receptor molecules so that they can respond appropriately to physiological signals within the patient. Further advantages of this approach may be that some applications may only require a one-time treatment, and that it may be possible to provide the stem cells in an encapsulated form, allowing confinement to a specific area and later retrieval, if required. Potential difficulties in the use of transplanted stem cells include rejection of the cells mediated by the immune response of the host and the challenge of controlling the differentiation of the cells to specific differentiated fates.

An advanced use of developmental biology-based therapeutics may involve the combined use of embryonic stem cells and developmentally important embryonic proteins. In these strategies, embryonic stem cells engineered to express specific developmental regulatory proteins may serve as self-renewing vehicles for gene therapies. These therapies may be targeted to specific tissues where the expressed proteins will enhance the potential of the stem cells and surrounding cells within the diseased/lost tissue to promote repair. In addition to their potential use as direct therapies and as vehicles for gene therapy, native and genetically engineered ES cells also may be useful tools in drug screening strategies, including the testing of embryonic proteins as therapeutic agents.

Future therapies may extend beyond the use of stem cells to the application of developmental biology to whole organ replacement. For example, researchers have made significant recent advances in the engineering of whole mammalian tissues, such as the *de novo* reconstitution of functional urinary bladders and arteries from canine and porcine cells, respectively [162, 163].

5.1 Sources of transplanted cells

Consideration of the source of transplanted cells is critical to their effectiveness as future therapeutic agents. Potential sources of transplanted cells for the treatment of human disease include autologous/autogeneic cells (from the same individual); allogeneic cells (from other individuals); and xeno-geneic cells (from non-human species). Each source of cells has advantages and disadvantages. Autogeneic cells are a perfect genetic match, and there-fore do not require strategies designed to avoid immunorejection of the cells. However, autogeneic cells are very likely to be in limited supply, may be hard to purify, and may be diseased.

Allogeneic cells also may be limited in supply and will likely require the use of immunosuppressive drugs to avoid rejection. Ethical concerns may limit or prohibit the direct use of human embryonic or foetal cells and tis-sues. The purification and culture of human or primate ES cells may provide a renewable "*in vitro*" source of pluripotent cells for transplantation and may circumvent some ethical concerns [164]. Thomson and colleagues recently have described the generation of long-lived human ES cell lines with normal genetic characteristics that have the capacity to differentiate into cell types of all three embryonic germ layers, including cartilage, bone, muscle, gan-glia, and gut cell phenotypes [165]. This publication has sparked both excite-ment at the potential therapeutic uses of transplantable cells derived from cultured human ES cells and also renewed debate of the ethics of using human derived cells of any kind. The potential power of this approach as a therapy was demonstrated recently by McKay and colleagues [166], who reported the successful use of ES cell-derived glial precursors in myelinating transplants in a rodent model system.

Xenogeneic cells, from primate or pig donor animals for example, may be more easily obtained than human cells, but are also likely to require the use of strategies to avoid rejection of the cells. Encapsulation of transplanted cells in devices that allow molecules to diffuse to and from the cells, but which prevent the entry of complement components and lymphocytes, may reduce or eliminate the need for general immunosuppression of the patient. Other strategies to avoid rejection of transplanted cells without immunosuppres-sion are being explored by companies such as Alexion and involve the use of donor cells from transgenic animals that express human immune regulatory molecules in order to inhibit or deceive the patient's immune system [163, 167]. Animals such as pigs may make good choices as donors because of their comparable size to humans, their similar physiology, and their relatively large litter sizes. Some studies have suggested that donor animals such as pigs, in addition to human and primate donors, may represent potential sources of infection with retroviruses such as the porcine endogenous retrovirus (PERV) (reviewed in [168]). Donor cells may therefore have to be screened before transplantation to avoid transmitting such viruses. However, a recent study by Paradis et al. [169], described the use of a battery of molecular techniques to analyze tissue and blood samples from 160 patients that had been exposed to living pig cells. These authors concluded that infection by PERV had not occurred in any of the patients. The ability to clone mammals such as sheep, cattle and mice [170-173] may also provide a homogeneous source of cells and organs for xenotransplantation in the future.

5.2   Cardiac cells

Cardiac disease is a major focus of research due to the prevalence of myocardiopathies and myocardial infarctions in the Western world. Recent experimental approaches have suggested that foetal cardiac cells may be used to replace damaged cardiac muscle in the treatment of heart disease. Field and colleagues have demonstrated that transplanted mouse or dog foetal cardiomyocytes can functionally populate the ventricular myocardium of recipient adult animals [174, 175]. By using foetal cardiac cells from transgenic animals expressing the beta-galactosidase enzyme as a marker, these researchers are easily able to identify donor cells in the hearts of recipient animals using colorimetric assays for enzyme activity. This group also has generated pure populations of cardiomyocytes from *in vitro* ES cell cultures and demonstrated that these cells also can be incorporated into working adult heart muscle [176]. Studies such as these will enable future protocols for the treatment of cardiac disease.

5.3   Haematopoietic stem cells

Haematopoietic stem cells (HSCs) are pluripotent cells that have the capacity to give rise to all cells of the haematopoietic system. They are first found in the yolk sac of the developing embryo and later in the foetal liver and the bone marrow. HSCs derived from the yolk sac, the foetal liver, umbilical cord blood, peripheral blood and bone marrow are all candidates for use as therapies to treat haematopoietic diseases, (auto)immune disorders and graft-*versus*-host disease. A major challenge in this field has been the identification of specific molecular markers of the true HSCs, allowing them to be distinguished from other haematopoietic (progenitor) cell types. Recent studies suggest that the VEGFR2/KDR receptor may be a useful cellular marker in defining the HSC cell type [177]. Intriguing studies also have demonstrated the plasticity of some stem cell populations and their ability to form diverse cell types. For example, Bjornson and colleagues showed that adult neural stem cells could even adopt haematopoietic fates when injected into irradiated mice [178].

Allogeneic bone marrow transplants are a potentially powerful therapy but often fail due to immunorejection and graft-*versus*-host disease (reviewed in [179, 180]). Broxmeyer and colleagues have demonstrated the promise of autologous or closely matched umbilical cord blood as a source of HSCs in the treatment of haematopoietic diseases, including anemias and leukaemias [179, 180]. Yolk sac stem cells (YS-HSCs) can be expanded *in vitro*, and transplanted YS-HSCs may be less immunoreactive than cord, bone or liver-derived HSCs since they lack expression of major histocompatability complex-associated antigens (reviewed in [181]). Systemix are investigating the potential use of YS-HSCs as therapies for a variety of blood disorders. Haematopoietic stem cells also may present both targets and vehicles for gene therapies of blood/immune diseases [179, 180].

5.4 Mesenchymal and other bone marrow stem cells

In addition to haematopoietic precursor cells, the adult bone marrow contains stem cells with the potential to differentiate into other cell fates. These include the mesenchymal stem cells (or marrow stromal cells, MSCs). MSCs can differentiate to form bone, cartilage, skeletal muscle, and adipocyte cell fates. The normal function of these cells may be to serve as a reserve of stem cells that have the capacity for regeneration of injured tissues after trauma or disease, or during aging. The multilineage potential of adult human MSCs was demonstrated by Pittenger and colleagues [182] who showed that MSCs could be maintained in stable, clonal culture and then induced to form specific daughter cell types, including cartilage, adipose and bone cells. Mesenchymal stem cells have potential for use in the treatment of soft tissue wounds, and tendon, cartilage and bone diseases including osteoporosis (reviewed in [183, 184]). For example, companies such as Osiris and MorphoGen are investigating the use of autologous MSCs, extracted from the bone marrow or other tissues of patients and expanded in culture, to repair joint surfaces in the treatment of arthritis or to restore damaged bone. A further use of MSCs might be as effective vehicles for gene therapy, whereby MSCs are engineered to express a therapeutic protein (such as a bone morphogenetic protein) and then are returned to the patient to repopulate the bone marrow and secrete the protein.

Recent studies also have revealed that haematopoietic and mesenchymal stem cells are not the only stem cells present in the bone marrow. Using rats as experimental models and genetically-marked donor cells, Petersen and colleagues [185] have demonstrated that cells of bone marrow origin can produce epithelial cells such as hepatic oval cells. This work, and that of others who have developed methods to purify and culture putative liver progenitor cells derived from the liver itself, offers promise for the future treatment of liver diseases [186, 187]. Further, the recent studies of Gussoni and colleagues of stem cells from bone marrow and muscle suggest that stem cells from diverse tissues may share many common biochemical properties [188].

5.5 Cells from the nervous system

Neural stem cells are being developed as therapies by companies such as NeuralStem Biopharmaceuticals for multiple diseases of the nervous system, including neurodegenerative diseases (Huntington's, Parkinson's, Alzheimer's), ALS, retinal degeneration, brain tumours, and myelination disorders [189–194]. Because the brain is an immunoprivileged site, implantation of embryonic neural stem cells to treat diseases of the brain may not require the use of immunosuppressive protocols that often complicate treatments involving other organs.

Snyder and colleagues [195] have successfully isolated stable clones of human foetal neural stem cells. These self-renewing clones were demonstrated to give rise to all types of neural lineages in culture. In addition, the stem cells were transplanted into the brains of newborn mice where they migrated appropriately to central nervous system regions and differentiated into multiple neural cell types [196]. Further, the human neural stem cells were capable of expressing foreign transgenes, demonstrating their potential as vehicles for gene therapy. This same research group has also demonstrated that even central nervous system diseases characterized by "global" neural degeneration might be amenable to stem cell neural transplantation [196]. They performed intracerebroventricular implantation of multipotent rodent neural stem cells into "shiverer" mice at birth. The oligodendrocytes of the shiverer mouse are dysfunctional because they lack myelin basic protein, a protein that is required for effective myelination. Shiverer mice exhibit a characteristic tremor. These mice therefore present an excellent experimental model for human diseases that result in extensive neural dysfunction. Shiverer mice receiving neural stem cells demonstrated widespread engraftment throughout the brain of myelin basic protein-positive oligodendrocyte descendant cells and some improvement of their symptoms [196]. Such studies may lead to future therapies for multiple sclerosis, cerebral palsy, Alzheimer's disease, and adrenoleukodystrophy.

Sources of neural stem cells for transplantation might not be limited to cells obtained from embryos. The occurrence of neurogenesis (the formation of new neurons) in adult rodent brains is widely accepted from the work of Altman and others (reviewed in [197]). It has been controversial, however, as to whether similar neurogenesis takes place in the adult primate brain. Recent work has demonstrated that this process does indeed occur in primates, including Old World monkeys and humans [198–200]. In a pivotal recent study, Gage and colleagues [198] examined the brains of cancer patients who had received diagnostic protocols involving the labeling of brain cells with bromodeoxyuridine. This compound marks actively dividing cells, and the researchers detected dividing cells in the dentate gyrus region of the hippocampus in all of the examined patients. In studies using macaque monkeys, others have observed similar patterns of neurogenesis [199]. In addition, the monkey studies suggested that the level of neurogenesis might decrease with age. Other laboratories have focused on identifying neural stem cells and on developing methods to purify and culture them. For example, one recent study has identified ependymal cells, cells of the neural tube lining, as having stem cell potential in the adult central nervous system [201]. The role of ependymal cells may be in providing new neural cells after injury. Another research group has isolated and characterized multipotent neural crest stem cells from foetal rats [202]. These cells can form functional neurons and glia after transplantation and exhibit self-renewal.

Successful remyelination has been observed following allogeneic and xenogeneic transplantation of oligodendrocyte astrocyte precursor cells into chemically- or impact-induced demyelinated lesions of the rat spinal cord [203, 204]. In human patients, foetal dopaminergic cells have been used to treat Parkinson's disease [205, 206], and similar cells obtained from foetal pigs (e.g. *Neurocell-PD*, Diacrin/Genzyme) are in clinical trials. Foetal pig brain cells expressing gamma-aminobutyric acid also are being examined in clinical trials in the treatment of Huntington's disease (e.g. *Neurocell-HD*, Diacrin/Genzyme). Other applications of embryonic neural cells include the use of cholinergic cells, obtained from the foetal adrenal medulla for example, as therapies for the treatment of Alzheimer's disease and as analgesics to combat pain.

6 Applications of developmental biology to animal agriculture

Animal agriculture is continually looking for ways to increase the efficiency of production of animal protein, specifically milk and meat. To date, most attention in this endeavor has focused on methods to increase the efficiency of conversion of feed to weight gain in the growing post-natal/post-hatch animal. Until recently, little or no attention was given to the animal before it was born or hatched. However, the embryonic and foetal period of development is forming an increasingly larger portion of an animal's lifetime from conception to market. For example, on average, broiler chickens go to market at 42 days of age after spending 21 days *in ovo*. This means that 33% of the lifetime of the broiler chicken grown for its meat is spent *in ovo*. A similar situation exists for cattle and swine. Pigs go to slaughter around 190 days of age and have a gestational period of approximately 114 days, so that about 37% of the lifetime of a pig in the swine industry is spent *in utero*. Beef cattle after 9 months of gestation have reached market weight at 20 months of age; 31% of their lifetime spent *in utero*. The embryonic/foetal period of development has just begun to be recognized as a time period that is potentially open to manipulation for increasing the efficiency of growth of the post-natal animal and for improving carcass characteristics of the animal at slaughter. In animal species, unlike in man, it is possible to consider the delivery of drugs directly to the developing embryo/foetus *in utero* or *in ovo*. In animal agriculture, therefore, the embryo/foetus itself can be considered a direct target for drug action creating a unique application of developmental biology to drug discovery. There are a number of advantages presented by drug delivery to the embryo. Firstly, it is possible to induce changes in the post-natal animal that would not be possible by post-natal/hatch drug delivery. For example, increasing muscle mass by increasing the total number of muscle fibers is only possible by manipulation *in utero* because in most mammalian species muscle fiber number is only labile during embryonic development and by birth the total number of fibers is fixed. Secondly, since embryonic development is a period of intense specification and differentiation, drug action is most likely targeted at a defined embryonic event that presents a defined window of opportunity for manipulation. The timing of drug delivery often needs to be precise, but the advantage is that the effect can often be irreversible leading to permanent changes in the developing embryo and permanent post-natal effects. For this reason, it is possible that a single administration of active agent would be sufficient to bring about the desired biological changes without a need for multiple dosing or long-term delivery.

In addition, the early administration of a drug, at least weeks if not months before the animal is slaughtered has the advantage of reducing the risk of residues in the tissues of the animal, particularly the meat: an ever present concern for meat producers. The indirect delivery of compounds to the developing mammalian embryo/foetus through the mother reduces this risk even further. In multiviviparous species, such as the pig, the delivery of pharmaceuticals to the mother that affect the entire offspring or litter allows drug delivery to multiple organisms through one single application.

In 1992, Embrex Inc. introduced the first automated egg injection system, the Inovoject system, to the USA which allowed for delivery of vaccines *in ovo* [207, 208]. Today more than 80% of broiler chickens are vaccinated *in ovo* against Marek's disease by delivery of the vaccine to the air sac of the day 18 developing chick embryo. Hence, a system is already in place and accepted by the industry for delivery of compounds *in ovo*. A procedure has been developed that enables injection prior to the onset of incubation without compromising embryo viability has opened up the window of embryonic development during incubation for intervention [209]. However, this field is still in its infancy with regard to the delivery of performance enhancing drugs. Two examples of such applications are the delivery of aromatase inhibitors and IGF-1 (insulin-like growth factor-1) *in ovo*. In the poultry industry, male birds are preferred over females since they grow faster and feed more efficiently. Chicken sexual dimorphism is thought to be the result of early embryonic exposure to different hormonal environments. The early embryonic gonads are bipotential and can develop as testes or ovary depending on the surrounding hormonal environment. High testosterone and low estradiol levels favor testes development and push development in the male direction. Several experimental paradigms exist for the induction of sex reversal in birds. Since females are the heterogametic sex in birds, gender selection by sperm sorting is not possible and the only way to make all male birds is to make females grow as males. Injection of aromatase inhibitors (AI, compounds that prevent estradiol biosynthesis from testosterone) have been shown to have dramatic sex-reversing effects on female chicks. A single treatment at day 5 of incubation was shown by Elbrecht and Smith [210] to cause testes production and spermatogenesis in female chickens. Similar results of *in ovo* injection of an aromatase inhibitor on producing a male phenotype in female birds have been reported by Johnston et al. [209]. Dewil et al. went on to show that when the AI vorozole was injected at day 6 of incubation, the treated female birds at 4 weeks post-hatch had reduced abdominal fat pad content [211]. Kocamis et al. have described positive effects after the delivery *in ovo* of recombinant IGF-1 [212]. Effects were greatest when the IGF-1 was delivered at day 1 or 4 of incubation where post-hatch feed efficiencies were improved for the first 3 weeks and live weights were increased in males.

For mammals, the embryo/foetus developing within the mother represents a challenge for drug delivery because the drug must have its effect across the placenta. Delivery to the mother can potentially occur *via* a number of routes including subcutaneous depots for long-term payouts, direct intravenous or intramuscular injection or orally. One example of drug delivery *in utero* that illustrates many of the features of embryonic drug delivery described earlier is the use of porcine somatotropin (pST) in gestating swine. Delivery of pST during days 15–45 of gestation in the pig leads to an increase in the number of muscle fibers in the developing foetus [213, 214]. Once a pig is born, the number of muscle fibers in any given muscle is effectively fixed, and the only way to increase muscle size (which translates into increased meat production) is by increasing the size of existing fibers, or muscle hypertrophy [215]. Increased muscle fiber number, or muscle hyperplasia, is a unique and complementary way to increase the muscle capacity of an animal. The increase in muscle fiber appears to lead to a permanent increase muscle size and meat characteristics such as loin eye area, in the post-natal animal up to market weight [216]. The mechanism of action of how pST delivery to the gestating sow leads to this effect is still uncertain, however, it is currently hypothesized that the increased maternal glucose concentration during somitogenesis leads to increased foetal hyperglycemia and raised foetal IGF-1 which affects the proliferation and differentiation of developing myofibers [217]. Although this application appears to show promise, the only large scale production trial of pST delivery *in utero* did not produce significant differences in growth or carcass characteristics of the treated animals, although there is some question as to whether post-natal nutrition was optimal enough to see the effect of treatment [218]. The recent discovery that ablation of function of GDF-8/myostatin, a muscle-specific conserved member of the TFGβ family of growth factors, leads to muscle hyperplasia has created a great deal of interest in animal agriculture [29]. This attention increased when it was found that natural mutations of the *myostatin* gene were the cause of the "double-muscling" phenotype in Belgian Blue and Piedmontese cattle [219–221]. These cattle, which have approximately 25% increased number of muscle fibers, have many desirable characteristics in terms of leanness and growth efficiency. Myostatin is expressed early during embryonic development and most likely functions during myogenesis as a negative regulator of muscle growth. To inhibit myostatin function pharmacologically to realise the hyperplastic muscle effects, it will be necessary to delivery myostatin antagonists *in utero* or *in ovo* and it can be expected that this application of developmental biology to drug discovery will continue to get attention in the near future.

7 Conclusions

Completion of the human genome project and the availability of genome information for model organisms will allow comprehensive analyses of the molecular nature of human diseases and the subsequent testing of the function of candidate genes. Novel therapeutic strategies will be developed for the treatment of injuries and major diseases such as cancer, heart disease, diabetes, neurodegenerative disorders, arthritis, infertility, and osteoporosis. These therapies may directly use multipotential stem cells, embryonic proteins, or will employ small molecules that target developmentally important pathways, to promote the functional repair or regeneration of diseased tissues. In addition, the genome itself will become a target: the reactivation and silencing of genes involved in development will be used to restore the normal gene expression profiles of diseased cells. It is clear that the increasing understanding of the molecular and cellular basis of eukaryotic development will provide important tools for the treatment of human diseases and will significantly impact animal agriculture.

Acknowledgement

We thank Dr. Pamela Crowell, Gretchen Parker and Kyle Sloop for constructive comments. We apologize to colleagues whose work is not referenced due to space constraints. Work in the laboratory of SJR is supported by grants from the National Science Foundation and the NRICGP/USDA.

References

1   J. Drews and S. Ryser: Drug Discovery Today 2, 365 (1997).
2   L.D. Hillier, G. Lennon, M. Becker, M.F. Bonaldo, B. Chiapelli, S. Chissoe, N. Dietrich, T. DuBuque, A. Favello, W. Gish et al.: Genome Res 6, 807 (1996).
3   V.E. Velculescu, L. Zhang, B. Vogelstein and K.W. Kinzler: Science 270, 484 (1995).
4   D. Stipp: Fortune, March 1997, 56.
5   M. Schena, D. Shalon, R.W. Davis and P.O. Brown: Science 270, 467 (1995).
6   E.A. Winzeler, D.R. Richards, A.R. Conway, A.L. Goldstein, S. Kalman, M.J. McCullough, J.H. McCusker, D.A. Stevens, L. Wodicka, D.J. Lockhart and R.W Davis: Science 281, 1194 (1998).
7   D. Ehrenstein: Science 277, 762 (1997).
8   S. Aldridge: Genetic Engineering News 18, 8 (1998).
9   S. Fields: Nature Genetics 15, 325 (1997).
10   P. Spence: Drug Discovery Today 3, 179 (1998).
11   S. Rastan and L.J. Beeley: Curr. Opin. Genet. Dev. 7, 777 (1997).
12   C.J. Rawlings and D.B. Searls: Curr. Opin. Genet. Dev. 7, 416 (1997).
13   G.L.G. Miklos and G. M. Rubin: Cell 86, 521 (1996).
14   R. Ainscough, S. Bardill, K. Barlow, V. Basham, C. Baynes, L. Beard, A. Beasley, M. Berks, J. Bonfield, J. Brown et al.: Science 282, 2012 (1998).
15   G. Ruvkun and O. Hobert: Science 282, 2033 (1998).
16   D.E. Bassett, M.S. Boguski, F. Spencer, R. Reeves, S-h. Kim, T. Weaver and P. Hieter: Nature Genetics 15, 339 (1997).
17   D.J. Grunwald: Science 274, 1634 (1996).
18   M. Granato and C. Nusslein-Volhard: Curr. Opin. Genet. Dev. 6, 461 (1996).
19   G. Vogel: Science 285, 901 (1999).
20   E.A. Winzeler E.A., D.D. Shoemaker, A. Astromoff, H. Liang, K. Anderson, B. Andre, R. Bangham, R. Benito, J.D. Boeke, H. Bussey et al.: Science 285, 901 (1999).
21   P.A. Sharp: Genes Dev. 13, 139 (1999).
22   S.R. Schwarze, A. Ho, A. Vocero-Akbani and S.F. Dowdy: Science 285, 1569 (1999).
23   Z. Galzie, A.R. Kinsella, and J.A. Smith: Biochem. Cell Biol. 75, 669 (1997).
24   D. Burke, D. Wilkes, T.L. Blundell and S. Malcolm: Trends Biochem. 23, 59 (1998).
25   A. Alevizopoulos and N. Mermod: Bioessays 19, 581 (1997).
26   B.L.M. Hogan: Genes Dev. 10, 1580 (1996).
27   M.R. Urist: J. Bone Min. Res. 12, 343 (1997).
28   A.C. McPherron, A.M. Lawler, and S.-J. Lee: Nature Genetics 22, 260 (1999).
29   A.C. McPherron, A.M. Lawler and S.J. Lee: Nature 387, 83 (1997).

30   J. Dong, D.F. Albertini, K. Nishimori, T.R. Kumar, N. Lu, and M.M. Matzuk: Nature *383*, 531 (1996).
31   L. Attisano and J.L. Wrana: Curr. Opin. Cell. Biol. *10*, 188 (1998).
32   K.W.Y. Cho and I.L. Blitz: Curr. Opin. Genet. Dev. *8*, 443 (1998).
33   D. St. Johnston and C. Nüsslein-Volhard: Cell *68*, 201 (1992).
34   M. Hammerschmidt, A. Brook and A.P. McMahon: Trends Genet. *13*, 14 (1997).
35   M.J. Bitgood, L. Shen and A.P. McMahon: Curr. Biol. *6*, 298 (1996).
36   B. St-Jacques, M. Hammerschmidt and A.P. McMahon: Genes Dev. *13*, 2072 (1999).
37   C. Chiang, Y. Litingtung, E. Lee, K.E. Young, J.L. Corden, H. Westphal and P.A. Beachy: Nature *383*, 407 (1996).
38   Y. Litingtung, L. Lei, H. Westphal and C. Chiang: Nature Genetics *20*, 58 (1998).
39   P.W. Ingham: Curr. Opin. Genet. Dev. *8*, 88 (1998).
40   R. L. Johnson and M. P. Scott: Curr. Opin. Genet. Dev. *8*, 450 (1998).
41   A.E. Oro, K.M. Higgins, Z. Hu, J.M. Bonifas, E.H. Epstein Jr. and M.P. Scott: Science *276*, 817 (1997).
42   J. Xie, M. Murone, S.-M. Luoh, A. Ryan, Q. Gu, C. Zhang, J.M. Bonifas, C.-W. Lam, M. Hynes, A. Goddard, A. Rosenthal et al.: *Nature* 391, 90 (1998).
43   M.R. Gailani and A.E. Bale: J. Natl. Cancer Inst. *89*, 1103 (1997).
44   W.P. Leenders: Int. J. Exp. Path. *79*, 339 (1998).
45   G. Neufeld, T. Cohen, S. Gengrinovitch and Z. Poltorak: FASEB J. *13*, 9 (1999).
46   I. Zachary: Int. J. Biochem. Cell Biol. *30*, 1169 (1998).
47   M. Paques, P. Massin and A. Gaudric: Diabetes Metab. *23*, 125 (1997).
48   J. Jonsson, L. Carlsson, T. Edlund and H. Edlund: Nature *371*, 606 (1994).
49   X. Luo, Y. Ikeda and K.L. Parker: Cell *77*, 481 (1994).
50   S.J.Rhodes, G.E. DiMattia and M.G Rosenfeld: Curr. Opin. Genet. Dev. *4*, 709 (1994).
51   P. Ducy, R. Zhang, V. Geoffroy, A.L. Ridall and G. Karsenty: Cell *89*, 747 (1997).
52   T. Komori, H. Yagi, S. Nomura, A. Yamaguchi, K. Sasaki, K. Deguchi, Y. Shimizu, R.T. Bronson, Y.H. Gao, M. Inada et al.: Cell *89*, 755 (1997).
53   D.C. Ludolph and S.F. Konieczny: FASEB J. *9*, 1595 (1995).
54   H.H. Arnold and B.N. Winter: Curr. Opin. Genet. Dev. *8*, 539 (1998).
55   D. Wang, M.J. Finegold, A. Bradley, C.N. Ou, S.V. Abdelsayed, M.D. Wilde, L.R. Taylor, D.R. Wilson and G.J. Darlington: Science *269*, 1108 (1995).
56   T.M. Loftus and M.D. Lane: Curr. Opin. Genet. Dev. *7*, 603 (1997).
57   P. Sarraf, E. Mueller, W.M. Smith, H.M. Wright, J.B. Kum, L.A. Aaltonen, A. de la Chapelle, B.M. Spiegelman and C. Eng: Mol. Cell *3*, 799 (1999).
58   M.L. Mucenski, K. McLain, A.B. Kier, S.H. Swerdlow, C.M. Schreiner, T.A. Miller, D.W. Pietryga, W.J. Scott Jr, S.S. Potter: Cell *65*, 677 (1991).
59   H. Lin and R. Grosschedl: Nature *376*, 263 (1995).
60   A.C. Perkins, A.H. Sharpe and S.H. Orkin: Nature *375*, 318 (1995).
61   P.P. Pandolfi, M.E. Roth, A. Karis, M.W. Leonard, E. Dzierzak, F.G. Grosveld, J.D. Engel and M.H. Lindenbaum: Nat. Genet. *11*, 40 (1995).
62   S.L. Nutt, A.M. Morrison, P. Dorfler, A. Rolink, M. Busslinger: EMBO J. *17*, 2319 (1998).
63   E.W. Scott, M.C. Simon, J. Anastasi and H. Singh: Science *265*, 1573 (1994).
64   M.M. Tondravi, S.R. McKercher, K. Anderson, J.M. Erdmann, M. Quiroz, R. Maki and S.L. Teitelbaum: Nature *386*, 81 (1997).
65   R.V. Pearse 2nd, D.W. Drolet, K.A. Kalla, F. Hooshmand, J.R. Bermingham Jr. and M.G. Rosenfeld: Proc. Natl. Acad. Sci. USA *94*, 7555 (1997).

66   D. Srivastava, T. Thomas, Q. Lin, M.L. Kirby, D. Brown and E.N. Olson: Nat. Genet. *16*, 154 (1997).

67   P. Riley, L. Anson-Cartwright and J.C. Cross: Na.t Genet. *18*, 271 (1998).

68   A.B. Firulli, D.G. McFadden, Q. Lin, D. Srivastava and E.N. Olson: Nat. Genet. *18*, 266 (1998).

69   J.D. Molkentin, Q. Lin, S.A. Duncan and E.N. Olson: Genes Dev. *11*, 1061 (1997).

70   I. Lyons, L.M. Parsons, L. Hartley, R. Li, J.E. Andrews, L. Robb, R.P. Harvey: Genes Dev. *9*, 1654 (1995).

71   C. Biben and R.P Harvey: Genes Dev. *11*, 1357 (1997).

72   H.M. Sucov, E. Dyson, C.L. Gumeringer, J. Price, K.R. Chien and R.M. Evans: Genes Dev. *8*, 1007 (1994).

73   M. Torres, E. Gomez-Pardo, G.R. Dressler and P Gruss: Development *121*, 4057 (1995).

74   J.A. Kreidberg, H. Sariola, J.M. Loring, M. Maeda, J. Pelletier, D. Housman and R. Jaenisch: Cell *74*, 679 (1993).

75   M.D. Shonemann, A.K. Ryan, R.J. McEvilly, S.M. O'Connell, C.A. Arias, K.A. Kalla, P. Li, P.E. Sawchenko and M.G. Rosenfeld: Genes Dev. *9*, 3122 (1995).

76   R.J. McEvilly, L. Erkman, L. Luo, P.E. Sawchenko, A.F. Ryan and M.G. Rosenfeld: Nature *384*, 574 (1996).

77   L. Erkman, R.J. McEvilly, L. Luo, A.K. Ryan, F. Hooshmand, S.M. O'Connell, E.M. Keithley, D.H. Rapaport, A.F. Ryan and M.G. Rosenfeld: Nature *381*, 603 (1996).

78   D. Phippard, L. Lu, D. Lee, J.C. Saunders and E.B. Crenshaw 3rd: J. Neurosci. *19*, 5980 (1999).

79   S.L. Pfaff, M. Mendelsohn, C.L. Stewart, T. Edlund and T.M. Jessell: Cell *84*, 309 (1996).

80   K. Sharma, H.Z. Sheng, K. Lettieri, H. Li, A. Karavanov, S. Potter, H. Westphal and S.L. Pfaff: Cell *95*, 817 (1998).

81   H. Li, D.P. Witte, W.W. Banford, B.J. Aronov, M. Weistein, S. Kaur, S. Wert, G. Singh, C.M. Schriener, J.A. Whitsett, W.J. Scott and S. Potter: EMBO J. *13*, 2876 (1994).

82   Y. Zhao, H.Z. Sheng, R. Amini, A. Grinberg, E. Lee, S. Huang, M. Taira and H. Westphal: Science *284*, 1155 (1999).

83   J.C. Grindley, D.R Davidson and R.E. Hill: Development *121*, 1433 (1995).

84   A. Stoykova, R. Fritsch, C. Walther and P Gruss: Development *122*, 3453 (1996).

85   J.L. Michaud, T. Rosenquist, N.R. May and C.M. Fan: Genes Dev. *12*, 3264 (1998).

86   J.R. Bermingham Jr., S.S. Scherer, S. O'Connell, E. Arroyo, K.A. Kalla, F.L. Powell and M.G. Rosenfeld: Genes Dev. *10*, 1751 (1996).

87   U. Ahlgren, S.L. Pfaff, T.M. Jessell, T. Edlund and H. Edlund: Nature *385*, 257 (1997).

88   B. Sosa-Pineda, K. Chowdhury, M. Torres, G. Oliver and P. Gruss: Nature *386*, 399 (1997).

89   L. St-Onge, B. Sosa-Pineda, K. Chowdhury, A. Mansouri and P. Gruss: Nature *387*, 406 (1997).

90   M. Sander, A. Neubuser, J. Kalamaras, H.C. Ee, G.R. Martin and M.S. German: Genes Dev. *11*, 1662 (1997).

91   H.Z. Sheng, K. Moriyama, T. Yamashita, H. Li, S.S. Potter, K.A. Mahon and H. Westphal: Science *278*, 1809 (1997).

92   S. Li, E.B. Crenshaw, III., E.J. Rawson, D.M. Simmons, L.W. Swanson and M.G. Rosenfeld: Nature *347*, 528 (1990).

93   M.W. Sornson, W. Wu, J.S. Dasen, S.E. Flynn, D.J. Norman, S.M. O'Connell, I. Gukovsky, C. Carrière, A.K. Ryan, A.P. and L. Miller et al.: Nature *384*, 327 (1996).

94   M.A. Rudnicki, T. Braun, S. Hinuma and R. Jaenisch: Cell *71*, 383 (1992).

95   Y. Nabeshima, K. Hanaoka, M. Hayasaka, E. Esumi, S. Li, I. Nonaka and Y. Nabeshima: Nature *364*, 532 (1993).

96   P. Hasty, A. Bradley, J.H. Morris, D.G. Edmondson, J.M. Venuti, E.N. Olson and W.H. Klein: Nature *364*, 501 (1993).

97   T. Braun, M.A. Rudnicki, H.H. Arnold, and R. Jaenisch: Cell *71*, 369 (1992).

98   E.N. Olson, H.H. Arnold, P.W. Rigby, and B.J. Wold: Cell *85*, 1 (1996).

99   B. Andersen, W.C. Weinberg, O. Rennekampff, R.J. McEvilly, J.R. Bermingham Jr, F. Hooshmand, V. Vasilyev, J.F. Hansbrough, M.R. Pittelkow, S.H. Yuspa and M.G. Rosenfeld: Genes Dev. *11*, 1873 (1997).

100   Q. Lin, J. Lu, H. Yanagisawa, R. Webb, G.E. Lyons, J.A. Richardson and E.N. Olson: Development *125*, 4565 (1998).

101   D.S. Latchman: Curr. Opin. Biotech. *8*, 713 (1997).

102   M.G. Peterson and V.R. Baichwal: TIBTECH *11*, 11 (1993).

103   S.A. Bustin and I.A.McKay: Brit. J. Biomed. Sci. *51*, 147 (1994).

104   T.R. Butt and S.K. Karathanasis: Gene Expression *4*, 319 (1995)

105   A. Heguy, A.A. Stewart, J.D. Haley, D.E. Smith and J.G. Foulkes: Gene Expression *4*, 337 (1995).

106   D.M.Harvey and C.T. Caskey: Curr. Opin. Chem. Biol. *2*, 512, (1998).

107   B.M. Forman, P. Tontonoz, J. Chen, R.P. Brun, B.M. Spiegelman and R.M. Evans: Cell *83*, 803 (1995).

108   K.B. Horwitz, T.A. Jackson, D.L. Bain, J.K. Richer, G.S. Takimoto and L. Tung: Mol. Endocrinol. *10*, 1167 (1996).

109   L. Xu, C.K. Glass and M.G. Rosenfeld: Curr. Opin. Genet. Dev. *9*, 140 (1997).

110   P.A. Wade, D. Pruss and A.P. Wolffe: Trends Biochem. Sci. *22*, 128 (1997).

111   M.J. Pazin and J.T. Kadonaga: Cell *89*, 325 (1997).

112   D. Vermaak and A.P. Wolffe: Dev. Genetics *22*, 1 (1998).

113   A.P. Wolffe and J.J. Hayes: Nuc. Acids Res. *27*, 711 (1999).

114   T.E. Spencer, G. Jenster, M.M. Burcin, C.D. Allis, J. Zhou, C.A. Mizzen, N.J. McKenna, S.A. Onate, S.Y. Tsai, M.J. Tsai and B.W. O'Malley: Nature *389*, 194 (1997).

115   J. Xu, Y. Qui, F.J. DeMayo, S.Y. Tsai, M.J. Tsai and B.W. O'Malley: Science *279*, 1922 (1998).

116   Y. Kamei, L. Xu, T. Heinzel, J. Torchia, R. Kurokawa, B. Gloss, S.C. Lin, R.A. Heyman, D.W. Rose, C.K. Glass and M.G. Rosenfeld: Cell *85*, 403 (1996).

117   H. Chen, R.J. Lin, R.L. Schiltz, D. Chakravarti, A. Nash, L. Nagy, M.L. Privalsky, Y. Nakatani and R.M. Evans: Cell *90*, 569 (1997).

118   T. Heinzel, R.M. Lavinsky, T.M. Mullen, M. Soderstrom, C.D. Laherty, J. Torchia, W.M. Yang, G. Brard, S.D. Ngo, J.R. Davie et al.: Nature *387*, 43 (1997).

119   J. Torchia, D.W. Rose, J. Inostroza, Y. Kamei, S. Westin, C.K. Glass and M.G. Rosenfeld: Nature *387*, 677 (1997).

120   R.T. Utley, K. Ikeda, P.A. Grant, J. Cote, D.J. Steger, A. Eberharter, S. John and J.L. Workman: Nature *394*, 498 (1998).

121   E. Korzus, J. Torchia, D.W. Rose,, L. Xu, R. Kurokawa, E.M. McInerney, T.M. Mullen, C.K. Glass and M.G. Rosenfeld: Science *279*, 703 (1998).

122   V.V. Ogryzko, R.L. Schiltz, V. Russanova, B.H. Howard and Y. Nakatani: Cell *87*, 953 (1996).

123   D. Chakravarti, V.J. LaMorte, M.C. Nelson, T. Nakajima, I.G. Schulman, H. Juguilon, M. Montminy and R.M. Evans: Nature *383*, 99 (1996).

124 C.L. Smith, S.A. Onate, M.J. Tsai and B.W. O'Malley: Proc. Natl. Acad. Sci. USA 93, 8884 (1996).

125 H. Kawasaki, R. Eckner, T.P. Yao, K. Taira, R. Chiu, D.M. Livingston and K.K. Yokoyama: Nature 393, 284 (1998).

126 V. Perissi, J.S. Dasen, R. Kurokawa, Z. Wang, E. Korzus, D.W. Rose, C.K. Glass and M.G. Rosenfeld: Proc. Natl. Acad. Sci. USA 96, 3652 (1999).

127 L. Xu, R.M. Lavinsky, J.S. Dasen, S.E. Flynn, E.M. McInerney, T.M. Mullen, T. Heinzel, D. Szeto, E. Korzus, R. Kurokawa et al.: Nature 395, 301 (1998).

128 P. Bailey, M. Downes, P. Lau, J. Harris, S. Chen, Y. Hamamori, V. Sartorelli and G.E.O. Muscat: Mol. Endocrinol. 13, 1155 (1999).

129 R.M. Lavinsky, K. Jepsen, T. Heinzel, J.Torchia, T.M. Mullen, R. Schiff, A.L. Del-Rio, M. Ricote, S. Ngo, J. Gemsch et al.: Proc. Natl. Acad. Sci. USA 95, 2920 (1998).

130 R.B. Lanz, N.J. McKenna, S.A. Onate, U. Albrecht, J. Wong, S.Y. Tsai, M.-J. Tsai and B.W. O'Malley: Cell 97, 17 (1999).

131 Y.B. Kim, K.H. Lee, K. Sugita, M. Yoshida and S. Horinouchi: Oncogene 18, 2461 (1999).

132 W. Feng, R.C. J. Ribeiro, R.L. Wagner, H. Nguyen, J.W. Apriletti, R.J. Fletterick, J.D. Baxter, P.J. Kushner and B.L.West: Science 280, 1747 (1998).

133 J.D. Norris, D. Fan, M.R. Stallcup and D.P. McDonnell: J. Biol. Chem. 273, 6679 (1998).

134 I. Zamir, J. Zhang and M.A. Lazar: Genes Dev. 11, 835 (1997).

135 R.J. Lin, L. Nagy, S. Inoue, W. Shao, W.H. Miller, Jr. and R.M. Evans: Nature 391, 811 (1998).

136 F. Grignani, S. De Matteis, C. Nervi, L. Tomassoni, V. Gelmetti, M. Cioce, M. Fanelli, M. Ruthardt, F.F. Ferrara, I. Zamir et al.: Nature 391, 815 (1998).

137 R.P Warrell, Jr., LZ. He, V. Richon, E. Calleja and P.P. Pandolfi: J. Natl. Cancer Inst. 90, 1621 (1998).

138 S. Eden, T. Hashimshony, I. Keshet, H. Cedar and AW. Thorne: Nature 394, 842 (1998).

139 P.A. Wade, A. Gegonne, P.L. Jones, E. Ballestar, F. Aubry and Wolffe: Nat. Genet. 23, 62 (1999).

140 D. Chen, H. Ma, H. Hong, S.S. Koh, S.-M. Huang, B.T. Schurter, D.W. Aswad and M.R. Stallcup: Science 284, 2174 (1999).

141 S.M. Jane and J.M. Cunningham: Brit. J. Haematol. 102, 415 (1998).

142 R.A. Swank and G. Stamatoyannopoulos: Curr. Opin. Genet. Dev. 8, 366 (1998).

143 A.F. Stewart, J. Suzow, T. Kubota, T. Ueyama and H.H. Chen: Circ. Res. 83, 43 (1998).

144 J.D. Molkentin and E.N. Olson: Circulation 96, 3833 (1997).

145 W.Y. Huang and C.C. Liew: J. Mol. Cell Cardiol. 30, 1673 (1998).

146 H.W. Lim and J.D. Molkentin: Nat. Med. 5, 246 (1999).

147 M.A. Sussman, H.W. Lim, N. Gude, T. Taigen, E.N. Olson, J. Robbins, M.C. Colbert, A. Gualberto, D.F. Wieczorek and J.D. Molkentin: Science 281, 1690 (1998).

148 R.A. Walsh: Circ. Res. 84, 741 (1999).

149 J.D. Molkentin, J.-R. Lu, C.L. Antos, B. Markham, J. Richardson, J. Robbins, S.R. Grant and E.N. Olson: Cell 93, 215 (1998).

150 S.V. Subramanian, C.G. Orosz and A.R.Strauch: Transplantation 65, 1652 (1998).

151 C. Depre, G.L. Shipley, W. Chen, Q. Han, T. Doenst, ML. Moore, S. Stepkowski, PJ. Davies and H. Taegtmeyer: Nat. Med. 4, 1269 (1998).

152 V.A. Zakian: Cell 91, 1 (1997).

153 J.W. Shay: J. Cell. Physiol. 173, 266 (1997).

154 S.E. Holt and J.W. Shay: J. Cell Physiol. 180, 10 (1999).

155   G. Nardone, M. Romano, A. Calabro, P.V. Pedone, I. de Sio, M. Persico, G. Budillon, C.B. Bruni, A. Riccio and R. Zarrilli: Hepatology *23*, 1304 (1996).

156   T. Andreu, T. Beckers, E. Thoenes, P. Hilgard and H. von Melchner: J. Biol. Chem. *273*, 13848 (1998).

157   G. Deng, A. Chen, J. Hong and H.S. Chae and Y.S. Kim: Cancer Res. *59*, 2029 (1999).

158   Y.W. Lin, C.H. Chen, G.T. Huang, P.H. Lee, J.T. Wang, D.S. Chen, F.J. Lu and JC. Sheu: Eur. J. Cancer *34*, 1789 (1998).

159   E.E. Cameron, K.E. Bachman, S. Myöhänen, J.G. Herman and S.B. Baylin: Nature Genetics *21*, 103 (1999).

160   L.M. Reid: Mol. Biol. Rep. *23*, 21 (1996).

161   D.L. Stocum, in: P. Ferretti and J. Geraudie (eds.): Cellular and molecular basis of regeneration: from invertebrates to humans, John Wiley and Sons Ltd., Chichester 1998, 411–450.

162   F. Oberpenning, J. Meng, J.J. Yoo and A. Atala: Nature Biotech. *17*, 149 (1999).

163   L.E. Niklason, J. Gao, W.M. Abbott, K.K. Hirshi, S. Houser, R. Marini and R. Langer: Science *284*, 489 (1999).

164   S.J. Wright: American Scientist *87*, 352 (1999).

165   J.A. Thomson, J. Itskovitz-Eldor, S.S. Shapiro, M.A. Waknitz, J.J. Swiergiel, V.S. Marshall and J.M. Jones: Science *282*, 1145 (1998).

166   O. Brüstle, K.N. Jones, R.D. Learish, K. Karram, K. Choudhary, O.D. Wiestler, I.D. Duncan and R.D.G. McKay: Science *285*, 754 (1999).

167   W.W. Hancock: Kidney Int. Supp. *58*, S36 (1997).

168   R.A. Weiss: Nature *391*, 327 (1998).

169   K. Paradis, G. Langford, Z. Long, W. Heneine, P. Sandstrom, W.M. Switzer, L.E. Chapman, C. Lockey, D. Onions, The XEN 111 Study Group and E. Otto: Science *285*, 1236 (1999).

170   K.H.S. Campbell, J. McWhir, W.A. Ritchie and I. Wilmut: Nature *380*, 64 (1996).

171   I. Wilmut, A.E. Schnieke, J. McWhir, A.J. Kind and K.H. Campbell: Nature 385, 810 (1997).

172   J.B. Cibelli, S.L. Stice, P.J. Golueke, J.J. Kane, J. Jerry, C. Blackwell, F., A. Ponce de León and J.M. Robl: Science *280*, 1256 (1998).

173   T. Wakayama, A.C.F. Perry, M. Zuccotti, K.R. Johnson and R. Yanagimachi: Nature *394*, 369 (1998).

174   M.H. Soonpaa, G.Y. Koh, M.G. Klug and L.J. Field: Science *264*, 98 (1994).

175   G.Y. Koh, S.J. Kim, M.G. Klug, K. Park, M.H. Soonpaa and L.J. Field: J. Clin. Invest. *96*, 2034 (1995).

176   M.G. Klug, M.H. Soonpaa, G.Y. Koh and L.J. Field: J. Clin. Invest. *98*, 216 (1996).

177   B. L. Ziegler, M. Valtieri, G. Almeida Porada, R. De Maria, R. Müller, B. Masella, M. Gabbianelli, I. Casella, E. Pelosi et al.: Science *285*, 1553 (1999).

178   C.R.R. Bjornson, R.L. Rietze, B.A. Reynolds, M.C. Magli and A.L. Vescovi: Science *283*, 534 (1999).

179   H.E. Broxmeyer, in: E.J. Freireich and H. Kantarjian (eds.): Molecular genetics and therapy of leukemia, Kluwer Academic, Boston 1996, 139–148.

180   L. Lu, R.N. Shen and H.E. Broxmeyer: Crit. Rev. Onc.-Hemat. *22*, 61 (1996).

181   R. Auerbach, H. Huang and L. Lu: Stem Cells *14*, 269 (1996).

182   M.F. Pittenger, A.M. Mackay, S.C. Beck, R.K. Jaiswal, R. Douglas, J.D. Mosca, M.A. Moorman, D.W. Simonetti, S. Craig and D.R. Marshak: Science *284*, 143 (1999).

183   S.P. Bruder, D.J. Fink and A.I. Caplan: J. Cell Biochem. *56*, 283 (1994).

184   D. Prockop: Science *276*, 71 (1997).

185   B.E. Petersen, W.C. Bowen, K.D. Patrene, W.M. Mars, A.K. Sullivan, N. Murase, S.S. Boggs, J.S. Greenberger and J.P. Goff: Science *284*, 1168 (1999).

186   M. Agelli, P. Dello Sbarba, E.D. Halay, R.A.D.E. Hixson and L.M. Reid: Histochem. J. *29*, 205 (1997).

187   S. Brill, I. Zvibel and L.M. Reid: Digest Dis. Sci. *44*, 364 (1999).

188   E. Gussoni, Y. Soneoka, C.D. Strickland, E.A. Buzney, M.K. Khan, A.F. Flint, L.M. Kunkel and R.C. Mulligan: Nature *401*, 390 (1999).

189   E.E. Baetge: Ann. New York Acad. Sci. *695*, 285 (1993).

190   F.H. Gage, J. Ray and L.J. Fisher: Ann. Rev. Neurosci. *18*, 159 (1995).

191   S.R. Whittemore, M.J. Eaton and S.M. Onifer: Adv. Neurology *72*, 113 (1997).

192   R. McKay: Science *276*, 66 (1997).

193   M. Mayer-Proschel, M.S. Rao and M. Noble: J. NIH Res. *9*, 31 (1997).

194   S.B. Dunnett and A. Björklund: Nature *399*, A32 (1998).

195   J.D. Flax, S. Aurora, C.Yang, C. Simonin, A.M. Wills, L.L. Billinghurst, M. Jendoubi, R.L. Sidman, J.H. Wolfe, S.U. Kim and E.Y. Snyder: Nature Biotech. *16*, 1033 (1998).

196   B.D. Yandava, L.L. Billinghurst and E.Y. Snyder: Proc. Natl. Acad. Sci. USA *96*, 7029 (1999).

197   S.A. Bayer: Ann. New York Acad. Sci. *457*, 163 (1983).

198   P.S. Eriksson, E. Perfilieva, T. Bjork-Eriksson, A.M. Alborn, C. Nordborg, D.A. Peterson and F.H. Gage: Nature Medicine *4*, 1313 (1998).

199   E. Gould, A.J. Reeves, M. Fallah, P. Tanapat, C.G. Gross and E. Fuchs: Proc. Natl. Acad. Sci. USA *96*, 5263 (1999).

200   E. Gould, A.J. Reeves, M.S.A. Graziano and C.G. Gross: Science *286*, 548 (1999).

201   C.B. Johansson, S. Momma, D.L. Clarke, M. Risling, U. Lendahl and J. Frisén: Cell *96*, 25 (1999).

202   S.J. Morrison, P.M. White, C. Zock and D.J. Anderson: Cell *96*, 737 (1999).

203   A.K. Groves, S.C. Barnett, R.J. Franklin, A.J. Crang, M. Mayer, W.F. Blakemore and M. Noble: Nature *362*, 453 (1993).

204   J. Rosenbluth, R. Schiff, W.L. Liang, G. Menna and W. Young: Exp. Neurol. *147*, 172 (1997).

205   A. Kupsch, W.H. Oertel, C.D. Earl and J. Sautter: J. Neur. Trans. Supp. *46*, 193 (1995).

206   C. French-Constant and G.A. Mathews: J. Neurol. *242* (Supp. 1), S29 (1994).

207   C.A. Ricks., A. Avakian, T. Bryan, R. Gildersleeve., E. Haddad., R. Ilich, S. King. L. Murray, P. Phelps, R. Poston et al.: Adv. Vet. Med. *41*, 495 (1999).

208   R.P. Gildersleeve, C.M. Hoyle, A.M. Miles, D.L. Murraym, C.A. Ricks, M.N. Secrest, C.J. Williams and C.L. Womack: J. Appl. Poultry Res. *2*, 337 (1993).

209   P.A. Johnston, H. Liu, T. O'Connell, P. Phelps, M. Bland, J. Tyczhowski, A. Kemper, T. Harding, A. Avakian, E. Haddad et al.: Poultry Sci. *76*, 165 (1997).

210   A. Elbrecht and R.G. Smith: Science *255*, 467 (1992).

211   E. Dewil, J. Buyse, J.D. Veldhuis., J. Mast, R. De Coster and E. Decuypere: Dom. Anim. Endocrinol. *15*, 115 (1998).

212   H. Kocamis, D.C. Kirkpatrick-Keller, H. Klandorf and J. Killefer: Poultry Sci. *77*, 1913 (1998).

213   C.M. Dwyer, J.M. Fletcher and N.C. Stickland: J. Anim. Sci. *71*, 3339 (1993).

214   C. Rehfeldt, I. Fiedler, R. Weikard, E. Kanitz and K. Ender: Biosci. Rep. *13*, 213 (1993).

215   N.C. Stickland: Meat Focus International, June 1995, 241.

216   R.L. Kelley, S.B. Jungst, T.E. Spencer, W.F. Owsley, C.H. Rahe and D.H. Mulvaney: Dom. Anim. Endocrinol. *12*, 83 (1995).

217   J.A. Sterle, T.C. Cantley, W.R. Lamberson, M.C. Lucy, D.E. Gerrard, R.L. Matteri and B.N. Day: J. Anim. Sci. *73*, 2980 (1995).

218   C.L. McLaughlin, C.S. Miner, M.T. Coffey, G. Pratt and C.A. Baile: J. Anim. Sci. *74* (Suppl.) 142 (1996).

219   R. Kambadur, M. Sharma, T.P.L. Smith and J.J. Bass: Genome Res. *7*, 910 (1997).

220   L. Grobet, L.J.R. Martin, D. Poncelet, D. Pirottin, B. Brouwers, J. Riquet, A. Schoeberlein, S. Dunner, F. Menissier, J. Massabanda et al.: Nature Genetics *17*, 71 (1997).

221   A.C. McPherron and S-J. Lee: Proc. Natl. Acad. Sci. USA *94*, 12457 (1997).

Index Vol. 54

Insulin sensitizers 195
Insulin 34, 50, 194
Insulin-like growth factor 237
Insulin-producing cells 221
Interleukin 34, 222
Inuline 19
Iometopane 104
Isoleucine 68, 134

Kainate receptors 156
Kainic acid 156
Kidney diseases 224
Kidney failure 226
Korsakoff's syndrome 124

Labetalol 9, 18
Learning 156
Leptin system 45
Leptin 34, 49, 53
Leu-enkephalin 128
Leukaemia, promyelocytic 235
Leukemia cells 72
Limbic hedonic systems 43
Lisinopril 19
Litoxetine 81
Lofepramine 111, 112

Magnesium ions 156
Mannitol 9, 18, 19, 21
Manzdiol 39
Maprotiline 111, 112
Marek's disease 246
Mazindol 71, 110
Mechano-receptors 33
Melanocortin 47, 134
Melanocyte-stimulating hormone 126
Meloxicam 8, 18
Memory 156
Metabolism of energy 34
Metallopeptidases 127
Metastasis 237
Metformin 194
Methotrexate 19
Methylscopolamine 9
Metoprolol 8, 17, 21
Monoamine transporter antagonists 71
Monoamines 39, 44
Morphine 127
Morphine-like peptides 124

Motilin 134
Multiple sclerosis 227
Mus musculus 218
Myelination disorders 243
Myocardial infarctions 241
Myocardiopathies 241
Myogenin 229
Myostatin 223, 248
Mysenchymal cells 242

Nadolol 9, 18
Naproxen 17
Natriuretic peptide 134
Nerve growing factor 132, 218
Neupogen 222
Neurobiology 124
Neurodegenerative diseases 156
Neuromodulators 124
Neuronal plasticity 156
Neuropathy 194
Neuropathy, diabetic 136
Neuropeptide receptors 125
Neuropeptide Y 44, 126
Neuropeptides 30, 35, 44, 121
Neuropeptides, synthesis 33
Neurotensin 126, 134, 144
Neurotransmitter systems 130
Neurotransmitters 30, 124
Neurotrophic factors 132
Neurotrophin 132
Neutropenia 224
Nevirapine 8, 17
Nicotine 8, 18
Nisoxetine 73, 78, 108
Nitroquipazine 81
N-Methyl-D-asparate 156
Noloxone 17
Nomifenisine 110
Noradrenalin 42
Norepinephrine transporters 70, 104
Norepinephrine 59
Norfluoxetine 73
Normoglycemia 194
Nortriptyline 111, 112
Norzimeldine 76
Noxiptiline 81
Nuclear proteins 228
Nucleus accumbens 35

Index of titles
Vol. 1–54 (1959–2000)

Impact of natural product research on drug discovery
23, 51 (1979)
Impact of state and society on medical research
35, 9 (1990)
Indole compounds
6, 75 (1963)
Indolstruktur, in Medizin und Biologie
2, 227 (1960)
Industrial drug research
20, 143 (1976)
Influenza virus, functional significance of the various components of
18, 253 (1974)
Insulin resistance, impaired glucose tolerance, and non-insulin-dependent diabetes, pathologic mechanisms and treatment: Current status and therapeutic possibilities
51, 33 (1998)
Interferons (Production and action): New insights into molecular mechanisms of gene regulation and expression
43, 239 (1994)
Ion and water transport in renal tubular cells
26, 87 (1982)
Ionenaustauscher, Anwendung in Pharmazie und Medizin
1, 11 (1959)
Isoprenoid biosynthesis via the mevalonate route, a novel target for antibacterial drugs
50, 135 (1998)
Isosterism and bioisosterism in drug design
37, 287 (1991)
Isotope, Anwendung in der pharmazeutischen Forschung
7, 59 (1964)

κ receptor, U-50,488 and the: A personalized account covering the period 1973 to 1990
52, 167 (1999)
κ receptor, U-50,488
53, 1 (1999)
Ketoconazole, a new step in the management of fungal disease
27, 63 (1983)

Leishmaniasis
18, 289 (1974)
Leishmaniasis, present status of
34, 447 (1990)
Leprosy, some neuropathologic and cellular aspects of
18, 53 (1974)
Leprosy in the Indian context, some practical problems of the epidemiology of
18, 25 (1974)
Leprosy, malaria and filariasis, new perspectives on the chemotherapy of
18, 99 (1974)
Leprosy, progress in the chemotherapy: Status, issues and prospects
34, 421 (1990)
Leukotriene antagonists and inhibitors of leukotriene biosynthesis
37, 9 (1991)
Levamisole
20, 347 (1976)
Light and dark as a "drug"
31, 383 (1987)
Lipophilicity and drug activity
23, 97 (1979)
Lokalanästhetika, Konstitution und Wirksamkeit
4, 353 (1962)
Luteinizing hormone regulators: Luteinizing hormone releasing hormone analogs, estrogens, opiates, and estrogen-opiate hybrids
42, 39 (1994)
Luteolytic agents in fertility regulation
40, 9 (1993)
Lysostaphin: Model for a specific enzymatic approach to infectious disease
16, 309 (1972)

Malaria, advances in chemotherapy
30, 221 (1986)
Malaria chemotherapy, repository antimalarial drugs
13, 170 (1969)
Malaria chemotherapy, antibiotics in
26, 167 (1982)
Malaria, eradication in India
18, 245 (1974)

Author and paper index
Vol. 1–54 (1959–2000)

Recent developments in the chemo-therapy of schistosomiasis *16*, 11 (1972)	S. Archer A. Yarinsky
Recent progress in the chemotherapy of schistosomiasis *18*, 15 (1974) Recent progress in research on narcotic antagonists *20*, 45 (1976)	S. Archer
Molecular geometry and mechanism of action of chemical carcinogens *4*, 407 (1962)	J. C. Arcos
Cell-kinetic and pharmacokinetic aspects in the use and further development of cancerostatic drugs *20*, 521 (1976)	M. von Ardenne
Molecular pharmacology, a basis for drug design *10*, 429 (1966) Reduction of drug action by drug combination *14*, 11 (1970)	E. J. Ariëns
Stereoselectivity and affinity in molecular pharmacology *20*, 101 (1976)	E. J. Ariëns J. F. Rodrigues de Miranda P. A. Lehmann
The pharmacology of caffeine *31*, 273 (1987)	M. J. Arnaud
Recent advances in central 5-hydroxytryptamine receptor agonists and antagonists *30*, 365 (1986)	Lars-Erik Arvidsson Uli Hacksell Richard A. Glennon
Drugs affecting the renin-angiotensin system *26*, 207 (1982)	R. W. Ashworth
Tetanus neonatorum *19*, 189 (1975) Tetanus in children *19*, 209 (1975)	V. B. Athavale P. N. Pai A. Fernandez P. N. Patnekar Y. S. Acharya
Toxicity of propellants *18*, 365 (1974)	D. M. Aviado
Polyamines as markers of malignancy *39*, 9 (1992)	Uriel Bachrach
Neuere Aspekte der chemischen Anthelminticaforschung *1*, 243 (1959)	J. Bally

Problems in preparation, testing and use of diphtheria, pertussis and tetanus vaccines *19*, 229 (1975)	D. D. Banker
Phosphodiesterase 4 (PDE4) inhibitors in asthma and chronic obstructive pulmonary disease *53*, 193 (1973)	Mary S. Barnette
Recent advances in electrophysiology of antiarrhythmic drugs *17*, 33 (1973)	A. L. Bassett A. L. Wit
Chirality and future drug design *41*, 191 (1993)	Sanjay Batra Manju Seth A. P. Bhaduri
Drugs for treatment of patients with high cholesterol blood levels and other dyslipidemias *43*, 9 (1994)	Harold E. Bays Carlos A. Dujovne
Stereochemical factors in biological activity *1*, 455 (1959)	A. H. Beckett
Natriuretic hormones II *45*, 245 (1995)	Elaine J. Benaksas E. David Murray, Jr. William J. Wechter
Molecular modelling and quantitative structure-activity analysis of anti-bacterial sulfanilamides and sulfones *36*, 361 (1991)	P. G. De Benedetti
Industrial research in the quest for new medicines *20*, 143 (1976) The experimental biologist and the medical scientist in the pharmaceutical industry *24*, 38 (1980)	B. Berde
Newer diuretics *2*, 9 (1960)	K. H. Beyer, Jr. J. E. Baer
Recent developments in 8-amino-quinoline antimalarials *28*, 197 (1984)	A. P. Bhaduri B. K. Bhat M. Seth
Studies on diphtheria in Bombay *19*, 241 (1975)	M. Bhaindarkar Y. S. Nimbkar
Bitoscanate in children with hookworm disease *19*, 6 (1975)	B. Bhandari L. N. Shrimali
Recent studies on genetic recombination in *Vibriocholerae* *19*, 460 (1975)	K. Bhaskaran

Interbiotype conversion of cholera vibrios by action of mutagens 19, 466 (1975)	P. Bhattacharya S. Ray
Experience with bitoscanate in hook-worm disease and trichuriasis in Mexico 19, 23 (1975)	F. Biagi
Analysis of symptoms and signs related with intestinal parasitosis in 5,215 cases 19, 10 (1975)	F. Biagi R. López J. Viso
Untersuchungen zur Biochemie und Pharmacologie der Thymoleptika 11, 121 (1968) The role of adipose tissue in the distribution and storage of drugs 28, 273 (1984)	M. H. Bickel
The β-adrenergic-blocking agents, pharmacology, and structure-activity relationships 10, 46 (1966)	J. H. Biel B. K. B. Lum
Prostaglandins 17, 410 (1973)	J. S. Bindra R. Bindra
In vitro models for the study of antibiotic activities 31, 349 (1987)	J. Blaser S. H. Zinner
The red blood cell membrane as a model for targets of drug action 17, 59 (1973)	L. Bolis
Epidemiology and public health. Importance of intestinal nematode infections in Latin America 19, 28 (1975)	D. Botero
Clinical importance of cardiovascular drug interactions 25, 133 (1981) Serum electrolyte abnormalities caused by drugs 30, 9 (1986)	D. Craig Brater
Update of cardiovascular drug interactions 29, 9 (1985)	D. Craig Brater Michael R. Vasko
Some practical problems of the epidemiology of leprosy in the Indian context 18, 25 (1974)	S. G. Browne
Brain neurotransmitters and the development and maintenance of experimental hypertension 30, 127 (1986)	Jerry J. Buccafusco Henry E. Brezenoff
Die Ionenaustauscher und ihre An-wendung in der Pharmazie und Medizin 1, 11 (1959)	J. Büchi

5-Hydroxytryptamine (5-HT)$_4$ receptors and central nervous system function: An update *49*, 9 (1997)	Richard M. Eglen
Drug-macromolecular interactions: Implications for pharmacological activity *14*, 59 (1970)	S. Ehrenpreis
Betrachtungen zur Entwicklung von Heilmitteln *10*, 33 (1966)	G. Ehrhart
Progress in malaria chemotherapy, Part I. Repository antimalarial drugs *13*, 170 (1969) New perspectives on the chemotherapy of malaria, filariasis and leprosy *18*, 99 (1974)	E. F. Elslager
Recent research in the field of 5-hydroxytryptamine and related indolealkylamines *3*, 151 (1961)	V. Erspamer
Recent advances in erythropoietin research *41*, 293 (1993)	James W. Fisher
The chemistry of DNA modification by antitumor antibiotics *32*, 411 (1988)	Jed. F. Fisher Paul A. Aristoff
Toward peptide receptor ligand drugs: Progress on nonpeptides *40*, 33 (1993)	Roger M. Freidinger
Transfer factor 1993: New frontiers *42*, 309 (1994)	H. Hugh Fudenberg Giancarlo Pizza
Drugs affecting serotonin neurons *35*, 85 (1990) Serotonin uptake inhibitors: Uses in clinical therapy and laboratory research *45*, 167 (1995)	Ray W. Fuller
Bacteriology at the periphery of the cholera pandemic *19*, 513 (1975)	A. L. Furniss
Emerging drug targets in the molecular pathogenesis of asthma *47*, 165 (1996)	Jeanne Fürst Jucker Gary P. Anderson
Iron and diphteria toxin production *19*, 283 (1975)	S. V. Gadre S. S. Rao
Effect of drugs on cholera toxin induced fluid in adult rabbit ileal loop *19*, 519 (1975)	B. B. Gaitonde P. H. Marker N. R. Rao
Drug action and assay by microbial kinetics *15*, 519 (1971)	E. R. Garrett

The use of quantum chemical methods to study molecular mechanisms of drug action 34, 9 (1990)	H.-D. Höltje M. Hense S. Marrer E. Maurhofer
Troglitazone and emerging glitazones: New avenues for potential therapeutic benefits beyond glycemic control 54, 235 (2000)	Hiroyoshi Horikoshi Toshihiko Hashimoto Toshihiko Fujiwara
Relationship of induced antibody titres to resistance to experimental human infection 19, 542 (1975)	R. B. Hornick R. A. Cash J. P. Libonati
Recent applications of mass spectrometry in pharmaceutical research 18, 399 (1974)	G. Horváth
Risk assessment problems in chemical oncogenesis 31, 257 (1987)	G. H. Hottendorf
Bacterial resistence to antibiotics: The role of biofilms 37, 91 (1991)	Brian D. Hoyle J. William Costerton
Recent developments in disease-modifying antirheumatic-drugs 24, 101 (1980)	I. M. Hunneyball
The pharmacology of homologous series 7, 305 (1964)	H. R. Ing
Progress in the experimental chemotherapy of helminth infections. Part. 1. Trematode and cestode diseases 17, 241 (1973)	P. J. Islip
Pharmacology of the brain: The hippocampus, learning and seizures 16, 211 (1972)	I. Izquierdo A. G. Nasello
Cholinergic mechanism – monoamines relation in certain brain structures 16, 334 (1972)	J. A. Izquierdo
The development of antifertility substances 7, 133 (1964)	H. Jackson
Development of novel anti-inflammatory agents: A pharmacological perspective on leukotrienes and their receptors 46, 115 (1996)	William T. Jackson Jerome H. Fleisch
Agents acting on central dopamine receptors 21, 409 (1977)	P. C. Jain N. Kumar
Recent advances in the treatment of parasitic infections in man 18, 191 (1974) The levamisole story 20, 347 (1976)	P. A. J. Janssen

Recent developments in cancer chemotherapy *25*, 275 (1981)	K. Jewers
Search for pharmaceutically interesting quinazoline derivatives: Efforts and results (1969–1980) *26*, 259 (1982)	S. Johne
Serotonin in migraine: Theories, animal models and emerging therapies *51*, 219 (1998)	Kirk W. Johnson Lee A. Phebus Marlene L. Cohen
A review of advances in prescribing for teratogenic hazards *29*, 121 (1985)	E. Marshall Johnson
A comparative of bitoscanate, bephenium hydroxynaphthoate and tetrachlor- ethylene in hookworm infection *19*, 70 (1975)	S. Johnson
Polyamines and cerebral ischemia *50*, 193 (1998)	T. David Johnson
Tetanus in Punjab with particular reference to the role of muscle relaxants in its management *19*, 288 (1975)	S. S. Jolly J. Singh S. M. Singh
Virulence-enhancing effect of ferric ammonium citrate on *Vibrio cholerae* *19*, 546 (1975)	I. Joó
Chemical teratogenesis *41*, 9 (1993) Chemical teratogenesis in humans: Biochemical and molecular mechanisms *49*, 25 (1997)	Mont R. Juchau
Drug molecules of marine origin *35*, 521 (1990) Alternative therapeutic modalities. Alternative medicine *47*, 251 (1996) Drug discovery: Past, present and future *50*, 9 (1998)	Pushkar N. Kaul
Toxoplasmosis *18*, 205 (1974)	B. H. Kean
The application of high-throughput screening to novel lead discovery *51*, 245 (1998)	Barry A. Kenny Mark Bushfield David J. Parry-Smith Simon Fogarty Mark Treherne
Tabellarische Zusammenstellung über die Substruktur der Proteine *16*, 364 (1972)	R. Kleine

Bioactive peptide analogs: *In vivo* and *in vitro* production *34*, 287 (1990)	Horst Kleinkauf Hans von Doehren
Enzymatic generation of complex peptides *48*, 27 (1997)	Horst Kleinkauf Hans von Doehren
Opiate receptors: Search for new drugs *36*, 49 (1991) Luteinizing hormone regulators: Luteinizing hormone releasing hormone analogs, estrogens, opiates, and estrogen-opiate hybrids *42*, 39 (1994) Novel and unusual nucleosides as drugs *48*, 195 (1997) Biomimicry as a basis for drug disovery *51*, 185 (1998)	Vera M. Kolb
Experimental evaluation of antituber- culous compounds, with special reference to the effect of combined treatment *18*, 211 (1974)	F. Kradolfer
The oxidative metabolism of drugs and other foreign compounds *17*, 488 (1973)	F. Kratz
Die Amidinstruktur in der Arzneistofforschung *11*, 356 (1968)	A. Kreutzberger
Present data on the pathogenesis of tetanus *19*, 301 (1975) Tetanus: general and pathophysiological aspects: Achievement, failures, perspectives of elaboration of the problem *19*, 314 (1975)	G. N. Kryzhanovsky
Lipophilicity and drug activity *23*, 97 (1979)	H. Kubinyi
Klinisch-pharmakologische Kriterien in der Bewertung eines neuen Antibiotikums. Grund- lagen und methodische Gesichtspunkte *23*, 327 (1978)	H. P. Kuemmerle
Regulation of NMDA receptors by ethanol *54*, 121 (2000)	Meena Kumari Maharaj K. Ticku
Recent advances in immunosuppressants *52*, 1 (1999)	Bijoy Kundu Sanjay K. Khare
Combinatorial chemistry: Polymer supported synthesis of peptide and nonpeptide libraries *53*, 89 (1999)	Bijoy Kundu Sanjay K. Khare Shiva K. Rastogi
Adrenergic receptor research: Recent developments *33*, 151 (1989)	George Kunos

Über neue Arzneimittel *1*, 531 (1959), *2*, 251 (1960), *3*, 369 (1961), *6*, 347 (1963), *10*, 360 (1966)	W. Kunz
Die Anwendung von Psychopharmaka in der psychosomatischen Medizin *10*, 530 (1966)	F. Labhardt
The bacterial cell surface and antimicrobial resistance *32*, 149 (1988)	Peter A. Lambert
Therapeutic measurement in tetanus *19*, 323 (1975)	D. R. Laurence
Clinical application of cytokines and immunostimulation and immunosuppression *39*, 167 (1992)	Betty Lee Thomas L. Ciardelli
Physicochemical methods in pharmaceutical chemistry I. Spectrofluorometry *6*, 151 (1963)	H. G. Leemann K. Stich Margrit Thomas
Biochemical acyl hydroxylations *16*, 229 (1972)	W. Lenk
Cholinesterase restoring therapy in tetanus *19*, 329 (1975)	G. Leonardi K. G. Nair F. D. Dastur
Perspective and overview of Chinese traditional medicine and contemporary pharmacology *47*, 131 (1996)	E. Leong Way Yong Qing-Liu Chieh-Fu Chen
The histamine H_3-receptor: A targeting for new drugs *39*, 127 (1992)	R. Leurs H. Timmerman
The medicinal chemistry and therapeutic potentials of the histamine H_3 receptor *45*, 107 (1995)	R. Leurs R.C. Vollinga H. Timmerman
Biliary excretion of drugs and other xenobiotics *25*, 361 (1981)	W. G. Levine
Structures, properties and disposition of drugs *29*, 67 (1985) Ribonucleotide reductase inhibitors as anti- cancer and antiviral agents *31*, 101 (1987) Fungal metabolites and Chinese herbal medicine as immunostimulants *34*, 395 (1990) Design and discovery of new drugs by stepping-up and stepping-down approaches *40*, 163 (1993)	Eric J. Lien

Immunopharmacological and biochemical bases of Chinese herbal medicine *46*, 263 (1996)	Eric J. Lien Arima Das Linda J. Lien
Physicochemical basis of the universal genetic codes – quantitative analysis *48*, 9 (1997)	Eric J. Lien Arima Das Partha Nandy Shijun Ren
In search of ideal antihypertensive drugs: Progress in five decades *43*, 43 (1994)	Eric J. Lien Hua Gao Linda L. Lien
Interactions between androgenic-anabolic steroids and glucocorticoids *14*, 139 (1970)	O. Linet
Drug inhibition of mast cell secretion *29*, 277 (1985)	R. Ludowyke D. Lagunoff
Reactivity of bentonite flocculation, indirect haemagglutination and Casoni tests in hydatid disease *19*, 75 (1975)	R. C. Mahajan N. L. Chitkara
Characteristics of catechol O-methyltransferase (COMT) and properties of selective COMT inhibitors *39*, 291 (1992)	P.T. Männistö I. Ulmanen K. Lundström J. Taskinen J. Tenhunen C. Tilgmann S. Kaakkola
Interaction of cancer chemotherapy agents with the mononuclear phagocyte system *35*, 487 (1990)	Alberto Mantovani
Mechanisms of fibrinolysis and clinical use of thrombolytic agents *39*, 197 (1992)	Maurizio Margaglione Elvira Grandone Giovanni Di Minno
Drugs affecting plasma fibrinogen levels. Implications for new anti-thrombotic strategies *46*, 169 (1996)	M. Margaglione E. Grandone F. P. Mancini G. Di Minno
Epidemiology of diphtheria *19*, 336 (1975)	L. G. Marquis
Biological activity of the terpenoids and their derivatives *6*, 279 (1963)	M. Martin-Smith T. Khatoon
Biological activity of the terpenoids and their derivatives – recent advances *13*, 11 (1969)	M. Martin-Smith W. E. Sneader
Antihypertensive agents 1962–1968 *13*, 101 (1969)	A. Marxer O. Schier

Fundamental structures in drug research – Part I *20*, 385 (1976) Fundamental structures in drug research – Part II *22*, 27 (1978) Antihypertensive agents 1969–1980 *25*, 9 (1981)	A. Marxer O. Schier
Relationships between the chemical structure and pharmacological activity in a series of synthetic quinuclidine derivatives *13*, 293 (1969)	M. D. Mashkovsky L. N. Yakhontov
Further developments in research on the chemistry and pharmacology of synthetic quinuclidine derivatives *27*, 9 (1983)	M. D. Mashkovsky L. N. Yakhontov M. E. Kaminka E. E. Mikhlina S. Ordzhonikidze
Role of neutrotransmitters in the central regulation of the cardiovascular system *35*, 25 (1990) Neurotransmitters involved in the central regulation of the cardiovascular system *46*, 43 (1996)	Robert B. McCall
On the understanding of drug potency 13, 123 (1971) The chemotherapy of intestinal nematodes *16*, 157 (1972)	J. W. McFarland
Non-steroidal menses-regulating agents: The present status *44*, 159 (1995)	P.K. Mehrotra Sanjay Batra A.P. Bhaduri
Zur Beeinflussung der Strahlen- empfindlichkeit von Säugetieren durch chemische Substanzen *9*, 11 (1966)	H.-J. Melching C. Streffer
Analgesia and addiction *5*, 155 (1963)	L. B. Mellett L. A. Woods
Comparative drug metabolism *13*, 136 (1969)	L. B. Mellett
The oral antiarrhythmic drugs *35*, 151 (1990)	Lisa Mendes Scott L. Beau John S. Wilson Philip J. Podrid
Mechanism of action of anxiolytic drugs *31*, 315 (1987)	T. Mennini S. Caccia S. Garattini
Pathogenesis of amebic disease *18*, 225 (1974)	M. J. Miller

Recent advances in cholera pathophysiology and therapeutics *19*, 563 (1975)	D. R. Nalin
Preparing the ground for research: Importance of data *18*, 239 (1974)	A. N. D. Nanavati
Computer-assisted structure – antileukemic activity analysis of purines and their aza and deaza analogs *34*, 319 (1990)	V. L. Narayanan Mohamed Nasr Kenneth D. Paull
Mechanism of drugs action on ion and water transport in renal tubular cells *26*, 87 (1982)	Yu. V. Natochin
Progesterone receptor binding of steroidal and nonsteroidal compounds *30*, 151 (1986)	Neelima M. Seth A. P. Bhaduri
Recent advances in drugs against hypertension *29*, 215 (1985)	Neelima B. K. Bhat A. P. Bhaduri
High resolution nuclear magnetic resonance spectroscopy of biological samples as an aid to drug development *31*, 427 (1987)	J. K. Nicholson Ian D. Wilson
Antibody response to two cholera vaccines in volunteers *19*, 554 (1975)	Y. S. Nimbkar R. S. Karbhari S. Cherian N. G. Chanderkar R. P. Bhamaria P. S. Ranadive B. B. Gaitonde
Surface interaction between bacteria and phagocytic cells *32*, 137 (1988)	L. Öhman G. Maluszynska K. E. Magnusson O. Stendahl
Die Chemotherapie der Wurmkrankheiten *1*, 159 (1959)	H.-A. Oelkers
Structural modifications patterns from agonists to antagonists and their application to drug design – A new serotonin(5HT$_3$)antagonist series *41*, 313 (1993)	Hiroshi Ohtaka Toshio Fujita
Serenics *42*, 167 (1994)	Berend Olivier Jan Mos Maikel Raghoeba Paul de Koning Marianne Mak

The 5-HT$_{1A}$ receptor and its ligands: structure and function 52, 103 (1999) Serotonin, dopamine and norepinephrine transporters in the central nervous system and their inhibitors 54, 59 (2000)	Berend Olivier Willem Soudijn Ineke van Wijngaarden
GABA-Drug interactions 31, 223 (1987)	Richard W. Olsen
Drug research and human sleep 22, 355 (1978)	I. Oswald
Effects of drugs on calmodulin-mediated enzymatic actions 33, 353 (1989)	Judit Ovádi
An extensive community outbreak of acute diarrhoeal diseases in children 19, 570 (1975)	S. C. Pal C. Koteswar Rao
Drug and its action according to Ayurveda 26, 55 (1982)	Madhabendra Nath Pal
Oligosaccharide chains of glycoproteins 32, 163 (1990)	Y. T. Pan Alan D. Elbein
Pharmacology of synthetic organic selenium compounds 36, 9 (1991)	Michael J. Parnham Erich Graf
Moral challenges in the organisation and management of drug research 42, 9 (1994)	Michael J. Parnham
3,4-Dihydroxyphenylalanine and related compounds 9, 223 (1966)	A. R. Patel A. Burger
Mescaline and related compounds 11, 11 (1968)	A. R. Patel
Experience with bitoscanate in adults 19, 90 (1975)	A. H. Patricia U. Prabakar Rao R. Subramaniam N. Madanagopalan
The impact of state and society on medical research 35, 9 (1990)	C. R. Pfaltz
Transfer factor in malignancy 42, 401 (1994)	Giancarlo Pizza Caterina De Vinci H. Hugh Fudenberg
Monoaminoxydase-Hemmer 2, 417 (1960)	A. Pletscher K. F. Gey P. Zeller
Antifungal therapy: Are we winning? 37, 183 (1991)	A. Polak P. G. Hartman

Epidemiology of pertussis *19*, 257 (1975)	J. A. Sa
Surgical amoebiasis *18*, 77 (1974)	A. E. de Sa
Role of beta-adrenergic blocking drug propranolol in severe tetanus *19*, 361 (1975)	G. S. Sainani K. L. Jain V. R. D. Deshpande A. B. Balsara S. A. Iyer
Studies on *Vibrio parahaemolyticus* in Bombay *19*, 586 (1975)	F. L. Saldanha A. K. Patil M. V. Sant
Leukotriene antagonists and inhibitors of leukotriene biosynthesis as potential therapeutic agents *37*, 9 (1991)	John A. Salmon Lawrence G. Garland
Pharmacology and toxicology of axoplasmic transport *28*, 53 (1984)	Fred Samson Ralph L. Smith J. Alejandro Donoso
Clinical experience with bitoscanate *19*, 96 (1975)	M. R. Samuel
Tetanus: Situational clinical trials and therapeutics *19*, 367 (1975)	R. K. M. Sanders M. L. Peacock B. Martyn B. D. Shende
Epidemiological studies on cholera in non-endemic regions with special reference to the problem of carrier state during epidemic and non-epidemic period *19*, 594 (1975)	M. V. Sant W. N. Gatlewar S. K. Bhindey
Epidemiological and biochemical studies in filariasis in four villages near Bombay *18*, 269 (1974)	M. V. Sant W. N. Gatlewar T. U. K. Menon
Hookworm anaemia and intestinal mal- absorption associated with hookworm infestation *19*, 108 (1975)	A. K. Saraya B. N. Tandon
The effects of structural alteration on the anti-inflammatory properties of hydrocortisone *5*, 11 (1963)	L. H. Sarett A. A. Patchett S. Steelman
The impact of natural product research on drug discovery *23*, 51 (1979)	L. H. Sarett
Aldose reductase inhibitors: Recent developments *40*, 99 (1993)	Reinhard Sarges Peter J. Oates

Drug nephrotoxicity – The significance of cellular mechanisms *41*, 51 (1993)	Robert J. Walker J. Paul Fawcett
Protease inhibitors as potential antiviral agents for the treatment of picornaviral infections *52*, 197 (1999)	Q. May Wang
Nicotine: An addictive substance or a therapeutic agent? *33*, 9 (1989)	David M. Warburton
Cell-wall antigens of *Vibrio cholerae* and their implication in cholera immunity *19*, 612 (1975)	Y. Watanabe R. Ganguly
Steroidogenic capacity in the adrenal cortex and its regulation *34*, 359 (1990)	Michael R. Watermann Evan R. Simpson
Antigen-specific T-cell factors and drug research *32*, 9 (1988)	David R. Webb
Where is immunology taking us? *20*, 573 (1976) Immunology in drug research *28*, 233 (1984)	W. J. Wechter Barbara E. Loughman
Natriuretic hormones *34*, 231 (1990)	W. J. Wechter Elaine J. Benaksas
The effects of NSAIDs and E-prosta-glandins on bone: A two signal hypothesis for the maintenance of skeletal bone *39*, 351 (1992)	William J. Wechter
Metabolic activation of chemical carcinogens *26*, 143 (1982)	E. K. Weisburger
A pharmacological approach to allergy *3*, 409 (1961) Adverse reactions of sugar polymers in animals and man *23*, 27 (1979) Biogenic amines and drug research *28*, 9 (1984)	G. B. West
A new approach to the medical interpretation of shock *14*, 196 (1970)	G. B. West M. S. Starr
Recent progress in understanding cholinergic function at the cellular and molecular levels *39*, 251 (1992)	V. P. Whittaker
Some biochemical and pharmacological properties of antiinflammatory drugs *8*, 321 (1965)	M. W. Whitehouse

Backlist

Vol. 41, 1993, 406 pp. ISBN 3-7643-2925-4

Mont J. Juchau: Chemical teratogenesis

Robert J. Walker and J. Paul Fawcett: Drug nephrotoxicity – The significance of cellular mechanisms

R. Sutherland: Bacterial resistance to β-lactam antibiotics: Problems and solutions

Noel W. Preston: Eradication by vaccination: The memorial to smallpox could be surrounded by others

Sanjay Batra, Manju Seth and A. P. Bhaduri: Chirality and future drug design

Wilhelm Schoner: Endogenous digitalis-like factors

James W. Fisher: Recent advances in erythropoietin research

Hiroshi Ohtaka and Toshio Fujita: Structural modification patterns from agonists to antagonists and their application to drug design – A new serotonin (5HT$_3$)-antagonist series

Vol. 42, 1994, 472 pp. ISBN 3-7643-2995-5

Michael J. Parnham: Moral challenges in the organization and management of drug research

Vera M. Kolb: Luteinizing hormone regulators: Luteinizing hormone releasing hormone analogs, estrogens, opiates, and estrogen-opiate hybrids

Shradha Sinha and Sudha Jain: Natural products as anticancer agents

A. Das, J. H. Wang and E. J. Lien: Carcinogenicity, mutagenicity and cancer preventing activities of flavonoids: A structure-system-activity relationship (SSAR) analysis

Berend Olivier, Jan Mos, Maikel Rayhoebar, Paul de Koning and Marianne Mak: Serenics

H. Hugh Fudenberg and Giancarlo Pizza: Transfer factor 1993: New frontiers

Giancarlo Pizza, Caterina de Vinci and H. Hugh Fudenberg: Transfer factor in malignancy

Vol. 43, 1994, 330 pp. ISBN 3-7643-5042-3

Harold E. Bays and Carlos Dujovne: Drugs for treatment of patients with high cholesterol blood levels and other dyslipidemias

Eric J. Lien, Hua Gao and Linda L. Lien: In search of ideal antihypertensive drugs: Progress in five decades

N. Seiler and C.L. Atanassov: The natural polyamines and the immune system

Shrada Sinha and Mukta Srivastava: Biologically active quinazolones

Mark P. Hayes and Kathryn C. Zoon: Production and action of interferons: New insights into molecular mechanisms of gene regulation and expression

Vol. 44, 1995, 342 pp. ISBN 3-7643-5149-7

George deStevens: Heterocyclic diversity: The road to biological activity

V. Zingel, C. Leschke and W. Schunack: Developments in Histamine H$_1$-receptor agonists

Paul D. Hoeprich: Antifungal chemotherapy

Richard M. Schultz: New antifolates in cancer therapy

P.K. Mehrotra, Sanjay Batra and A.P. Bhaduri: Non-steroidal menses-regulating agents: The present status

Anil K. Saxena and Mridula Saxena: Developments in anticonvulsants

Vol. 45, 1995, 386 pp. ISBN 3-7643-5212-4

Vijendra K. Singh: Neuropeptides as native immune modulators

Margaret E. Gnegy: Calmodulin: Effects of cell stimuli and drugs on cellular activation

S. P. Gupta: Recent advances in benzodiazepine (BZR) binding studies

R. Leurs, R.C. Vollinga and H. Timmerman: The medicinal chemistry and therapeutic potentials of ligands of the histamine H$_3$ receptor

Ray W. Fuller: Serotonin uptake inhibitors: Uses in clinical therapy and in laboratory research

Nissim Claude Cohen and Vincenzo Tschinke: Generation of new-lead structures in computer-aided drug design

Elaine J. Benaksas, E. David Murray, Jr. and William J. Wechter: Natriuretic hormones II

Indra Dwivedy and Suprabhat Ray: Recent developments in the chemotherapy of osteoporosis

Vol. 46, 1996, 329 pp. ISBN 3-7643-5298-1

Norman K. Hollenberg and Steven W. Graves: Endogenous sodium pump inhibition: Current status and therapeutic opportunities

Robert B. McCall: Neurotransmitters involved in the central regulation of the cardiovascular system

William T. Jackson and Jerome H. Fleisch: Development of novel anti-inflammatory agents: A pharmacologic perspective on leukotrienes and their receptors

M. Margaglione, E. Grandone, F.P. Mancini and G. Di Minno: Drugs affecting plasma fibrinogen levels. Implications for new antithrombotic strategies

N. Seiler, A. Hardy and J.P. Moulinoux: Aminoglycosides and polyamines: Targets and effects in the mammalian organism of two important groups of natural aliphatic polycations

James Claghorn and Michael D. Lesem: Recent developments in antidepressant agents

Eric J. Lien, Arima Das and Linda L. Lien: Immunopharmacological and biochemical bases of Chinese herbal medicine

Vol. 47, 1996, 346 pp. ISBN 3-7643-5299-X

Kurt R. H. Repke, Kathleen J. Sweadner, Jürgen Weiland, Rudolf Megges and Rudolf Schön: In search of ideal inotropic steroids: Recent progress

Silvano Sozzani, Paola Allavena, Paul Proost, Jo Van Damme and Alberto Mantovani: Chemokines as targets for pharmacological intervention

J. Paul Hieble and Robert R. Ruffolo, Jr: Subclassification and nomenclature of α_1- and α_2-adrenoceptors

E. Leong Way, Yong Qing Liu and Chieh-Fu Chen: Perspective and overview of Chinese traditional medicine and contemporary pharmacology

Jeanne Fürst Jucker and Gary P. Anderson: Emerging drug targets in the molecular pathogenesis of asthma

Gaetano Cardi, Thomas L. Ciardelli and Marc S. Ernstoff: Therapeutic applications of cytokines for immunostimulation and immunosuppression: An update

Pushkar N. Kaul: Alternative therapeutic modalities. Alternative medicine

Leo E. Hollister and Enrique S. Garza-Trevino: Calcium channel blockers in psychiatry

Vol. 48, 1997, 288 pp. ISBN 3-7643-5671-5

Eric J. Lien, Arima Das, Partha Nandy and Shijun Ren: Physicochemical basis of the universal genetic codes – quantitative analysis

Horst Kleinkauf and Hans von Döhren: Enzymatic generation of complex peptides

Iradj Hajimohamadreza and J. Mark Treherne: The role of apoptosis in neurodegenerative diseases

Esteban Domingo, Luis Menéndez-Arias, Miguel E. Quiñones-Mateu, Africa Holguín, Mónica Gutiérrez-Rivas, Miguel A. Martínez, Josep Quer, Isabel S. Novella and John J. Holland: Viral quasispecies and the problem of vaccine-escape and drug-resistant mutants

Vijendra K. Singh: Immunotherapy for brain diseases and mental illnesses

Shijun Ren and Eric J. Lien: Natural products and their derivatives as cancer chemopreventive agents

Deborah S. Hartman and Olivier Civelli: Dopamine receptor diversity: Molecular and pharmacological perspectives

Vera M. Kolb: Novel and unusual nucleosides as drugs

Vol. 49, 1997, 373 pp. ISBN 3-7643-5672-3

Richard M. Eglen: 5-Hydroxytryptamine (5-HT)4 receptors and central nervous system function: An update

Mont R. Juchau: Chemical teratogenesis in humans: Biochemical and molecular mechanisms

Gillian Edwards and Arthur H. Weston: Recent advances in potassium channel modulation

Helen Wise: Neuronal prostacyclin receptors

M.D. Murray and D. Craig Brater: Effects of NSAIDs on the kidney

Olivier Valdenaire and Philippe Vernier: G protein coupled receptors as modules of interacting proteins: A family meeting

Annemarie Polak: Antifungal therapy, an everlasting battle

Vol. 50, 1998, 373 pp. ISBN 3-7643-5821-1

P.N. Kaul: Drug discovery: Past, present and future

G. Edwards and A.H. Weston: Endothelium-derived hyperpolarizing factor – a critical appraisal

M. Rohmer: Isoprenoid biosynthesis via the mevalonate-independent route, a novel target for antibacterial drugs

R.W. Rockhold: Glutamatergic involvement in psychomotor stimulant action

T.D. Johnson: Polyamines and cerebral ischemia

J.M. Colacino and K.A. Staschke: The identification and development of antiviral agents for the treatment of chronic hepatitis B virus infection

Vol. 51, 1998, 330 pp. ISBN 3-7643-5822-X

Shijun Ren and Eric J. Lien: Development of HIV protease inhibitors: A survey

Nicholas C. Turner and John C. Clapham: Insulin resistance, impaired glucose tolerance and non-insulin-dependent diabetes, pathologic mechanisms and treatment: Current status and therapeutic possibilities

P.N. Kaul: Drug discovery: Past, present and future

G. Edwards and A.H. Weston: Endothelium-derived hyperpolarizing factor – a critical appraisal

M. Rohmer: Isoprenoid biosynthesis via the mevalonate-independent route, a novel target for antibacterial drugs

R.W. Rockhold: Glutamatergic involvement in psychomotor stimulant action

T.D. Johnson: Polyamines and cerebral ischemia

J.M. Colacino and K.A. Staschke: The identification and development of antiviral agents for the treatment of chronic hepatitis B virus infection

Vol. 52, 1999, 280 pp. ISBN 3-7643-5979-X

Bijoy Kundu and Sanjay K. Khare: Recent advances in immunosuppressants

Vishnu J. Ram and Atul Goel: Present status of hepatoprotectants

Berend Olivier, Willem Soudijn and Ineke van Wijngarden: The $5HT_{1A}$ receptor and its ligands: structure and function

Jacob Szmuszkovicz: U-50,488 and the κ receptor: A personalized account covering the period of 1973–1990

Q. May Wang: Protease inhibitors as potential antiviral agents for the treatment of picornaviral infections

Vol. 53, 1999, 290 pp. ISBN 3-7643-6028-3

Jacob Szmuszkovicz: U-50,488 and the κ receptor: Part II: 1991–1998

Satya P. Gupta: Quantitative structure-activity relationships of antihypertensive agents

Bijoy Kundu, Sanjay K. Khare and Shiva K. Rastogi: Combinatorial chemistry: Polymer supported synthesis of peptide and nonpeptide libraries

Paul Spence: From genome to drug – optimising the drug discovery process

Mary S. Barnette: Phosphodiesterase 4 (PDE4) inhibitors in asthma and chronic obstructive pulmonary disease (COPD)